AF710722

PATIENT CARE MANAGEMENT

A LAB WORKBOOK FOR PRESCRIPTION PRACTICE

THIRD EDITION

PATIENT CARE MANAGEMENT

A LAB WORKBOOK FOR PRESCRIPTION PRACTICE

THIRD EDITION

RICHARD FINKEL, PharmD
Clinical Assistant Professor
Pharmaceutical Sciences
College of Pharmacy
Nova Southeastern University
Fort Lauderdale, Florida

Wolters Kluwer | Lippincott Williams & Wilkins
Health
Philadelphia • Baltimore • New York • London
Buenos Aires • Hong Kong • Sydney • Tokyo

Acquisitions Editor: David Troy
Product Manager: Andrea M. Klingler
Marketing Manager: Shauna Kelley
Designer: Joan Wendt
Compositor: Absolute Service, Inc.

Third Edition
Copyright © 2013 Lippincott Williams & Wilkins, a Wolters Kluwer business
351 West Camden Street
Baltimore, MD 21201

Two Commerce Square
2001 Market Street
Philadelphia, PA 19103

Printed in China

All rights reserved. This book is protected by copyright. No part of this book may be reproduced or transmitted in any form or by any means, including as photocopies or scanned-in or other electronic copies, or utilized by any information storage and retrieval system without written permission from the copyright owner, except for brief quotations embodied in critical articles and reviews. Materials appearing in this book prepared by individuals as part of their official duties as U.S. government employees are not covered by the above-mentioned copyright. To request permission, please contact Lippincott Williams & Wilkins at Two Commerce Square, 2001 Market Street, Philadelphia, PA 19103, via e-mail at permissions@lww.com, or via website at lww.com (products and services).

9 8 7 6 5 4

Library of Congress Cataloging-in-Publication Data

Finkel, Richard, PharmD.
Patient care management : a lab workbook for prescription practice / Richard Finkel. — 3rd ed.
p. ; cm.
Rev. ed. of: Patient care management lab : a workbook for prescription practice / Richard Finkel. 2nd ed. c2008.
Includes bibliographical references and index.
ISBN 978-1-4511-1346-4 (alk. paper)
I. Finkel, Richard, PharmD. Patient care management lab. II. Title.
[DNLM: 1. Drug Prescriptions—Problems and Exercises. 2. Drug Interactions--Problems and Exercises. 3. Pharmacy—Problems and Exercises. QV 18.2]

615.4076—dc23

2011040558

INSERT CIP DATA HERE

DISCLAIMER

Care has been taken to confirm the accuracy of the information present and to describe generally accepted practices. However, the authors, editors, and publisher are not responsible for errors or omissions or for any consequences from application of the information in this book and make no warranty, expressed or implied, with respect to the currency, completeness, or accuracy of the contents of the publication. Application of this information in a particular situation remains the professional responsibility of the practitioner; the clinical treatments described and recommended may not be considered absolute and universal recommendations.

The authors, editors, and publisher have exerted every effort to ensure that drug selection and dosage set forth in this text are in accordance with the current recommendations and practice at the time of publication. However, in view of ongoing research, changes in government regulations, and the constant flow of information relating to drug therapy and drug reactions, the reader is urged to check the package insert for each drug for any change in indications and dosage and for added warnings and precautions. This is particularly important when the recommended agent is a new or infrequently employed drug.

Some drugs and medical devices presented in this publication have U.S. Food and Drug Administration (FDA) clearance for limited use in restricted research settings. It is the responsibility of the health care provider to ascertain the FDA status of each drug or device planned for use in his or her clinical practice.

To purchase additional copies of this book, call our customer service department at (800) 638-3030 or fax orders to (301) 223-2320. International customers should call (301) 223-2300.

Visit Lippincott Williams & Wilkins on the Internet: http://www.lww.com. Lippincott Williams & Wilkins customer service representatives are available from 8:30 am to 6:00 pm, EST.

To Rose Capizzi Finkel and Albert (Abraham) Finkel,
my mother and father, the Finkel family,
and in honor of our great students.

PREFACE

Patient Care Management: A Lab Workbook for Prescription Practice, Third Edition, was designed specifically for the contemporary pharmacy student. The primary purpose of this workbook is to train students to think of prescriptions as a component of the whole spectrum of patient care that includes profiles, lifestyles, allergies, gender, disease states, and other historical notes. This workbook is meant to be practical and to provide the student with the opportunity to fill prescriptions as well as to monitor for hidden problems and counsel the patient and/or caregiver.

Each chapter consists of true cases. Every case is drawn from a real-life patient history as adapted from the many profiles contributed by pharmacists, including the author. The prescriptions were written by licensed prescribers. (The names of the patients and prescribers have been changed. Similarities to any person or persons, living or dead, are coincidental.)

This workbook provides examples of cases that contain full patient histories, partial case histories, or no case histories. When the case history information is incomplete, the student must interview the patient, caregiver, or prescriber to determine relevant information. This omission of data reflects conditions in real practice, especially in the retail or community setting, where actual patient histories are sometimes incomplete.

The patient's body mass index (BMI) in kilograms per meters squared (kg/m^2) is entered on some cases. When absent, the pharmacist (student) should obtain the height and weight and calculate the BMI.

What Is New in This Edition

All the prescriptions in this book have been reviewed for currency, and many have been updated. In addition, many new prescriptions have been added to each chapter. Another significant change is that "Appendix B: Puzzles and Problems," has been updated. The 44 prescriptions in this appendix exemplify prescriptions or drug orders that are difficult to decipher or that, if filled as written, could cause serious harm to the patient. This appendix strives to alert students to the fact that medications are sometimes unclearly or incorrectly ordered. When confronted with unclear or incorrect orders, the pharmacist assesses the situation and, if necessary, intervenes appropriately. Therefore, this workbook will contribute to future pharmacists' ability to detect and prevent medication errors in a challenging and constantly changing health care system.

Organization of the Manual

The workbook is organized into chapters arranged by various disease states. Each chapter can be completed in one or two 3-hour sessions, or the materials can be used in whatever time frame is available. Included in each chapter are the following:

- Objectives: Successful review of the prescription cases in the chapter should prepare the student to master the objectives for the subject area.
- Drug List: List of medications relevant to the chapter.
- Drug Hot Points: Summaries of key characteristics and concerns associated with the drugs covered in the chapter. They serve as brief references and are not intended to be comprehensive.
- Questions to Be Answered in Preparation for Lab: Before working on the profile/prescription cases, students should have background knowledge of the drugs and conditions included in the chapter. Competency should be demonstrated by correctly answering the questions in this section.
- Profile/Prescription Cases: The profile/prescription cases are the core of *Patient Care Management: A Lab Workbook for Prescription Practice, Third Edition*. Each profile provides the medical/drug history of the patient and is associated with new prescriptions to be dispensed. In reading the prescriptions and referencing the patient profile, students assume the role of practicing pharmacists. Practical concerns of filling the prescriptions and possible complications associated with various drugs or dosages in the patient profile should be considered.

Prescriptions from Appendices A and B can be used by the instructor for additional practice or as replacement prescriptions, per the instructor's preference. Appendix A contains 85 supplemental prescriptions, whereas (as mentioned previously) Appendix B contains 44 prescriptions that are particularly difficult to decipher or that, if filled as written, could cause serious harm to the patient.

Teaching Tools

This workbook includes patients' profiles, lifestyles, allergies, gender, disease states, and drug interactions as teaching tools. Each chapter in the book is organized to correspond to a particular disease state that is amenable to pharmaceutical care (such as hypertension, cardiovascular, geriatrics, pain management, gastroenterology, genitourinary, infectious disease, and diabetes). Students have the opportunity to practice real cases in a safe environment, allowing them to gain a deeper understanding of issues involved in medication therapy management. Taking into account ethical and legal considerations regarding dispensing medications while addressing patient needs should also be discussed. This workbook also allows pharmacy students to obtain an appreciation for the traditional and evolving community practice setting. The knowledge acquired from the use of *Patient Care Management: A Lab Workbook for Prescription Practice, Third Edition,* can be useful in any setting and can be beneficial not only to pharmacy students, but also to students in other health care professions, such as pharmacy technicians, physicians, physician assistants, nurses, and nurse practitioners.

Medication Therapy Management

An important new section in each chapter involves questions and comments to be directed to the "patient" or to the caregiver. These examples are drawn from the author's interactions with community pharmacy clients based on 55 years of practice. They now are referred to as part of MTM, or medication therapy management. Clients in the community or retail settings need more active counseling and direction from registered pharmacists and pharmacy technicians than ever before. Conditions in the health care setting have changed. Pharmacists and pharmacy technicians have inherited the thrilling role of managing the health care of our patients. *Patient Care Management: A Lab Workbook for Prescription Practice, Third Edition,* is designed to illustrate to our students that their education is now appropriate for this important task. This will allow students as well as practicing pharmacists and technicians to do what we all wanted when we took on the role of patient care managers.

Student Responsibilities

Prerequisites or corequisites for this course should include pharmacodynamics, therapeutics, law, calculations, and pharmacokinetics. To maximize learning, each student must complete the product worksheet (after the "Acknowledgments" section of the front matter of this book) for the relevant drug(s) and master the material prior to attending corresponding sessions. The student should complete each question in the "Questions to Be Answered in Preparation for Lab" before the laboratory session.

Information sources such as *Facts and Comparisons, Drug Information Handbook by Lexi-Comp, and Clinical Pharmacology* should be utilized. Sources of information for nonprescription products can be found in the following: *Nonprescription Product Therapeutics* (W. Steven Pray) and *Handbook of Nonprescription Drugs* (APhA). Sources of principles of pharmacology are available in *Lippincott's Illustrated Reviews: Pharmacology, 5th Edition* (R. Harvey).

Instructor's Manuals

For faculty adopting the book, two instructor's manuals—one geared toward instructors of pharmacy students and one geared toward instructors of pharmacy technician students—can be accessed at http://thepoint.lww.com/finkel3e.

ACKNOWLEDGMENTS

This workbook is used in Patient Care Management, a course that has been taught at Nova Southeastern University, Fort Lauderdale, Florida, since 1989.

The course was created by the author and eight other practicing pharmacists under the direction of Dr. John Triplett, PhD, whose vision initiated the course. The workbook was encouraged by former chancellor and founder of the Health Professions Division, Dr. Morton Terry; current chancellor and the author's mentor and preceptor, Dr. Fred Lippman; Dean Emeritus Bill Hardigan; Dean Dr. Andrés Malavé; Dr. Appu Rathinavelu; and Department Chair Dr. Michelle Clark.

Enhancements were contributed by the following colleagues: Lillian Arce, PharmD; Kathy Fuller, PharmD; Jose Rey, PharmD; Sami Shafiq, PharmD; Tracy Hunter, PhD; and Jorge Varela, PharmD.

I am appreciative that Nova Southeastern University provided resources and time for the project to be completed.

I would also like to acknowledge my partnership with Andrea Klingler and David Troy of Lippincott Williams & Wilkins.

Our pharmacy students at Nova Southeastern University are the driving force of this book. Without our students, there would be no patient care management book. I thank them for allowing us to be a part of their lives.

COLLEGE OF PHARMACY

PATIENT CARE MANAGEMENT LAB DRUG PRODUCT WORKSHEET

To be completed in the student's handwriting and mastered before laboratory session

Generic Name:			Therapeutic Class:
Brand Name:			Dosage Forms/Strengths:
Major Indications:			Dosage Range/Frequency:
Mechanism of Action:			
Contraindications:			
Significant Side Effects:			
Drug-Herbal-Food Interactions:			
Legal Classification: (✓)	Rx	DEA Schedule II-III-IV-V	OTC
Storage Requirements: (✓) Cool/Dry/Dark/Refrigerate: 36–46° F (2–8° C)			
Special Patient Information(Counseling):			Alternate Drug(s) That Can Achieve Similar Outcomes:
			Alternate Drug Class or Class(es):
Student Name:			Lab Date:

BASIC GENERAL MEDICATION THERAPY MANAGEMENT QUESTIONS

How are you?
Did your doctor tell you what to expect from the medication?
How did the doctor say to take your medication?
Is your medication helping?
What type of lifestyle and dietary changes did the doctor recommend?
Do you have any questions for me at this time?
Do you know what you are taking this medication for?
Are you taking any weight loss products?
Do you take any health-food–related products of any kind?
Are you taking any herbal products?
Do you take any nonprescription drugs or OTCs from us or any other store, business, friend, or the Internet?
Did your doctor tell you what to do if you forget to take your medication?
Are you taking any other prescription drugs from other pharmacies, the Internet, friends, or physician samples?
Did you ever have a rash or difficulty breathing with any medication?
Do you take anything, even if it is not a medication?
If you drink alcohol or smoke, do you plan to discontinue using these now?
Are you doing any exercise or physical activity, such as walking, jogging, yoga, and so forth?

CONTENTS

CHAPTER **1**

CARDIOVASCULAR, Part 1 1

CHAPTER **2**

CARDIOVASCULAR, Part 2 35

CHAPTER **3**

GERIATRICS 79

CHAPTER **4**

PAIN AND CONTROLLED DRUGS 111

CHAPTER **5**

DRUGS FOR NEOPLASTIC DISORDERS AND IMMUNOSUPPRESSANTS . . 141

CHAPTER **6**

GASTROENTEROLOGY 167

CHAPTER **7**

GENITOURINARY 197

CHAPTER **8**

ANTIMICROBIALS 225

CHAPTER **9**

MENTAL HEALTH, Part 1 255

CHAPTER **10**

MENTAL HEALTH, Part 2 285

CHAPTER **11**

MUSCLE RELAXANTS AND NONSTEROIDAL ANTI-INFLAMMATORY DRUGS 317

CHAPTER **12**

CHRONIC OBSTRUCTIVE PULMONARY DISEASE AND ASTHMA 345

CHAPTER **13**

OPHTHALMICS 373

CHAPTER **14**

DIABETES 399

CHAPTER **15**

MISCELLANEOUS PRODUCTS 427

APPENDIX A

Supplemental Prescriptions 456

APPENDIX B

Puzzles and Problems 500

ABBREVIATIONS . . . . . Inside Back Cover

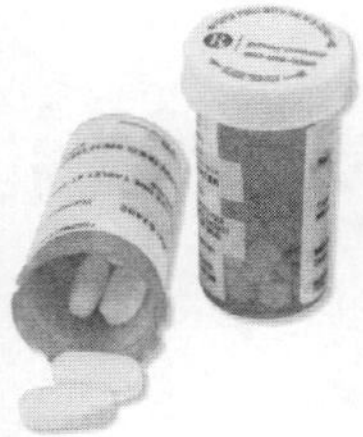

• CARDIOVASCULAR, PART I

1

UPON COMPLETION OF THIS CHAPTER, THE STUDENT WILL BE ABLE TO:

- discuss the various strengths of nitroglycerin with patients so that they understand the relative potencies of these products.
- explain the importance of compliance when taking antihypertensive medications.
- counsel patients on the proper use of topical formulations of nitroglycerin.
- counsel patients receiving Coumadin and/or digoxin therapy as to the risks involved when other prescription and nonprescription medications are taken (salicylates, antacids, herbals, etc.).
- discuss the relationship between PT and INR.
- discuss appropriate dosing of diuretics as related to the time of the day.
- recognize and discuss electrolyte imbalance problems associated with diuretic therapy.
- counsel patients as to the methods for minimizing gastrointestinal irritation associated with oral potassium supplementation.
- discuss digoxin overdose and toxicity (low pulse, GI upset, etc.).
- explain the use of Digibind in treating digoxin toxicity.
- advise the person using medications to improve blood circulation that it will take some time for results to be achieved.

DRUG LIST

Aggrenox
Aldactone
Aldomet
BiDil
Coreg
Coumadin
Digoxin
Dyazide
Hydrochlorothiazide
Inderal
Inspra
Isosorbide (dinitrate and mononitrate)
KCl
Lasix
Lopressor/Toprol XL
Nitroglycerin
Persantine
Plavix
Pletal
Ranexa
Tenormin
Trental

• DRUG HOT POINTS

Aggrenox
200-mg extended-release dipyridamole with 25-mg aspirin
Antiplatelet action is the result of both drugs

Aldactone
Compare with Inspra (eplerenone)
HTN dose and cirrhosis dose
Potassium sparing
Watch salt substitutes

Aldomet
Counsel on side effects
Importance of blood tests
Can be used to treat HTN in pregnant patients
Included on the Beers list

BiDil
Isosorbide dinitrate and hydralazine hydrochloride
For treatment of heart failure as an adjunct to standard therapy in self-identified black patients

Coreg (carvedilol)
Nonselective beta- & alpha-1 blocker
CHF indication
Take BID with food to avoid orthostasis

Coumadin
Colors vs. strengths
No salicylates (Rx or OTC)
Food counseling: *Consistent* intake of green leafy vegetables: Brussels sprouts, spinach, etc.
Limit intake of acetaminophen (APAP) to a total of not more than 2 g per day

Digoxin
Slows and strengthens the heart
Watch absorption by OTC and Rx meds
Digitalis toxicity and treatment
Adjust dose for age and gender
Renally excreted

Dyazide
Compare with Maxzide and Maxzide-25
Potassium-sparing plus potassium-wasting diuretic

Hydrochlorothiazide (HCTZ)
Decreases Na^+, K^+, Mg^{2+}; increases Ca^{2+}
Dosing: 12.5 to 25 mg/day
Potassium-wasting: monitor other meds
Compare with Lozol and Hygroton

Inderal
Side-effect profile: counseling
Migraine prophylaxis, treatment for HTN, heart rhythm disturbances, akathisia; other uses
Nonselective: bronchospasm warning
Monitor: depression (lipophilic)
Membrane-stabilizing effect
Compare with other beta-blockers
May mask hypoglycemia symptoms
Compare with Corgard (nadolol) and Visken (pindolol)

Isosorbide
Dosing: nitrate-free interval
Isordil: dinitrate; SL, tabs, Tembids, caps
ISMO: mononitrate; BID, 7 hours apart
Imdur: extended-release mononitrate
Contraindicated with Viagra-type products

KCl/Potassium Chloride
K-Dur: can be mixed in water to drink
Compliance: must be taken as ordered
Important part of drug regimen
Dilute liquids, follow with water
Take with food (GI upset)
Do not crush (Slow-K, Klor-Con 10)

• DRUG HOT POINTS (*continued*)

Lasix
Contrast loop diuretics with thiazides
Decreases Na^+, K^+, Mg^{2+}, Ca^{2+}
Compliance with potassium Rx (KCl, etc.)
Compare potency and action to Bumex & Demadex

Lopressor (metoprolol tartrate)
Beta 1-selective in low doses
Not as lipophilic as Inderal
Toprol XL: long-acting formulation (metoprolol succinate)

Nitroglycerin
Strengths (mg/grain equivalents)
Storage: original glass container
Patch application
First-pass effect (PO vs. others)
Do not shake Nitrolingual Pumpspray
Contraindicated with Viagra-type products

Persantine
Adjunct to coumarin anticoagulants in the prevention of thromboembolic complications of cardiac valve replacement
May be inappropriate for the elderly

Plavix
Inhibits platelet aggregation
Mechanism, counseling
Compare with aspirin
Caution: metabolized to active metabolite by CYP-450 2C19 enzyme; inhibitors can reduce therapeutic effect

Pletal
Role in treating intermittent claudication
90 to 100 days to see effect
Compare with Trental

Ranexa
Indicated to treat chronic angina
500 mg BID and increase to 1000 mg, based on clinical symptoms
Metabolized by CYP3A and CYP2D6

Tenormin
One daily dose
Selectivity in low doses
Not lipophilic

• QUESTIONS TO BE ANSWERED IN PREPARATION FOR CHAPTER 1 LAB

- Which vitamin does warfarin affect?
- Why, in most cases, should we advise our clients to avoid aspirin products while taking Coumadin?
- Which food products contain a substance that may inhibit the therapeutic effect of warfarin?
- Your client has forgotten one dose of Coumadin. The next day, he calls you and asks whether he should take a double dose. What would your answer be?
- A person who has been stabilized on warfarin presents you with a new prescription for itraconazole 100-mg caps for the treatment of a fungal skin infection. What would you do?
- Explain the action of digoxin as a:
  - positive inotrope
  - negative chronotrope
- What are the two diuretics contained in Dyazide and Maxzide?
- Which nonselective beta-blocker is most lipophilic?
- Which beta-blocker would most likely cause CNS side effects?
- Why would atenolol be more appropriate than propranolol for use in a patient with COPD?
- What is a possible advantage of Inspra over spironolactone?
- Why is immediate-release (IR) dipyridamole included on the Beers list?
- What is the mechanism of action of Trental?
- Why should you advise the person who is just starting to take Trental that it may take as long as 3 months for the full therapeutic effect to start in the treatment of his leg cramps?
- What is the advantage of Pletal over Trental?
- What are the mechanisms of action and the cautions for the use of Plavix?
- What are the advantages of Plavix over Ticlid?
- Visken (pindolol) has ISA. What does that mean?
- What is the therapeutic rationale for prescribing a beta-blocker with ISA?
- What are the storage requirements for nitroglycerin SL tablets?
- What is the difference in pharmacokinetics between Ismo and Isordil?
- What is the difference in dosing between ISMO and Isordil?
- How does spironolactone work as a diuretic when used to treat HTN?
- Explain the mechanism of action of spironolactone when used to treat a patient who has cirrhosis with ascites.
- Explain the sites of action of furosemide (Lasix) and HCTZ.
- How do Lasix and HCTZ affect the renal elimination of calcium?
- Why should we counsel our clients to take Coreg with food?
- How many milligrams of KCl (mol wt 74.5) are contained in one K-Dur 20 mEq tablet?
- How many milliequivalents of KCl are contained in each 15 mL of KCl 10% liquid?
- What would be the outcome if a person were taking a regimen of both digoxin and furosemide without a source of potassium?
- How many milliliters of digoxin oral solution are equal in potency to one tablet of digoxin 0.125 mg?
- Describe the boxed warning for warfarin.
- Describe the boxed warnings for beta-blockers.
- Why is Aldomet (methyldopa) included on the Beers list?
- What is the Beers list?
- What is BMI?
- How is BMI calculated?

• CARDIOVASCULAR, PART 1, MEDICATION THERAPY MANAGEMENT QUESTIONS AND COMMENTS

- I notice that your lab results show low amounts of potassium in your body. Did your doctor mention any foods or medications for you to take?
- I notice that your lab results show low amounts of sodium in your body. Did your doctor mention any foods or medications for you to take?
- Have you experienced any light-headedness after taking your new blood pressure medicine?
- When you take your blood pressure medications, are you able to stand very slowly to avoid becoming dizzy?
- Did your doctor mention that caffeine in coffee and other drinks could raise your blood pressure?
- I notice that your skin appears to be dry. Have you been able to drink enough water each day? Water is better for your body than other drinks.
- Did your doctor mention a diet called the "DASH" diet? Let's talk about it.
- Did your doctor tell you to take your "nitro" patch off after wearing it for 12 hours?
- You are taking a "blood thinner" called warfarin. Are you aware of the importance of taking the same consistent amount of green leafy vegetables each week?
- Did the doctor tell you to avoid herbal or natural remedies when taking this medication?
- In addition, if you take Tylenol in any form, do not exceed 2000 mg (4 of the 500-mg tablets) in any day.
- Are you aware that OTC pain and fever medications called "NSAIDs" increase the risk of raising your blood pressure? I can give you a list of the most popular products to avoid. Some examples are aspirin, ibuprofen, and naproxen sodium, which are available in many forms and names.
- If you are smoking or drinking alcohol, would you like to discuss some very easy methods of slowly tapering down or decreasing them? This would have a good effect on your health.
- I notice that your lab results indicate that your liver is giving you problems. Do you take any OTC pain or fever products with the name of acetaminophen, APAP, nonaspirin, or Tylenol alone or in combination? In addition, do you drink any alcohol?
- Your medication for chest pressure is called "nitrate." It might cause a headache. Did your doctor say that a small dose (one 500-mg tablet) of Tylenol or acetaminophen taken four times a day, when needed, might help?
- Your medicine is a "beta-blocker." It is important that you stay with it and take it exactly as prescribed. It is critical that if the doctor stops it, the medicine must be slowly reduced over a 2-week period.
- Your new medicine is Plavix. Please take it exactly as prescribed. Do not take any nonprescription (OTC) pills of any kind without asking us first. Some pain medications might cause an adverse reaction when taken with Plavix.
- Additionally, please look at your arms and legs each day. If you see unusual dark blue or purple marks, contact your physician.
- Please call us to allow us to advise you before you take any nonprescription drugs along with Plavix.
- Pletal is your medicine to increase blood flow to your lower part of the body. It might take a few weeks to start working. Please do not stop taking it without telling your doctor or contacting us.

1.1

PT. NAME: **GRACE PHILLIPS** | AGE: **79** | GENDER: **F** | DX: **SPASTIC COLON, HTN, CHF** | ADDRESS: **54 NORTH AVE.** | ALLERGY: **PCN** | WEIGHT: **133** | HX: **SMOKER FOR LIFE** | BMI: **21.5**

MEDICATION	SIG.	PRESCRIBER	ORIG. DATE	REFILL DATE	REFILL DATE	REFILL DATE	REFILL DATE
Robitussin 120 mL	5 mL tid prn cough	Sauls	11/20	1/5			
Bentyl 10 mg #C	1 tid prn	Sauls	2/20				
HCTZ-25 mg #30	1 q am	Sauls	12/15	1/20	2/20		
Lanoxin 0.25 mg #30	1 q am	Sauls	12/15	1/20	2/20		

Dr. Alfred Sauls
151212 S. High Rd., Chicago, IL 23875
954-555-1300

Name Grace Phillips Date 3/20

Address 54 North Ave. Age 79

℞

Aggrenox #60

i PO B.I.D

Refills 5

Dr. Alfred Sauls

1.1a

Dr. Alfred Sauls
151212 S. High Rd., Chicago, IL 23875
954-555-1300

Name Grace Phillips Date 3/20

Address 54 North Ave. Age 79

℞

Nitrodur 0.6 mg

#30

1 patch on 8 PM off 10 PM qd

Refill 6 times

Dr. Alfred Sauls

1.1b

1.2

PT. NAME: **FRED LONG**	GENDER: **M**	ADDRESS: **3 EAST CT.**	WEIGHT: **160**	BMI: **27**
AGE: **80**	DX: **EDEMA, HTN, DEMENTIA**	ALLERGY: **NKA**	HX: **SEDENTARY LIFESTYLE**	

MEDICATION	SIG.	PRESCRIBER	ORIG. DATE	REFILL DATE	REFILL DATE	REFILL DATE	REFILL DATE
HCTZ 25 mg #50	1 q am	Thomas	5/11	8/20			
K-Dur 10 mEq #50	1 q am	Thomas	5/11	10/20			
Robitussin Syr 4 oz	1 tsp tid prn	Thomas	5/18				
Tylenol No. 3 #12	1 q 4–6 h prn tooth pain	Griffin	11/15				

Dr. Erin Thomas
988 North Ridge, New York, NY 88364
813-555-7554

Name Fred Long Date 12/15

Address 3 East Ct. Age 80

℞

Lasix 20mgm
#CC
Sig: tab i daily

Refills 2

Dr. Erin Thomas

1.2a

Dr. Erin Thomas
988 North Ridge, New York, NY 88364
813-555-7554

Name Fred Long Date 12/15

Address 3 East Ct. Age 80

℞

K-Dur 20mEq
#30
Take i p.o. QD

Refills 2

Dr. Erin Thomas

1.2b

1.3

PT. NAME: **MARVIN ADAMS** | AGE: **66** | GENDER: **M** | DX: **HIGH CHOLESTEROL, HTN, OA, SKIN FUNGAL INFECTION** | ADDRESS: **7 SOUTH ST.** | ALLERGY: **NKA** | WEIGHT: **177** | HX: **SOCIAL DRINKER** | BMI: **27**

MEDICATION	SIG.	PRESCRIBER	ORIG. DATE	REFILL DATE	REFILL DATE	REFILL DATE	REFILL DATE
Questran Powder 378 g can	1 scoop bid	Griffin	12/8	2/27			
HCTZ 25 mg #50	1 q am	Griffin	1/8	2/27			
Mycolog cr 15 g	Apply tid ud	Griffin	1/9				

Dr. Doug Griffin
7611 147th Terrace, Monterey, CA 38411
705-555-6644

Name Marvin Adams Date 3/7

Address 7 South St. Age 66

℞

KCl 10mEq

#100

Sig 1 bid

Refills 4

Dr. Doug Griffin

1.3a

Dr. Doug Griffin
7611 147th Terrace, Monterey, CA 38411
705-555-6644

Name Marvin Adams Date 3/7

Address 7 South St. Age 66

℞

(60)

Extra strength Tyl.

Refills sig i q3-4h prn

Dr. Doug Griffin

1.3b

1.4

PT. NAME: **BOB THOMAS** AGE: **73**
GENDER: **M** DX: **STOMACH PROBLEMS, HTN, CHF**
ADDRESS: **894 WEST ROAD** ALLERGY: **NKA**
WEIGHT: **126** BMI: **20**

MEDICATION	SIG.	PRESCRIBER	ORIG. DATE	REFILL DATE	REFILL DATE	REFILL DATE	REFILL DATE
Zantac 150 mg #60	1 bid	Weiss	2/16	3/1			
Capoten 12.5 mg #60	1 bid	Weiss	2/16				
Furosemide 20 mg #60	1 bid	Weiss	2/16				

Dr. Barry Weiss
901 Sheridan St., Austin, TX 90902
874-555-9000

Name Bob Thomas Date 3/16

Address 894 West Rd. Age 73

℞

Lasix 40 mg
Tabs ii po q AM
#60

Refills 3

Dr. Barry Weiss

1.4a

Dr. Barry Weiss
901 Sheridan St., Austin, TX 90902
874-555-9000

Name Bob Thomas Date 3/16

Address 894 West Rd. Age 73

℞

Lanoxin
Lanoxin 0.125 mg
#100
i po QOD
1 po

Refills 3

Dr. Barry Weiss

1.4b

1.5

PT. NAME: **LOU SMITH** | GENDER: **M** | ADDRESS: **2 TALLAHASSEE CT.** | WEIGHT: **155** | BMI: **25**

AGE: **75** | DX: **ASTHMA, HTN, DEPRESSION, ANGINA, LEG CRAMPS WHILE WALKING** | ALLERGY: **NKA**

MEDICATION	SIG.	PRESCRIBER	ORIG. DATE	REFILL DATE	REFILL DATE	REFILL DATE	REFILL DATE
Trental 400 mg #C	1 tid with food	Robins	11/15	12/31	2/9		
HCTZ 25 mg #C	1 qd am	Robins	12/10	2/14			
Prozac 10 mg #30	1 q am	Robins	11/15	12/14	1/14	2/10	
Proventil HFA spray 6.7 g	2 puffs tid prn	Robins	12/16	1/15	2/9		

Dr. Calvin Robins
7823 Tea Rose Trail, Miami, FL 44718
463-555-8000

Name Lou Smith Date 2/15

Address 2 Tallahassee Ct. Age 75

℞

TENORMIN 50mg
Disp: 100
Sig ½ qHS for blood pressure

Refills 1

Dr. Calvin Robins

1.5a

Dr. Calvin Robins
7823 Tea Rose Trail, Miami, FL 44718
463-555-8000

Name Lou Smith Date 2/15

Address 2 Tallahassee Ct. Age 75

℞

NTG [illegible] SL
prn CP
#25

Refills 1

Dr. Calvin Robins

1.5b

1.6

PT. NAME: **LEWIS GREEN** GENDER: **M** ADDRESS: **6 PENNSYLVANIA AVE. NW** WEIGHT: **148** BMI: **27**
AGE: **68** DX: **GERD, HTN, ANGINA** ALLERGY: **PCN** HX: **ETOH**

MEDICATION	SIG.	PRESCRIBER	ORIG. DATE	REFILL DATE	REFILL DATE	REFILL DATE	REFILL DATE
Capoten 25 mg #C	1 tid	Thomas	12/8	2/28			
HCTZ 25 mg #30	1 q am	Thomas	2/8	3/8	4/7		
Pepcid 20 mg #60	1 bid	Thomas	2/2	3/1	4/2		
Robitussin DM 4 oz	1 tsp qid	OTC	12/10	12/15	12/30	1/10	2/15

Dr. Erin Thomas
988 North Ridge, New York, NY 88364
813-555-7554

Name Lewis Green Date 4/18

Address 6 Pensylvania Ave NW Age 68

℞

SL nitro
1/150
prn
chestpain
#100

Refills 6

Dr. Erin Thomas

1.6a

Dr. Erin Thomas
988 North Ridge, New York, NY 88364
813-555-7554

Name Lewis Green Date 4/18

Address 6 Pennsylvania Ave NW Age 68

℞

Digoxin 0.125mg
#100
i po Qd
Skip Sunday

Refills 6

Dr. Erin Thomas

1.6b

1.7

PT. NAME: **MORTON WALKER** GENDER: **M** ADDRESS: **564 CAPITOL AVE.** WEIGHT: **152** BMI: **22**
AGE: **82** DX: **CHF, ANGINA, HTN, EDEMA** ALLERGY: **NKA**

MEDICATION	SIG.	PRESCRIBER	ORIG. DATE	REFILL DATE	REFILL DATE	REFILL DATE	REFILL DATE
Lasix 40 mg #90	1 tid	Griffin	8/1	9/2	10/3	11/4	12/15
Lanoxin 0.125 mg #30	1 qod	Griffin	8/3	10/4	12/5		
Halcion 0.25 mg #15	1/2 tab hs prn	Griffin	10/3	11/4			

Dr. Doug Griffin
7611 147th Terrace, Monterey, CA 38411
705-555-6644

Name Morton Walker Date 12/16

Address 564 Capitol Ave Age 82

℞

NTG SL 0.4 mg
Sig: SL 1 prn for CP
Disp: #1

Refills 4

Dr. Doug Griffin

1.7a

Dr. Doug Griffin
7611 147th Terrace, Monterey, CA 38411
705-555-6644

Name Morton Walker Date 12/16

Address 564 Capitol Ave Age 82

℞

K Dur 20 mEq
#15
Sig 1/2 tab daily

Refills 4

Dr. Doug Griffin

1.7b

1.8

PT. NAME: **ART JOHNSON**	GENDER: **M**	ADDRESS: **321 WEST ROAD**	WEIGHT: **185**	BMI: **29**
AGE: **66**	DX: **ANGINA, HTN, BPH, DM, OA, GOUT**	ALLERGY: **NKA**	HX: **OVEREATER**	

MEDICATION	SIG.	PRESCRIBER	ORIG. DATE	REFILL DATE	REFILL DATE	REFILL DATE	REFILL DATE
Colchicine 0.6 mg #90	1 qd	Sauls	8/5	11/2			
Tylenol No. 3 #50	1 q 4–6 h prn	Sauls	8/1	12/10			
Glyburide 5 mg #30	1 qd	Sauls	8/5	9/7	10/8	11/9	12/8
Dyazide #90	1 qd	Sauls	12/10				

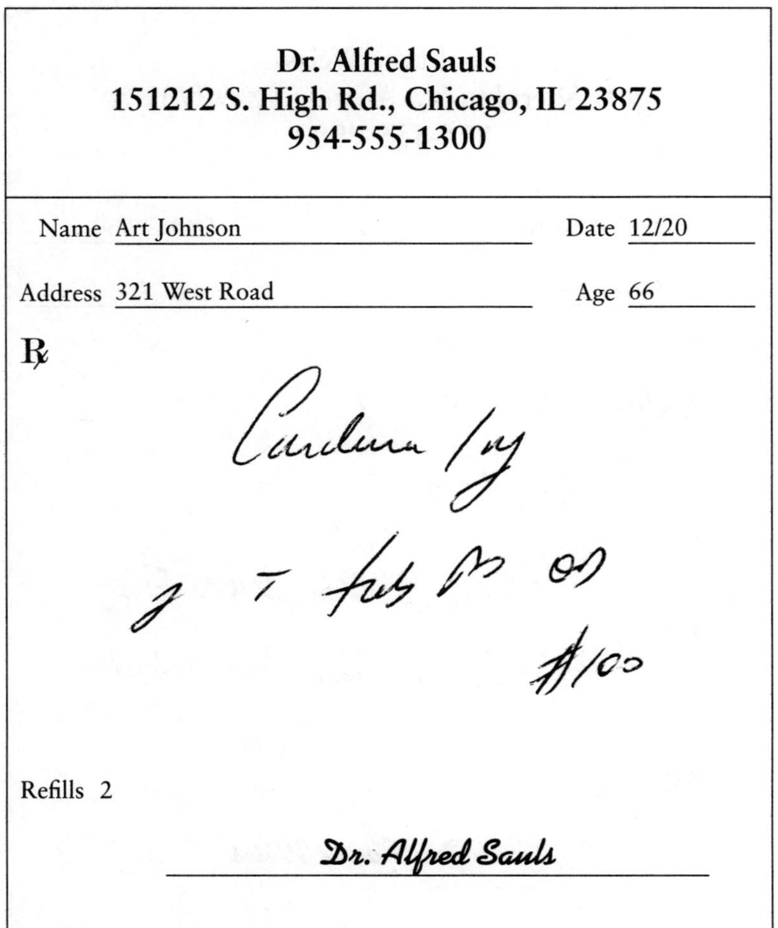

Dr. Alfred Sauls
151212 S. High Rd., Chicago, IL 23875
954-555-1300

Name Art Johnson Date 12/20
Address 321 West Road Age 66

℞

Cardura 1mg
i T tab po qd
#100

Refills 2

Dr. Alfred Sauls

1.8a

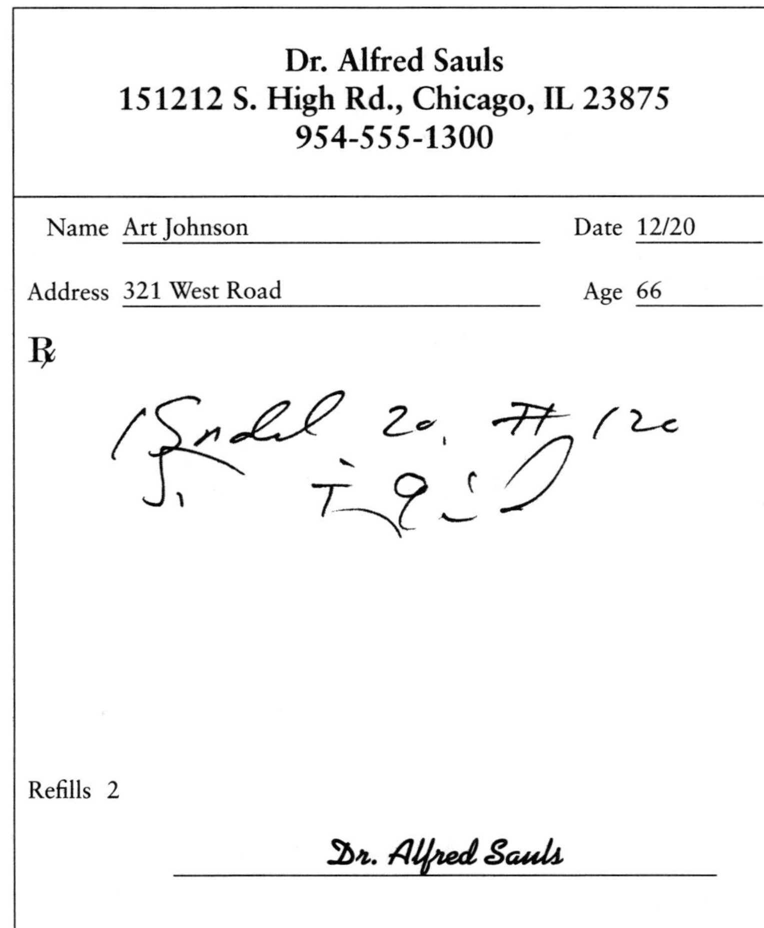

Dr. Alfred Sauls
151212 S. High Rd., Chicago, IL 23875
954-555-1300

Name Art Johnson Date 12/20
Address 321 West Road Age 66

℞

Inderal 20, #120
Si T qid

Refills 2

Dr. Alfred Sauls

1.8b

1.9	PT. NAME: **ARNOLD HARRIS** AGE: **72**	GENDER: **M** DX: **HTN, A-FIB, TENSION HEADACHE**	ADDRESS: **566 EAST CT.** ALLERGY: **NKA**	WEIGHT: **170**	BMI: **24**

MEDICATION	SIG.	PRESCRIBER	ORIG. DATE	REFILL DATE	REFILL DATE	REFILL DATE	REFILL DATE
Warfarin 5 mg #90	I q am	Weiss	8/5	12/6			
Fioricet #50	I bid prn	Weiss	8/5	12/15			
Lasix 40 mg #90	I bid	Weiss	8/10	11/1			

Dr. Barry Weiss
901 Sheridan St., Austin, TX 90902
874-555-9000

Name Arnold Harris Date 12/30

Address 566 East Ct. Age 72

℞

Digoxin 0.125 mg

i tab qd

#60

Refills 3

Dr. Barry Weiss

1.9a

Dr. Barry Weiss
901 Sheridan St., Austin, TX 90902
874-555-9000

Name Arnold Harris Date 12/30

Address 566 East Ct. Age 72

℞

Coumadin 5 mg

#100

Sig: ii tabs q. Mon, Wed. Fri

i tab q Tue, Thurs Sat &

Sun.

Refill NR times

Dr. Barry Weiss

1.9b

1.10

PT. NAME: **MARGARET ADAMS**	GENDER: **F**	ADDRESS: **23 SOUTH ST.**	WEIGHT: **140**	BMI: **24**
AGE: **72**	DX: **HTN, ANGINA**	ALLERGY: **NOT ON FILE (ASK FOR ALLERGIES)**		

MEDICATION	SIG.	PRESCRIBER	ORIG. DATE	REFILL DATE	REFILL DATE	REFILL DATE	REFILL DATE
K-Dur 20 mEq #60	1 bid	Robins	10/3	12/4			
NTG 1/150 gr (0.4 mg) #C	1 sl prn	Robins	10/1	11/2	12/10		
Lasix 40 mg #60	1 bid	Robins	10/3	12/15			

Dr. Calvin Robins
7823 Tea Rose Trail, Miami, FL 44718
463-555-8000

Name Margaret Adams Date 12/21

Address 23 South St. Age 72

℞

Inderal 20 mg
T po BID
#100

Refills 5

Dr. Calvin Robins

1.10a

Dr. Calvin Robins
7823 Tea Rose Trail, Miami, FL 44718
463-555-8000

Name Margaret Adams Date 12/21

Address 23 South St. Age 72

℞

Nitro ointment 2%
5g : apply 2" q8h

Refills 5

Dr. Calvin Robins

1.10b

1.11

PT. NAME: **BRET HARRIS**	GENDER: **M**	ADDRESS: **145 NORTH AVE.**	WEIGHT: **156**	BMI: **27**
AGE: **74**	DX: **HTN, ANGINA**	ALLERGY: **NKA**	HX: **SOCIAL DRINKER**	

MEDICATION	SIG.	PRESCRIBER	ORIG. DATE	REFILL DATE	REFILL DATE	REFILL DATE	REFILL DATE
NTG 1/150 gr (0.4 mg) #C	1 sl prn	Thomas	10/1	11/2	12/10		
Dyazide #30	1 q am	Thomas	10/1	11/2	12/1		

Dr. Erin Thomas
988 North Ridge, New York, NY 88364
813-555-7554

Name Bret Harris Date 12/23

Address 145 North Ave. Age 74

℞

① Lopressor 50mg #30 Sig ½ tab bid
② Lasix 40mg #30 Sig 1 tab QD
③ K-dur 20meq #30 Sig 1 tab QD
④ Ecotrin 325mg #30 Sig 1 tab QD.

Refills 1

Dr. Erin Thomas

1.11a

Dr. Erin Thomas
988 North Ridge, New York, NY 88364
813-555-7554

Name Bret Harris Date 12/23

Address 145 North Ave. Age 74

℞

Nitrostat 0.4 mg
#100
1 tablet under tongue as needed.

Refills 1

Dr. Erin Thomas

1.11b

1.12

PT. NAME: **MARY ADAMS** GENDER: **F** ADDRESS: **325 IRIS BLVD.** WEIGHT: **135** HEIGHT: **5′** BMI: **26**
AGE: **75** DX: **HTN, CHF, ANGINA, RHINORRHEA** ALLERGY: **NKA** HX: **SMOKER FOR 30 YEARS; QUIT SMOKING 5 YEARS AGO**

MEDICATION	SIG.	PRESCRIBER	ORIG. DATE	REFILL DATE	REFILL DATE	REFILL DATE	REFILL DATE
Digoxin 0.125 mg #90	1 q am	Griffin	8/1	11/5			
HCTZ 25 mg #90	1 q am	Griffin	8/1	11/5			
Claritin 10 mg #30	1 q am	OTC	9/5	10/20			

Dr. Doug Griffin
7611 147th Terrace, Monterey, CA 38411
705-555-6644

Name Mary Adams Date 12/15

Address 325 Iris Blvd. Age 75

℞

Ismo 20mg
Disp #C
Sig i po BID

Cardene 30mg
Disp #C
Sig [illegible]

Refills 3

Dr. Doug Griffin

1.12a

Dr. Doug Griffin
7611 147th Terrace, Monterey, CA 38411
705-555-6644

Name Mary Adams Date 12/15

Address 325 Iris Blvd. Age 75

℞

Nitrostat 1/150
i SL chest pain
#100

Refills 3

Dr. Doug Griffin

1.12b

1.13

PT. NAME: **MICHELLE ROBINS**	GENDER: **F**	ADDRESS: **452 HALL ST.**	WEIGHT: **120** HEIGHT: **5′ 3″**
AGE: **75**	DX: **HTN, CHF, ASTHMA, ANGINA, LDL-C: 150 mg/dL**	ALLERGY: **TOMATO**	HX: **SMOKER FOR 25 YEARS; 1 PACK/DAY; QUIT SMOKING 3 YEARS AGO**

MEDICATION	SIG.	PRESCRIBER	ORIG. DATE	REFILL DATE	REFILL DATE	REFILL DATE	REFILL DATE
NTG SL 1/150 gr (0.4 mg) #25	1 sl prn	Sauls	10/5				
Capoten 12.5 mg #60	1 bid	Sauls	10/5				
ProAir HFA 8.5 g	use bid prn	Sauls	8/1	9/2	10/3		

Dr. Alfred Sauls
151212 S. High Rd., Chicago, IL 23875
954-555-1300

Name Michelle Robins Date 11/1

Address 452 Hall Street Age 75

℞

HCTZ 25mg
i po qd
#50

Refills 4

Dr. Alfred Sauls

1.13a

Dr. Alfred Sauls
151212 S. High Rd., Chicago, IL 23875
954-555-1300

Name Michelle Robins Date 11/1

Address 452 Hall Street Age 75

℞

[illegible]
20 mg qd
qd #60

Refills 4

Dr. Alfred Sauls

1.13b

1.14

PT. NAME: **LARRY JONES** GENDER: **M** ADDRESS: **688 GREEN ST.** WEIGHT: **150** BMI: **26**
AGE: **65** DX: **HTN, ANGINA, ASTHMA** ALLERGY: **NKA** HX: **STILL SMOKES 1 PACK/DAY**

MEDICATION	SIG.	PRESCRIBER	ORIG. DATE	REFILL DATE	REFILL DATE	REFILL DATE	REFILL DATE
Theophylline SR 300 mg #60	1 bid	Weiss	10/1	12/3			
Proventil HFA spray 6.7 g	Use tid prn	Weiss	10/1	10/20	11/15		
Lasix 40 mg #30	1 q am	Weiss	8/1	11/1	12/1		
Halcion 0.125 mg #30	1 q am	Weiss	6/1	7/3	8/2	9/1	

Dr. Barry Weiss
901 Sheridan St., Austin, TX 90902
874-555-9000

Name Larry Jones Date 12/14
Address 688 Green St. Age 65

℞
Inderal 20 mg
po q 8h
#60

Refills 5

Dr. Barry Weiss

1.14a

Dr. Barry Weiss
901 Sheridan St., Austin, TX 90902
874-555-9000

Name Larry Jones Date 12/14
Address 688 Green St. Age 65

℞
Catapres TTS II patch
#4
Sig: Apply weekly

Refills 5

Dr. Barry Weiss

1.14b

1.15 PT. NAME: **MATTHEW BAKER** AGE: **80** GENDER: **M** DX: **HTN, DM, ANGINA** ADDRESS: **845 FANTASTIC ST.** ALLERGY: **PCN** WEIGHT: **142** HX: **SOCIAL DRINKER** BMI: **23**

MEDICATION	SIG.	PRESCRIBER	ORIG. DATE	REFILL DATE	REFILL DATE	REFILL DATE	REFILL DATE
Inderal 40 mg #90	1 tid	Robins	10/1				
Lasix 40 mg #30	1 qd	Robins	10/1				
Robitussin Syr 4 oz	5 mL tid prn cough	Robins	8/1	9/2	10/3		
NTG 1/150 gr (0.4 mg) #25	prn	Robins	8/5				
DiaBeta 5 mg #30	1 qd	Robins	6/1	7/2	10/5		

Dr. Calvin Robins
7823 Tea Rose Trail, Miami, FL 44718
463-555-8000

Name Matthew Baker Date 10/23

Address 845 Fantastic Street Age 80

℞

Nitropatch 0.4 mg
(30)

M: daily

Refills 2

Dr. Calvin Robins

1.15a

Dr. Calvin Robins
7823 Tea Rose Trail, Miami, FL 44718
463-555-8000

Name Matthew Baker Date 10/23

Address 845 Fantastic Street Age 80

℞

Tenormin 50 mg
#100

Sig: i T QD [illegible]

Refills 2

Dr. Calvin Robins

1.15b

1.16 PT. NAME: **ROSE BAKER** AGE: **70** GENDER: **F** DX: **HTN, ANGINA, OA** ADDRESS: **89 DEXTER AVE.** ALLERGY: **NKA** WEIGHT: **150** HEIGHT: **5′ 2″** HX: **OVERWEIGHT MOST OF HER LIFE**

MEDICATION	SIG.	PRESCRIBER	ORIG. DATE	REFILL DATE	REFILL DATE	REFILL DATE	REFILL DATE
NTG 1/150 gr (0.4 mg) #C	I sl prn	Thomas	10/1	11/1	12/2	1/3	
ASA 81 mg #36	I q am to thin blood	Thomas	10/1	11/5	12/6		
Isordil 10 mg #90	I tid ac	Thomas	10/1	11/2	12/4	1/5	
Motrin 400 mg #90	I tid for arthritis	Thomas	10/1	11/2	12/5	1/8	
Sudafed 30 mg #C	I bid for sinus prn	Weiss	12/20				

Dr. Erin Thomas
988 North Ridge, New York, NY 88364
813-555-7554

Name Rose Baker Date 1/18
Address 89 Dexter Ave. Age 70

℞
Lopressor 50 mg
Sig: i po daily

#100

Refills 3

Dr. Erin Thomas

1.16a

Dr. Erin Thomas
988 North Ridge, New York, NY 88364
813-555-7554

Name Rose Baker Date 1/18
Address 89 Dexter Ave. Age 70

℞
Zestril 10 mg
Sig: i po daily

#60

Refills 3

Dr. Erin Thomas

1.16b

1.17	PT. NAME: **HENRIETTA SMITH**	GENDER: **F**	ADDRESS: **564 CAPITOL AVE.**	WEIGHT: **198**	BMI: **32**
	AGE: **68**	DX: **HTN, LIVER CIRRHOSIS**	ALLERGY: **NKA**	HX: **SMOKER, ETOH**	

MEDICATION	SIG.	PRESCRIBER	ORIG. DATE	REFILL DATE	REFILL DATE	REFILL DATE	REFILL DATE
No medications on file: Ask patient for medication history							

Dr. Doug Griffin
7611 147th Terrace, Monterey, CA 38411
705-555-6644

Name Henrietta Smith Date 8/14

Address 564 Capitol Ave. Age 68

℞

Lasix 60mg ī po qd 20mg
tablets 3 po qd
Mitte 100

Refills 0

Dr. Doug Griffin

1.17a

Dr. Doug Griffin
7611 147th Terrace, Monterey, CA 38411
705-555-6644

Name Henrietta Smith Date 8/14

Address 564 Capitol Ave. Age 68

℞

Aldactone 25mg IV cq
po bid Mitte 240

Refills 0

Dr. Doug Griffin

1.17b

1.18

PT. NAME: **JOHN BRILL**	GENDER: **M**	ADDRESS: **548 NORTH AVE.**	WEIGHT: **180**	HEIGHT: **5′ 9″**
AGE: **73**	DX: **BPH, HTN, OA, LEG CRAMPS, GERD, NAUSEA, ANXIETY, CONSTIPATION**	ALLERGY: **NKA**	HX: **RETIRED**	

MEDICATION	SIG.	PRESCRIBER	ORIG. DATE	REFILL DATE	REFILL DATE	REFILL DATE	REFILL DATE
Quinine Sulfate 324 mg #60	1 hs prn	Adams	9/26	11/21	12/18		
Losartan 100 mg #90	1 qd	Adams	6/14	9/8	12/10		
Metoprolol 50 mg #45	1/2 tab qd	Adams	7/5	9/3	11/1		
Nexium 40 mg #30	1 q am, 60 min ac bkfst	Adams	6/22	8/30	9/26	11/20	

Dr. Jill Adams
3388 S. High Rd., Chicago, IL 23875
954-555-7777

Name John Brill Date 12/21

Address 548 North Ave Age 73

℞

① XANAX 0.25mg #90 Sig 1 tab tid
② Colace 100mg #60 Sig 1 tab bid
③ NORVASC 10mg # 30 Sig 1 tab QD

LABEL

Refill ① times

Dr. Jill Adams

1.18a

Dr. Jill Adams
3388 S. High Rd., Chicago, IL 23875
954-555-7777

Name John Brill Date 12/21

Address 548 North Ave Age 73

℞

Tigan Caps 300 mg
disp # 6
Sig. T q 4-6 h prn nausea

Refills 3x

Dr. Jill Adams

1.18b

1.19

PT. NAME: **LEONARD GRILLO**	GENDER: **M**	ADDRESS: **3888 FRANKLIN BLVD.**	WEIGHT: **155**	BMI: **24**
AGE: **79**	DX: **HTN, OA, SEBORRHEA, DIARRHEA**	ALLERGY: **NKA**	HX: **ETOH, SMOKER**	

MEDICATION	SIG.	PRESCRIBER	ORIG. DATE	REFILL DATE	REFILL DATE	REFILL DATE	REFILL DATE
Ketoconazole 2% shampoo	Apply ud	Wells	11/23				
Lomotil tablets #30	1 tab tid prn	Salls	7/20	9/13			
Ultracet 37.5/325 mg #30	1 tab q 4–6 h prn pain	Salls	7/20	8/20	9/5	10/12	11/15

Dr. Barry Salls
22 NW 3 Ave.
Miami, FL 33162
305-888-5567

Name Leonard Grillo Date 12/21

Address 3888 Franklin Blvd. Age 79

℞

Cardizem 60 mg
#200

Sig: i PO BID

Label yes

Refill 3

Dr. Barry Salls

1.19a

Dr. Barry Salls
22 NW 3 Ave.
Miami, FL 33162
305-888-5567

Name Leonard Grillo Date 12/21

Address 3888 Franklin Blvd. Age 79

℞

Vasotec 2.5 mg #200
two Hundred

i PO qd.

Label

Refill 5

Dr. Barry Salls

1.19b

1.20

PT. NAME: **BRYAN COOKE** AGE: **70**
GENDER: **M** DX: **HTN, HIGH LIPIDS, SKIN IRRITATION**
ADDRESS: **8 NO. EVERGLADES DR.** ALLERGY: **PCN**
WEIGHT: **149** HX: **PART-TIME CLERK**
HEIGHT: **5′ 3″**

MEDICATION	SIG.	PRESCRIBER	ORIG. DATE	REFILL DATE	REFILL DATE	REFILL DATE	REFILL DATE
Coreg 3.125 mg #60	1 bid	Rich	9/4	10/5	11/3	12/1	
Caduet 5/20 mg #30	1 qd	Rich	9/4	10/5	11/3		
Vitamin D 1000 IU #90	1 qd	Rich	9/4	10/3	11/5	12/7	

Dr. Al Rich
66 White St.
Baltimore, MD 44499
444-595-2212

Name Bryan Cooke Date 12/21

Address 8 No. Everglades Dr. Age 70

℞

Caduet 10/20 mg
ī po qd
#30

Diovan 160mg
ī po qd
#30

❏ Label

Refill X3 times

Dr. Al Rich

1.20a

Dr. Nancy Jerus
61 White St.
Baltimore, MD 44499
444-595-9998

Name Bryan Cooke Date 12/21

Address 8 No. Everglades Dr. Age 70

℞

Kenalog 1% Cream
Disp ī tube
2g apply BID

❏ Label

Refill 3 times

Dr. Nancy Jerus

1.20b

1.21

PT. NAME: **SHARON ROSEN** AGE: **80** GENDER: **F** DX: **ANGINA, HTN** ADDRESS: **55 NW GREEN TERR.** ALLERGY: **NKA** WEIGHT: **113** HX: **EX-SMOKER** BMI: **22**

MEDICATION	SIG.	PRESCRIBER	ORIG. DATE	REFILL DATE	REFILL DATE	REFILL DATE	REFILL DATE
NTG 0.4 mg #100	1 sl prn C.P.	Green	5/5				
Aldactone 25 mg #60	1 bid	Green	5/5	6/30	9/6	11/8	
Aggrenox caps #60	1 bid	Green	6/9	7/8	8/11		

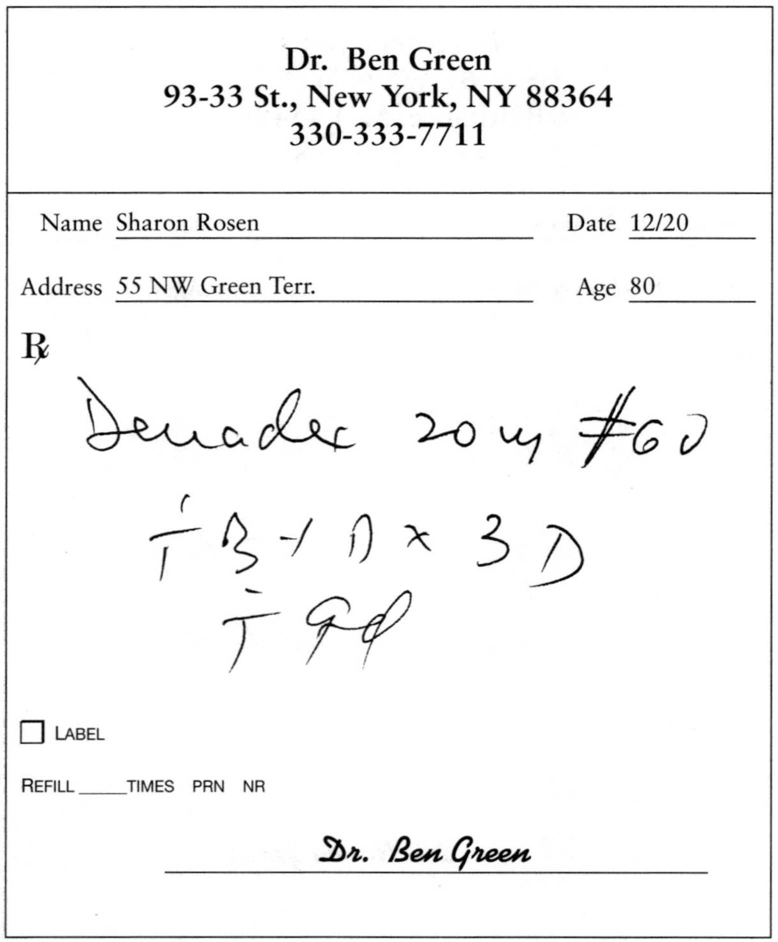

Dr. Ben Green
93-33 St., New York, NY 88364
330-333-7711

Name Sharon Rosen Date 12/20

Address 55 NW Green Terr. Age 80

℞

Demadex 20 mg #60
i B-1 D x 3 D
i qd

☐ LABEL

REFILL _____ TIMES PRN NR

Dr. Ben Green

1.21a

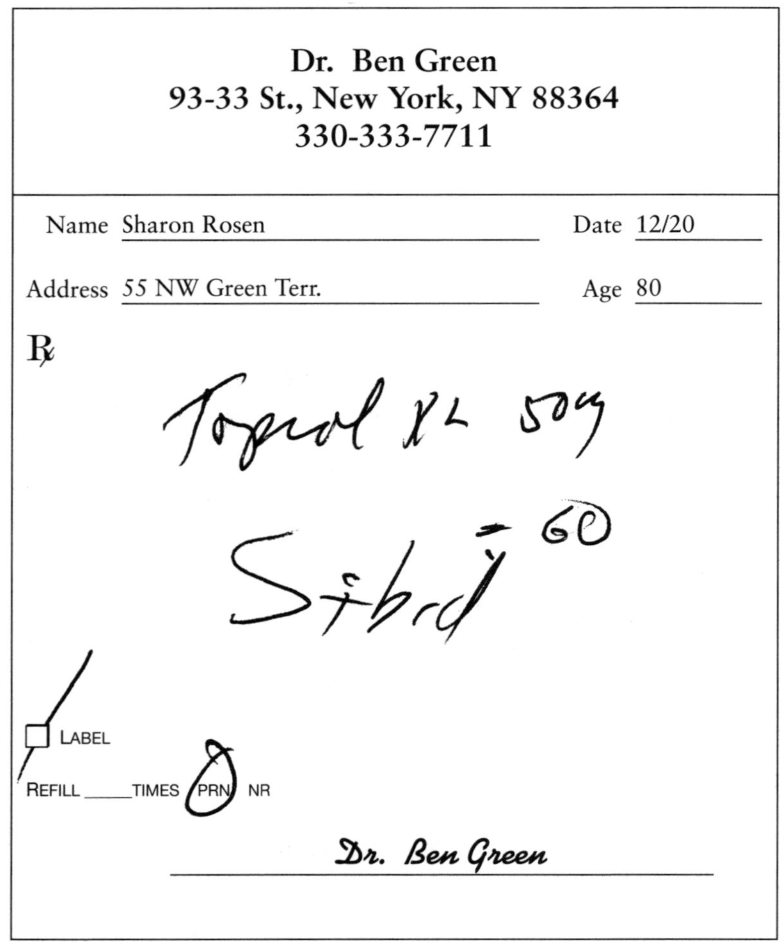

Dr. Ben Green
93-33 St., New York, NY 88364
330-333-7711

Name Sharon Rosen Date 12/20

Address 55 NW Green Terr. Age 80

℞

Toprol XL 50 mg
Sig i bid #60

☑ LABEL

REFILL _____ TIMES PRN NR

Dr. Ben Green

1.21b

1.22

PT. NAME: **SHELDON NANE**	GENDER: **M**	ADDRESS: **60 MELLOW AVE.**	WEIGHT: **105**	BMI: **20**
AGE: **92**	DX: **OPEN-ANGLE GLAUCOMA, HTN, UTI, HEARTBURN, BPH**	ALLERGY: **SULFA, ERYTHROMYCIN**	HX: **EX-SMOKER**	

MEDICATION	SIG.	PRESCRIBER	ORIG. DATE	REFILL DATE	REFILL DATE	REFILL DATE	REFILL DATE
Flomax 0.4 mg #30	1 cap at 8 pm qd	Nash	10/4	11/25			
Protonix 40 mg #30	1 qd 60 min ac bkfst	Mone	4/1	8/30			
Xalatan 0.005% 2.5 mL	1 drop ou qd	Ng	10/30	12/16			
Trusopt 2% 10 mL	1 drop ou bid ud	Ng	6/4	8/14	10/26		

Dr. David Nathan
55 SW 20 Ave., San Diego, CA 44718
463-555-8441

Name Sheldon Nane Date 12/21

Address 60 Mellow Ave. Age 92

℞

Cardizem CD 120 #100

T po

Refills

Dr. David Nathan

1.22a

Dr. David Nathan
55 SW 20 Ave., San Diego, CA 44718
463-555-8441

Name Sheldon Nane Date 12/21

Address 60 Mellow Ave. Age 92

℞

HCTZ 25mg

#30

T po QD

Dr. David Nathan

1.22b

1.23

PT. NAME: **BILL ROSS** GENDER: **M** ADDRESS: **50 CANAL ST.** WEIGHT: **121** BMI: **20**

AGE: **73** DX: **HTN, GOUT, TYPE 2 DM, GERD, URINARY IRRITATION** ALLERGY: **NKA** HX: **SEDENTARY LIFESTYLE**

MEDICATION	SIG.	PRESCRIBER	ORIG. DATE	REFILL DATE	REFILL DATE	REFILL DATE	REFILL DATE
Zyloprim 100 mg #90	I qd	Cesar	8/2	11/14			
Coumadin 2.5 mg #90	I qd	Cesar	8/2	11/14			
Diovan 80 mg #90	I qd	Cesar	9/19				
Bumex 0.5 mg #180	I bid	Cesar	6/1	8/8	10/2	11/12	
Plavix 75 mg #90	I qd	Cesar	6/1	9/14	11/2		
Omeprazole 20 mg #42	prn	OTC	7/5	8/20	10/5	11/20	

Dr. Ray Cesar
800 No. Circle Dr., Orlando, FL 48488
705-555-6630

Name Bill Ross Date 12/21

Address 50 Canal St. Age 73

℞

Isoptin SR 180 mg
1/2 po qd
#30

☐ Label

Refill 2 times PRN

Dr. Ray Cesar

1.23a

Dr. Ray Cesar
800 No. Circle Dr., Orlando, FL 48488
705-555-6630

Name Bill Ross Date 12/21

Address 50 Canal St. Age 73

℞

Pyridium 100 mg
(i) BID

#30

Dr. Ray Cesar

1.23b

1.24

PT. NAME: **GRACE FULLER** AGE: **82** GENDER: **F** DX: **TYPE 2 DM, ANGINA, HTN, CHF, DEPRESSION, HIGH LIPID** ADDRESS: **3300 TAFT ST.** ALLERGY: **STRAWBERRIES** WEIGHT: **148** HX: **OVEREATER** BMI: **28**

MEDICATION	SIG.	PRESCRIBER	ORIG. DATE	REFILL DATE	REFILL DATE	REFILL DATE	REFILL DATE
Digoxin 0.125 mg #30	1 qd	Walker	10/12				
Lexapro 10 mg #30	1 qd	White	10/1	11/2	12/1		
Crestor 5 mg #30	1 qd	Walker	9/4	10/3	11/3	12/1	
Glyburide 2.5 mg #30	1 q am	Walker	10/2	11/3	12/6		

Dr. Al Walker
33 DeKalb Ave, Brooklyn, NY 11201
812-333-8863

Name Grace Fuller Date 12/20

Address 3300 Taft St. Age 82

℞

Lasix 20mg
#20

Sig 1 PRN swell

☐ Label

Refill ______ times

Dr. Al Walker

1.24a

Dr. Al Walker
33 DeKalb Ave, Brooklyn, NY 11201
812-333-8863

Name Grace Fuller Date 12/20

Address 3300 Taft St. Age 82

℞

Nitrodur .4mg
#30

Sig apply in AM
off in PM

REFILL 0 TIMES

Dr. Al Walker

1.24b

1.25	PT. NAME: **HAL GRANT**	GENDER: **M**	ADDRESS: **566 EAST CT.**	WEIGHT: **149**	HEIGHT: **5′ 1″**
	AGE: **77**	DX: **TYPE 2 DM, OA, ANGINA, HYPOTHYROID, HTN, GUM INFECTION, HEARTBURN, PERIPHERAL ARTERY DISEASE**		ALLERGY: **ERYTHROMYCIN**	HX: **SMOKES CIGARS**

MEDICATION	SIG.	PRESCRIBER	ORIG. DATE	REFILL DATE	REFILL DATE	REFILL DATE	REFILL DATE
Tylenol No. 3 #30	1 tab tid	Meisel, DDS	8/30	10/28	11/29		
Plavix 75 mg #60	1 qd	Rhodes	10/31	12/1			
Synthroid 50 mcg #60	1 q am	Rhodes	8/19	10/19	12/20		
Prandin 2 mg #90	1 tid	Rhodes	9/5	10/4	11/6	12/8	

Dr. John Rhodes
3030 Garret Parkway
Dallas, TX 68696
440-444-1123

Name Hal Grant Date 12/21

Address 566 East Ct. Age 77

℞

		MG./CC	QUAN.	TIMES REFILL
℞1	ZANTAC 150	150 MG	60	(0) 1 2 3 4 5
SIG.	T B.I.D AM + HS			
℞2	[illegible] ADALAT 30CC		30	0 1 2 3 4 5
SIG.	ONCE DAILY			
℞3	NITRO DUR 0.2 MG	0.2	30	0 1 2 3 4 5
SIG.	1 T HS			

Dr. John Rhodes

1.25a

Dr. Harris Meisel, DDS
44 Grove Drive
Dallas, TX 68696
440-444-7696

Name Hal Grant Date 12/21

Address 566 East Ct. Age 77

℞

Cephalexin 500 mg

Disp: Pulv. #18

Sig: 2 pulv stat, then 1 tid starting tomorrow

☐ Label

Refill - 0 - (1) - 2 - 3 - 4 - PRN

Dr. Harris Meisel, DDS

1.25b

1.26

PT. NAME: **HARRIS EPSTEIN**	GENDER: **M**	ADDRESS: **33 W. AVE.**	WEIGHT: **150**	HEIGHT: **5′ 10″**
AGE: **71**	DX: **HTN, STROKE, ALZHEIMER'S DISEASE, HYPERCHOLESTEROL, INSOMNIA, AGITATION**		ALLERGY: **NKA**	HX: **SMOKER FOR 20 YEARS; SMOKES 2 PACKS/DAY**

MEDICATION	SIG.	PRESCRIBER	ORIG. DATE	REFILL DATE	REFILL DATE	REFILL DATE	REFILL DATE
Zocor 40 mg #30	1 qd	Alvarez	2/9	5/31	9/22		
Aricept 5 mg #30	1 hs	Blum	3/9	6/3			
Aricept 10 mg #30	1 hs	Blum	8/4				
Norvasc 5 mg #30	1 qd	Alvarez	2/9	4/8	6/9	9/2	
Seroquel 25 mg #30	1 hs qd	Blum	9/5				

Dr. Raul Alvarez
66 N. Arce Ave.
Houston TX 44099
233-555-7789

Name Harris Epstein Date 10/3

Address 33 W. Ave. Age 71

℞

AGGRENOX

i cap PO BID

c̄ meals

#60

☐ Label

Refill - 0 - (1) - 2 - 3 - 4 - PRN

Dr. Raul Alvarez

1.26a

Dr. Joyce Levy, DDS
82 S. Marsh Lane
Houston, TX 44099
233-919-9944

Name Harris Epstein Date 10/3

Address 33 W. Ave. Age 71

℞

Vicodin

Disp #20

Sig i tab q6h

prn pain

Refills NR

Dr. J. Levy, DDS

DEA# AL1234563

1.26b

1.27

PT. NAME: **ALICE CARDIFF** GENDER: **F** ADDRESS: **88 NORTH AVE.** WEIGHT: **144** BMI: **33**

AGE: **79** DX: **ANGINA, HTN, DYSLIPIDEMIA, CONSTIPATION, ANXIETY, POST MI** ALLERGY: **NKA**

MEDICATION	SIG.	PRESCRIBER	ORIG. DATE	REFILL DATE	REFILL DATE	REFILL DATE	REFILL DATE
Plavix 75 mg #30	I qd	Garcia	6/20	7/19	8/21	9/22	
Simvastatin 20 mg #30	I hs	Garcia	6/23	7/22	10/22		
Xanax 0.5 mg #60	I bid	Garcia	9/21	10/25			
Norvasc 5 mg #30	I qd	Garcia	9/21	10/20			
Isosorbide MN 30 mg #60	I bid	Garcia	6/20	7/21	8/21	9/20	10/20
Metoprolol Succinate ER 25 mg #60	I bid	Garcia	9/21	10/20			

Dr. Alfredo Garcia
12 S. High Rd. Chicago, IL 23875
954-555-1654

Name Alice Cardiff Date 10/29

Address 88 North Ave. Age 79

℞

RANEXA 500 mg

#60

1 BID

Refills 3 X

Dr. Alfredo Garcia

1.27a

Dr. Alfredo Garcia
12 S. High Rd. Chicago, IL 23875
954-555-1654

Name Alice Cardiff Date 10/29

Address 88 North Ave. Age 79

℞ MIRALAX™
Polyethylene Glycol 3350, NF Powder

☐ **Dispense one 255 g bottle**
Sig: Use as Directed

☒ **Dispense one 527 g bottle**
Sig: Use as Directed

☐ Label

Refill 3 times PRN NR

Do Not Substitute ☐

Dr. Alfredo Garcia

1.27b

1.28 PT. NAME: **JOAN KENNEDY** AGE: **78** GENDER: **F** DX: **CHF, TYPE 2 DM, HTN, HYPERTHYROID, OA** ADDRESS: **500 SE 2ND ST.** ALLERGY: **NKA** WEIGHT: **118** HX: **YEARS OF "NERVES" AND DIARRHEA** HEIGHT: **5′ 4″**

MEDICATION	SIG.	PRESCRIBER	ORIG. DATE	REFILL DATE	REFILL DATE	REFILL DATE	REFILL DATE
Lanoxin 0.125 mg #90	1 qd	Hauber	7/1	10/2			
Vasotec 10 mg #90	1 bid	Hauber	8/2	9/15			
Celebrex 100 mg #30	1 qd	Hauber	9/15				
HCTZ 25 mg #45	1/2 tab q am with OJ	Hauber	8/2				
Glyburide 5 mg #30	1 q am	Hauber	5/6	6/4	7/8	8/2	9/30

Dr. Don Hauber
7600 Orange Ave., Fresno, CA 38411
705-555-6944

Name Joan Kennedy Date 10/10

Address 500 SE 2nd St. Age 78

℞

Plavix 75
Sig: 1 daily
#30

Refills PRN

Dr. Don Hauber

1.28a

Dr. Alan Limmer
9091 Orange Ave., Fresno, CA 38411
705-555-0001

Name Joan Kennedy Date 10/10

Address 500 SE 2nd St. Age 78

℞

#30 Tapazole 10mg
Sig: 1/2 bid

Refills X 3

Dr. Alan Limmer

1.28b

1.29 PT. NAME: **ERNIE PEZZONI** AGE: **74** GENDER: **M** ADDRESS: **45 10TH ST.** DX: **INTERMITTENT CLAUDICATION, HTN, CONJUNCTIVITIS, HIGH HOMOCYSTEINE LEVELS, CONSTIPATION** WEIGHT: **145** ALLERGY: **ASA** BMI: **23** HX: **ATHLETE ALL HIS LIFE; CONSTIPATED FOR YEARS**

MEDICATION	SIG.	PRESCRIBER	ORIG. DATE	REFILL DATE	REFILL DATE	REFILL DATE	REFILL DATE
Bacitracin Ophthalmic Ointment	Apply ud to affected eye	Dooner	12/2				
Norvasc 5 mg #30	1 qd	Ariola	8/25	9/23	10/24	11/26	12/27
Toprol XL 25 mg #30	1 qd	Ariola	8/25	9/23	10/24	11/26	12/27
Fleet Saline Enema 118 mL #3	1 qd rectally prn	OTC	7/22	9/23	10/9	11/2	12/1

Dr. Alfonso Ariola
1345 Victory Place
E. Brunswick, NJ 33399
585-868-1010

Name Ernie Pezzoni Date 12/28

Address 45 10th Street Age 74

℞ Pletal 50 mg

#60

i B.I.D.

☒ Label

Refill 60 times PRN NR

Dr. Alfonso Ariola

1.29a

Dr. Alfonso Ariola
1345 Victory Place
E. Brunswick, NJ 33399
585-868-1010

Name Ernie Pezzoni Date 12/28

Address 45 10th Street Age 74

℞ Foltx tabs

#XXX

Sig: i daily

Refills 3

Dr. Alfonso Ariola

1.29b

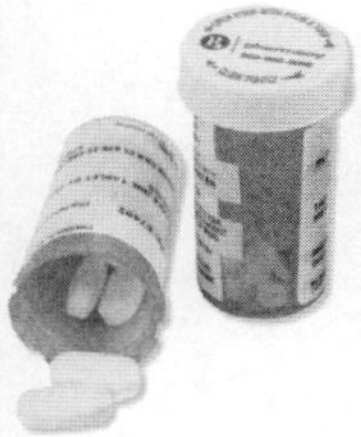

2 • CARDIOVASCULAR, PART 2

UPON COMPLETION OF THIS CHAPTER,
THE STUDENT WILL BE ABLE TO:

- advise patients taking antihypertensive agents and diuretics on dietary restrictions, mild exercise, and lifestyle modifications.
- explain to patients the importance of avoiding salt and salt substitutes when taking ACE inhibitors.
- counsel patients on the importance of continuing their antihypertensive medications.
- discuss the occurrence of postural hypotension associated with vasodilator therapy and recommend appropriate methods to diminish this effect.
- discuss differences in side effect profiles associated with the therapeutic use of calcium channel-blocking agents (verapamil/diltiazem/nifedipine).
- counsel patients regarding food (grapefruit) and drug interactions.
- demonstrate a working knowledge of the classification of antiarrhythmic agents, including the ion channels that are blocked and the results of their actions.

DRUG LIST

ACE Inhibitors
A II receptor antagonists
Antiarrhythmic agents
Apresoline
Caduet
Cardizem
Catapres
Hytrin/Cardura/Minipress
Lipitor/Lescol/Pravachol/Zocor/Crestor/Livalo
Lopid, Tricor, Questran, Niaspan, Vytorin, Zetia, Trilipix
Lotrel
Procardia
Tekturna
Verapamil

• DRUG HOT POINTS

Apresoline
Arteriolar vasodilator
Drug-induced SLE symptoms (high doses)

Caduet
Blood pressure and lipid treatment in a single product

Capoten
Inhibits A II formation, reduces aldosterone
Monitor side effects: cough
Potassium sparing
ACE inhibitors are not for pregnant patients

Cardizem
Action: between verapamil & nifedipine
Counsel: compliance
Counsel: diet, exercise
Some constipation
Tablets: regular and LA

Catapres
Apply patches once a **week**
2 patches: 1 with drug, 1 overlay
Do not stop medication
Side effects: dry mouth, constipation
Counseling for side effects
Other uses for clonidine

Cholestyramine (Questran)
Place in water, drink, pour more water on same glass and drink
Caution: constipation
May interfere with other meds
Two formulations: regular and light

Cordarone (amiodarone)
Long half-life, thyroid (↑ or ↓)
Interactions with digoxin and warfarin
Caution: cough, eye exams
Compare with Betapace, Betapace AF

Hytrin/Cardura/Minipress
Long-acting, alpha-1 antagonists
Two uses: BPH & HTN (not initial therapy)
Caution: OTC meds: urinary obstruction

Lipitor/Lescol/Pravachol/Zocor/Crestor/Livalo
Lowers LDL-C and total cholesterol
Caution: muscle pain (myositis, myalgia, potential for rhabdomyolysis)
Compare with Niaspan, Vytorin, Zetia
Compare potencies within "statin" class

Lopid
30 minutes before food, BID
Lowers triglycerides
Compare with Tricor and Trilipix

Losartan (Cozaar)
Mechanism of action to treat HTN
Blocks AT II at type AT_1 receptor
Also in combination with diuretics
Cozaar and Hyzaar: compare with Diovan, Avapro, Atacand, and other ARBs
ARBs are not for pregnant patients

Lotrel
Blood pressure control via two different mechanisms of action

Procardia
Potent peripheral vasodilator
Potential for pedal edema, dizziness, and gingival enlargement
Compare with Norvasc, DynaCirc, Plendil, Sular, Cardene
Counsel: grapefruit juice interaction

Quinidine
Grains vs. mg (200 mg = 3 gr)
Digoxin: quinidine interaction
Caution: quinine/quinidine confusion

• DRUG HOT POINTS (*continued*)

Tambocor (flecainide)
Mechanism, cautions, counseling
BID should be every 12 hours
Class Ic antiarrhythmic: compare with Rythmol

Tekturna (aliskiren)
Direct renin inhibitor
Indicated for treatment of hypertension
Pregnancy warnings
Reduces plasma renin activity

Vasotec (enalapril)
Potential for hyperkalemia
Caution: salt substitutes (KCl)
Prodrug
Watch for cough
Compare with other ACE inhibitors (lisinopril, ramipril, etc.)
ACE inhibitors commonly combined with HCTZ

Verapamil (Calan, Isoptin)
Side effect profile: constipation
Tablet SR: with food
Covera-HS, Verelan, Verelan PM
Digoxin/verapamil interaction
Compare with Procardia & Cardizem

• QUESTIONS TO BE ANSWERED IN PREPARATION FOR CHAPTER 2 LAB

- What is the mechanism of action of terazosin in the treatment of BPH?
- Describe the mechanism for the tachycardia that may occur with Procardia.
- Explain why hyperkalemia can occur with the use of Capoten.
- Why would a client taking Prinivil present with swelling of the mouth and tongue?
- Which specific part of the vasculature is affected by Apresoline?
- Explain the action of hydralazine in the treatment of CHF.
- Why should a patient **not** suddenly stop taking Catapres? The answer must explain the outcome.
- Explain the proposed mechanism of action of Catapres in the treatment of hypertension. The answer must include the receptor involved and the action of Catapres at the receptor.
- Why would a patient who is taking Procardia and using Nitro-Dur patches experience headache and dizziness?
- A doctor prescribes the following prescription: captopril 6.25 mg Sig: 1 tablet TID. Explain how you would fill the prescription.
- A patient taking Hytrin 2 mg qd for the treatment of BPH presents a prescription to you for dicyclomine for abdominal cramps. What would you do?
- Which autonomic receptors are being affected by the dicyclomine?
- Which class of calcium channel blockers causes the most peripheral vasodilation?
- Why would a person experience dizziness on taking the first dose of Hytrin or Cardura?
- A pregnant patient presents a prescription to you for Capoten to treat her hypertension. Why is this drug contraindicated for her? What is the pregnancy category in the third trimester? Which agent would be more appropriate to treat her hypertension?
- Which "statin" drug is the most potent, milligram for milligram?
- Name two class Ic antiarrhythmic agents.
- Which channels are blocked by members of the class I antiarrhythmic agents?
- What is the meaning of the initials "TTS" in Catapres TTS patches?
- Which "statin" is not metabolized at all by the CYP-450 system?
- How many milligrams of Zocor would be equal to 10 mg of Lipitor in lowering LDL-C?
- Explain the cause of dry mouth and constipation that occurs in many patients who take clonidine.
- Explain the differences in channel blockade between the various classes of antiarrhythmic agents.
- Describe the mechanism by which the following agents cause hyperkalemia:
  - spironolactone
  - Zestril
- You receive the following prescription: Tambocor 100 mg. The instruction is 1 tablet QID. What would you do?
- Which calcium channel blocker is most likely to cause constipation?
- You receive the following prescription: Cardizem CD 300 mg Sig: 1 capsule QID. What would you do?
- A prescription for gemfibrozil (Lopid) reads "Take one tablet BID." Should the patient take it before, with, or after food?
- Your client has been taking Zocor. He complains of muscle pain in his arms. If drug related, what could be the problem?
- Your client presents a prescription for one of the "statin" drugs for the treatment of high cholesterol. He mentions that he takes his morning medicines with grapefruit juice. What is the nature of the potentially serious food–drug interaction in this case?
- Your customer is taking Catapres 0.2-mg tabs PO bid for the treatment of hypertension. He says that he is going to stop the pills because he is feeling okay. He also says that the pills cause dry mouth. How would you advise this person?

• QUESTIONS TO BE ANSWERED IN PREPARATION FOR CHAPTER 2 LAB *(continued)*

- How do ACE inhibitors work in the treatment of CHF and HTN?
- Describe an additional antihypertensive mechanism of ACE inhibitors involving bradykinin.
- Explain the difference in the actions of ACE inhibitors and angiotensin receptor blockers.
- Describe the classification system for antiarrhythmic agents with the members of each group: which channels are blocked, the indications of each agent, and side-effect profiles.
- What is the advantage of combining an ACE inhibitor or an ARB (angiotensin receptor blocker) with HCTZ in one tablet?
- Compare Trilipix to Tricor.

• CARDIOVASCULAR, PART 2, MEDICATION THERAPY MANAGEMENT QUESTIONS AND COMMENTS

- Your medication for heart rhythm is prescribed twice a day. Did your doctor tell you to take the pills 12 hours apart?
- You are taking a pill called Procardia. Did the prescriber say that you should visit your dentist frequently for teeth cleanings? It is important when taking this medication.
- Are you aware that when you take this medicine called a "statin," you should visit your doctor at recommended intervals for blood tests? Also, if you experience any unusual muscle pain, please contact us or your prescriber.
- Your father is receiving a new pill called an "alpha-blocker." It will help his urine flow and blood pressure. However, during the first week, ask him to stand up very slowly to avoid becoming dizzy.
- You are receiving a new medicine called a "clonidine patch." Please remember that the medicine is in the small pink patch. The larger one is a cover for the small one. That will protect the medicine-containing patch for the whole week when it must be worn.
- Your prescription for clonidine will probably make your mouth dry and cause some constipation. Please do not stop the medicine. If you have questions, we can recommend sugarless gum and or appropriate laxatives.
- Your new blood pressure medication is called an "ACE inhibitor." It is an effective medication. Remember to drink adequate amounts of water each day. If you experience an annoying dry cough, please contact us or your doctor.
- Your doctor has prescribed Apresoline or hydralazine for your patient. It is important that he stands up very slowly and takes all his other medicines. Some of them will help this medication work well.
- Your doctor has prescribed an ACE inhibitor for you, for blood pressure control. Because you are of childbearing age, it is important for me to ask you the following: Are you or do you plan to get pregnant? If so, I must contact the doctor to consult with him. This medication must not be taken by a pregnant patient.
- Your doctor has prescribed a medication called an ARB. Did the prescriber tell you to avoid salt substitutes? They contain potassium, and this medication might combine with a salt substitute to cause too much potassium in your body.
- I realize that you are taking many medications at different times of the day. I would recommend that you place the week's supply in a plastic daily reminder container that we carry. It will let you know when to take each one or more of your medicines. They must be put into the plastic container by a trained nurse or pharmacist.
- I notice that you have a new prescription for Lotrel, and you have been taking a medicine called Altace. Did the doctor tell you to stop Altace? It contains similar medicine that is in Lotrel.
- Your cardiovascular system will enjoy a small amount of movement. Too much sitting could be bad for your body. Did your doctor recommend short but frequent daily walks?

2.1

PT. NAME: **ROSE BAKER**	GENDER: **F**	ADDRESS: **544 BURNS ST.**	WEIGHT: **140**	HEIGHT: **5′**
AGE: **70**	DX: **HTN, ANGINA**	ALLERGY: **MILK**		

MEDICATION	SIG.	PRESCRIBER	ORIG. DATE	REFILL DATE	REFILL DATE	REFILL DATE	REFILL DATE
NTG 1/150 gr (0.4 mg) #C	I sl prn	Griffin	6/4	8/3			
ASA 81 mg #36	I q am to thin blood	Griffin	6/4	7/5			
Isordil 10 mg #90	I tid	Griffin	6/4	7/8			

Dr. Doug Griffin
7611 147th Terrace, Monterey, CA 38411
705-555-6644

Name Rose Baker Date 8/5

Address 544 Burns Street Age 70

℞

Norvasc 5 mg
#30
Sig: i po qd

Refills 4

Dr. Doug Griffin

2.1a

Dr. Doug Griffin
7611 147th Terrace, Monterey, CA 38411
705-555-6644

Name Rose Baker Date 8/5

Address 544 Burns Street Age 70

℞

Verapamil SR 240 mg
#100
1/2 po bid

Refills 0

Dr. Doug Griffin

2.1b

2.2

PT. NAME: **ABRAHAM WALKER**	GENDER: **M**	ADDRESS: **821 ALBERTY CIRCLE**	WEIGHT: **150**	BMI: **24**
AGE: **75**	DX: **ANGINA, HTN, POST MI**	ALLERGY: **NKA**		

MEDICATION	SIG.	PRESCRIBER	ORIG. DATE	REFILL DATE	REFILL DATE	REFILL DATE	REFILL DATE
Lanoxin 0.125 mg #30	1 q am	Sauls	10/1	11/3			
HCTZ 25 mg #30	1 q am	Sauls	10/1	11/4			
Apresoline 25 mg #60	1 bid	Sauls	10/1	11/10			
OTC EC ASA 81 mg #C	1 q am	Sauls	10/1	11/2			

Dr. Alfred Sauls
151212 S. High Rd., Chicago, IL 23875
954-555-1300

Name Abraham Walker Date 11/15

Address 821 Alberty Cir. Age 75

℞

K-Dur 20 meq

#100 A.D

Refills 0

Dr. Alfred Sauls

2.2a

Dr. Alfred Sauls
151212 S. High Rd., Chicago, IL 23875
954-555-1300

Name Abraham Walker Date 11/15

Address 821 Alberty Cir. Age 75

℞

[illegible]

#100

[illegible]

Refills 0

Dr. Alfred Sauls

2.2b

2.3	PT. NAME: **HARRY ROBINS**	GENDER: **M**	ADDRESS: **195 DEXTER AVE.**	WEIGHT: **162**	HEIGHT: **5′ 5″**
	AGE: **82**	DX: **HTN, ANGINA, BPH**	ALLERGY: **NKA**		

MEDICATION	SIG.	PRESCRIBER	ORIG. DATE	REFILL DATE	REFILL DATE	REFILL DATE	REFILL DATE
Tenormin 25 mg #30	I q am	Weiss	4/6				
Furosemide 40 mg #30	I qd	Weiss	4/6				
NTG 0.4 mg SL #C	I sl prn	Weiss	4/6				

Dr. Barry Weiss
901 Sheridan St., Austin, TX 90902
874-555-9000

Name Harry Robins Date 4/7

Address 195 Dexter Ave. Age 82

℞

Hytrin 1 mg
i po QHS x3d
Then, ii po QHS x5d
Then iiii QHS
#[illegible] (12)

Refills 2

Dr. Barry Weiss

2.3a

Erica Jones, DDS
100 First St., Austin, TX 90902
874-555-9123

Name Harry Robins Date 4/7

Address 195 Dexter Ave. Age 82

℞

Amoxicillin 500mg
Disp: Caps #4
Sig: 4 caps 1hr before appt.

Refills 2

Dr. Erica Jones, DDS

2.3b

2.4

PT. NAME: **MARGARET BAKER** AGE: **79** | GENDER: **F** | DX: **HTN, ANGINA** | ADDRESS: **12 CAPITOL AVE.** | ALLERGY: **NKA** | WEIGHT: **122** | HX: **SMOKES 1 PACK/WEEK** | HEIGHT: **5′ 2″**

MEDICATION	SIG.	PRESCRIBER	ORIG. DATE	REFILL DATE	REFILL DATE	REFILL DATE	REFILL DATE
K-Dur 20 mEq #60	1 bid	Robins	12/2				
NTG 1/150 gr (0.4 mg) #C	1 sl prn	Robins	8/4				
Monoket 20 mg #60	1 q 12 h	Robins	12/2				
Furosemide 40 mg #60	1 bid	Robins	12/2				

Dr. Calvin Robins
7823 Tea Rose Trail, Miami, FL 44718
463-555-8000

Name Margaret Baker Date 12/20

Address 12 Capitol Ave. Age 79

℞

Cardizem 60 mg
Sig: i po TID
A/W

Refills 3

Dr. Calvin Robins

2.4a

Dr. Calvin Robins
7823 Tea Rose Trail, Miami, FL 44718
463-555-8000

Name Margaret Baker Date 12/20

Address 12 Capitol Ave. Age 79

℞

Vasotec 2.5 mg
#100
i BID

Refills 3

Dr. Calvin Robins

2.4b

2.5

PT. NAME: **JOAN ADAMS**	GENDER: **F**	ADDRESS: **854 GREEN ST.**	WEIGHT: **150**	HEIGHT: **5′ 3″**
AGE: **80**	DX: **HTN, ANGINA, TINEA PEDIS, ANXIETY, HIGH LDL-C**	ALLERGY: **NKA**	HX: **ETOH**	

MEDICATION	SIG.	PRESCRIBER	ORIG. DATE	REFILL DATE	REFILL DATE	REFILL DATE	REFILL DATE
Miconazole cream 2% 30 g	Apply bid prn itch	Thomas	3/7				
Lasix 40 mg #30	I q am	Thomas	4/10				
Xanax 0.25 mg #30	I q hs—prn only	Thomas	1/20	2/19			
Nitro-Dur 0.2 mg/hr #30	I qd ud	Thomas	4/10				

Dr. Erin Thomas
988 North Ridge, New York, NY 88364
813-555-7554

Name Joan Adams Date 4/20

Address 854 Green St. Age 80

℞

Procardia 60 XL #100
take i q day

Refills 1

Dr. Erin Thomas

2.5a

Dr. Erin Thomas
988 North Ridge, New York, NY 88364
813-555-7554

Name Joan Adams Date 4/20

Address 854 Green St. Age 80

℞

Zocor 20 mg
#30
Sig. i PO QD

Refills 0

Dr. Erin Thomas

2.5b

2.6

PT. NAME: **LISA ADAMS**	GENDER: **F**	ADDRESS: **53 IRIS BLVD.**	WEIGHT: **102**	HEIGHT: **5′ 1″**
AGE: **80**	DX: **HTN, CHF, A-FIB**	ALLERGY: **NKA**	HX: **RETIRED TEACHER, SOCIALLY ACTIVE**	

MEDICATION	SIG.	PRESCRIBER	ORIG. DATE	REFILL DATE	REFILL DATE	REFILL DATE	REFILL DATE
Lanoxin 0.25 mg #30	I qd	Griffin	6/4	8/14			
KCl 20 mEq #60	I bid	Griffin	6/4	8/14			

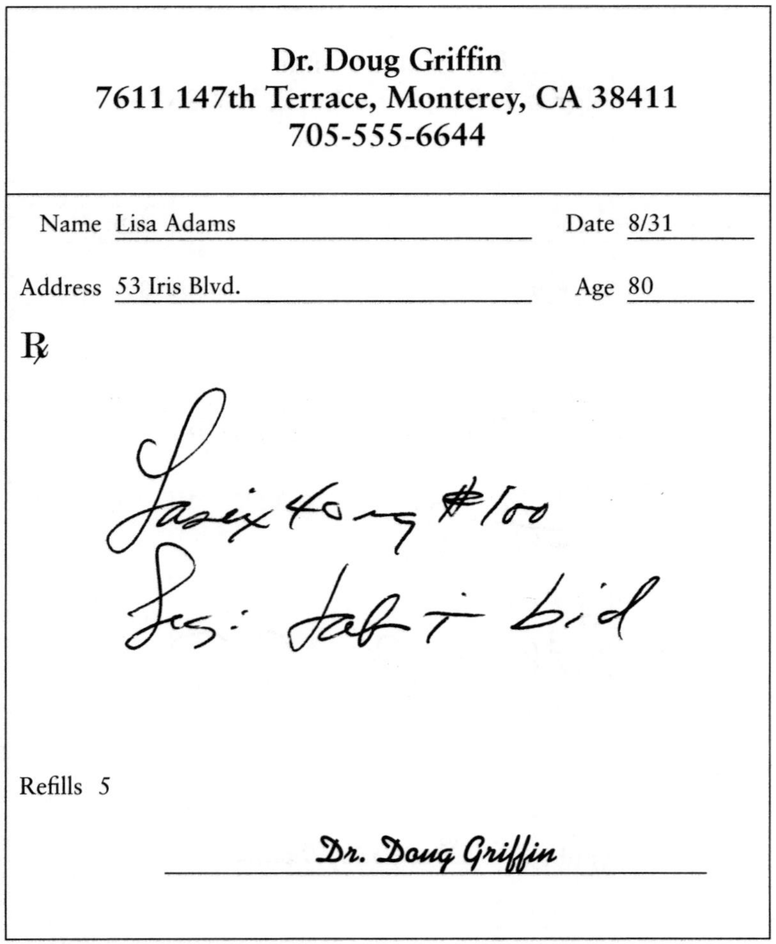
Dr. Doug Griffin
7611 147th Terrace, Monterey, CA 38411
705-555-6644

Name Lisa Adams Date 8/31

Address 53 Iris Blvd. Age 80

℞

Lasix 40 mg #100
Sig: tab i bid

Refills 5

Dr. Doug Griffin

2.6a

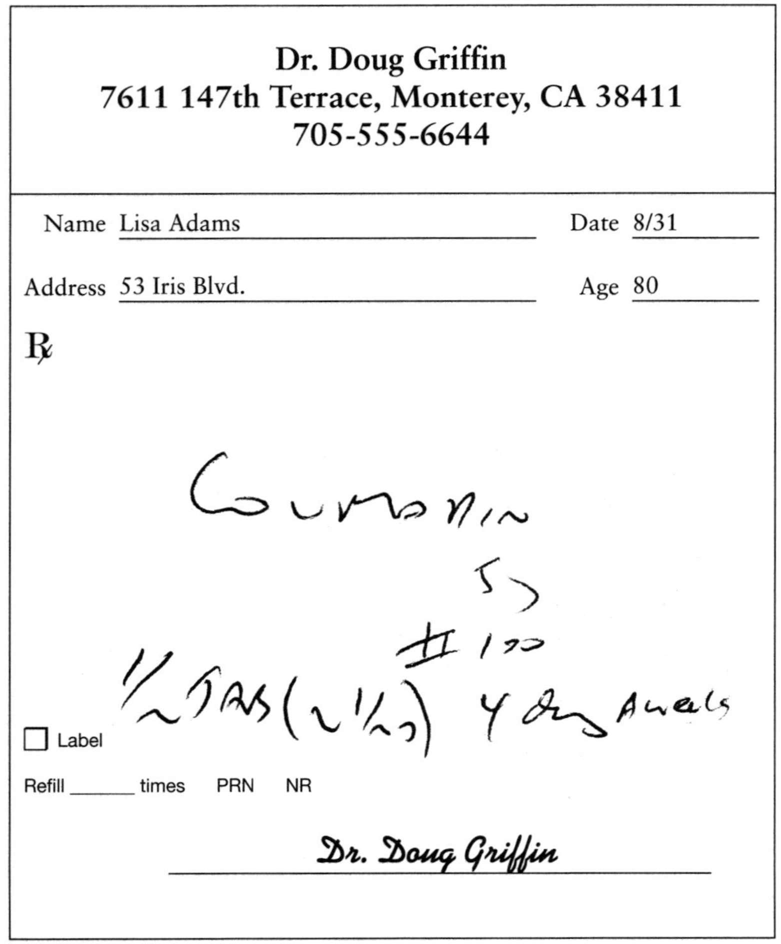
Dr. Doug Griffin
7611 147th Terrace, Monterey, CA 38411
705-555-6644

Name Lisa Adams Date 8/31

Address 53 Iris Blvd. Age 80

℞

Coumadin
5 mg
#100
1/2 TAB (2 1/2 mg) 4 day A meals

☐ Label

Refill ______ times PRN NR

Dr. Doug Griffin

2.6b

2.7

PT. NAME: **JOHN ADAMS** | GENDER: **M** | ADDRESS: **5577 BLACK DR.** | WEIGHT: **147** | HEIGHT: **5′ 4″**

AGE: **75** | DX: **HTN, CHF, TYPE 2 DM, ANGINA** | ALLERGY: **NKA** | HX: **RETIRED, DATES, PLAYS GOLF**

MEDICATION	SIG.	PRESCRIBER	ORIG. DATE	REFILL DATE	REFILL DATE	REFILL DATE	REFILL DATE
Lanoxin 0.25 mg #30	1 q am	Sauls	4/6				
DiaBeta 5 mg #30	1 q am	Sauls	4/6				

Dr. Alfred Sauls
151212 S. High Rd., Chicago, IL 23875
954-555-1300

Name John Adams Date 4/8

Address 5577 Black Dr. Age 75

℞

NTG 1/150
100
1 tablet SL prn
chest pain

Norvasc 5mg
~~100~~ #120
1 tablet po qd

Refills 0

Dr. Alfred Sauls

2.7a

Dr. Alfred Sauls
151212 S. High Rd., Chicago, IL 23875
954-555-1300

Name John Adams Date 4/8

Address 5577 Black Dr. Age 75

℞

accupril 20 mg
disp# 30
Sig: one a daily
label Blood pressure
medicine

Refills 0

Dr. Alfred Sauls

2.7b

2.8

PT. NAME: **DAN SMITH** | GENDER: **M** | ADDRESS: **642 JAFFREY CIR.** | WEIGHT: **134** | BMI: **24**
AGE: **81** | DX: **ANGINA, HTN, TYPE 2 DM, OA** | ALLERGY: **PCN** | HX: **SMOKER**

MEDICATION	SIG.	PRESCRIBER	ORIG. DATE	REFILL DATE	REFILL DATE	REFILL DATE	REFILL DATE
NTG 0.4 mg SL #25	I prn sl	Weiss	4/10				
Naprosyn 500 mg #30	I bid	Weiss	3/28	4/10			
Restoril 15 mg #30	I hs	Weiss	2/5	3/20	4/30	5/30	
Precose 50 mg #90	I with 1st bite of each meal	Weiss	6/4				

Dr. Barry Weiss
901 Sheridan St., Austin, TX 90902
874-555-9000

Name Dan Smith   Date 6/12

Address 642 Jaffrey Cir.   Age 81

℞

Capoten 12.5mg
#100
1/2 BID

Refills 4

Dr. Barry Weiss

2.8a

Dr. Barry Weiss
901 Sheridan St., Austin, TX 90902
874-555-9000

Name Dan Smith   Date 6/12

Address 642 Jaffrey Cir.   Age 81

℞

Maxzide-25
#100
i 9 Am for B.P.

Refills 1

Dr. Barry Weiss

2.8b

2.9 PT. NAME: **MARIA GREEN** AGE: **28** GENDER: **F** DX: **HTN, THIRD TRIMESTER PREGNANCY, CONSTIPATION** ADDRESS: **1 EAGLE RUN** ALLERGY: **PCN** WEIGHT: **APPEARS OVERWEIGHT** HX: **FIRST PREGNANCY**

MEDICATION	SIG.	PRESCRIBER	ORIG. DATE	REFILL DATE	REFILL DATE	REFILL DATE	REFILL DATE
Prenatal vitamins with folic acid #C	As directed	Robins	3/1				

Dr. Calvin Robins
7823 Tea Rose Trail, Miami, FL 44718
463-555-8000

Name Maria Green Date 5/1

Address 1 Eagle Run Age 28

℞

Captopril 50mg
#100

Sig: i BID

Refills 1

Dr. Calvin Robins

2.9a

Dr. Calvin Robins
7823 Tea Rose Trail, Miami, FL 44718
463-555-8000

Name Maria Green Date 5/1

Address 1 Eagle Run Age 28

℞

Miralax,
Disp 255g,
Sig: i capful in glass of
water every night

☐ LABEL

REFILL ____ TIMES PRN NR

Dr. Calvin Robins

2.9b

2.10

PT. NAME: **MARGARET JONES** AGE: **77** GENDER: **F** DX: **HTN, SKIN FUNGAL INFECTION, NERVES** ADDRESS: **977 IBIS LANE** ALLERGY: **PCN** WEIGHT: **158** HX: **SOCIAL DRINKER, DENIES ALCOHOL ABUSE** HEIGHT: **5′ 6″**

MEDICATION	SIG.	PRESCRIBER	ORIG. DATE	REFILL DATE	REFILL DATE	REFILL DATE	REFILL DATE
Lotrisone Cr. 45 g	ud prn	Thomas	6/5	9/4			
Ativan 0.5 mg #30	1 hs prn sleep	Thomas	6/9	9/2			

Dr. Erin Thomas
988 North Ridge, New York, NY 88364
813-555-7554

Name Margaret Jones Date 9/15

Address 977 Ibis Lane Age 77

℞

Vasotec 5 mg.

Sig: i bid

#100

Refills 2

Dr. Erin Thomas

2.10a

Dr. Erin Thomas
988 North Ridge, New York, NY 88364
813-555-7554

Name Margaret Jones Date 9/15

Address 977 Ibis Lane Age 77

℞

Verapamil 120 mg

Sig: i bid

#100

Refills 2

Dr. Erin Thomas

2.10b

2.11

PT. NAME: **MARY PHILLIPS** GENDER: **F** ADDRESS: **684 HURRICANE ALLEY** WEIGHT: **160** HEIGHT: **5′ 7″**
AGE: **84** DX: **HTN, ANEMIA, INSOMNIA** ALLERGY: **NKA** HX: **HAPPILY MARRIED GRANDMOTHER**

MEDICATION	SIG.	PRESCRIBER	ORIG. DATE	REFILL DATE	REFILL DATE	REFILL DATE	REFILL DATE
Zolpidem 5 mg #30	I hs	Griffin	4/5				
$FeSO_4$ 325 mg #C	I tid ac	Griffin	3/20				
Furosemide 40 mg #60	I bid	Griffin	5/6				

Dr. Doug Griffin
7611 147th Terrace, Monterey, CA 38411
705-555-6644

Name Mary Phillips Date 5/31

Address 684 Hurricane Alley Age 84

℞

Procardia XL 30
Sig T daily
#30

Refills 3

Dr. Doug Griffin

2.11a

Dr. Doug Griffin
7611 147th Terrace, Monterey, CA 38411
705-555-6644

Name Mary Phillips Date 5/31

Address 684 Hurricane Alley Age 84

℞

Accupril 10 mg
#30
T QD

Refills 3

Dr. Doug Griffin

2.11b

2.12

PT. NAME: **JIM LEWIS** GENDER: **M** ADDRESS: **1984 GREEN ST.** WEIGHT: **144** HEIGHT: **5′ 3″**
AGE: **79** DX: **HTN, ANGINA, TYPE 2 DM, CHF, GUM INFECTION** ALLERGY: **PCN** HX: **VERY SEDENTARY**

MEDICATION	SIG.	PRESCRIBER	ORIG. DATE	REFILL DATE	REFILL DATE	REFILL DATE	REFILL DATE
Furosemide 40 mg #30	I q am	Sauls	3/4	4/2			
Glyburide 5 mg #30	I q am	Sauls	3/4				
Digoxin 0.25 mg #30	I q am	Sauls	3/4	4/2			
NTG 1/150 gr (0.4 mg) #100	I sl prn	Sauls	4/2				

Dr. Alfred Sauls
151212 S. High Rd., Chicago, IL 23875
954-555-1300

Name Jim Lewis Date 4/9

Address 1984 Green St. Age 79

℞

Zestril 10 mg
Ⓣ T q PM
#C

Refills 0

Dr. Alfred Sauls

2.12a

Dr. Karen David, DDS
400 No. High Rd., Chicago, IL 23875
954-444-9871

Name Jim Lewis Date 4/9

Address 1984 Green St. Age 79

℞

Augmentin 500 mg
#21
T PO TID

Dr. Karen David, DDS

2.12b

2.13

PT. NAME: **SHIRLEY HARRIS**	GENDER: **F**	ADDRESS: **774 FANTASTIC ST.**	WEIGHT: **182**	BMI: **34**
AGE: **62**	DX: **HTN, TYPE 2 DM, ANGINA**	ALLERGY: **NKA**	HX: **OBESE ALL HER LIFE**	

MEDICATION	SIG.	PRESCRIBER	ORIG. DATE	REFILL DATE	REFILL DATE	REFILL DATE	REFILL DATE
Glucophage 500 mg #50	I tid	Weiss	3/6				
NTG 0.3 mg SL #C	I sl prn	Weiss	3/6				

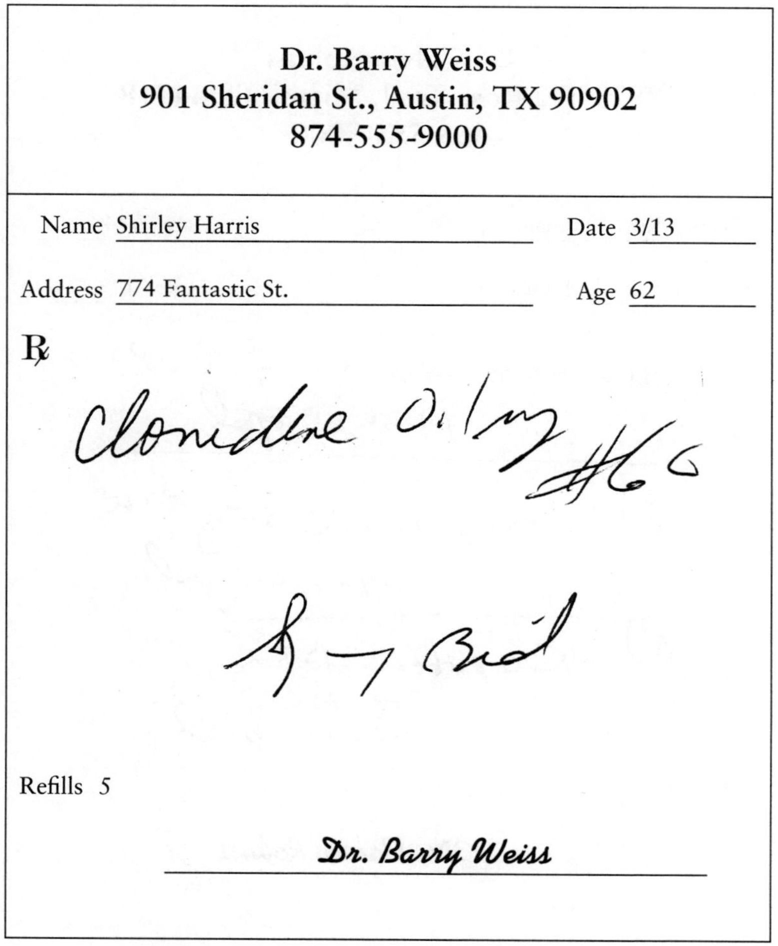
Dr. Barry Weiss
901 Sheridan St., Austin, TX 90902
874-555-9000

Name Shirley Harris Date 3/13

Address 774 Fantastic St. Age 62

℞

Clonidine 0.1 mg #60

[illegible]

Refills 5

Dr. Barry Weiss

2.13a

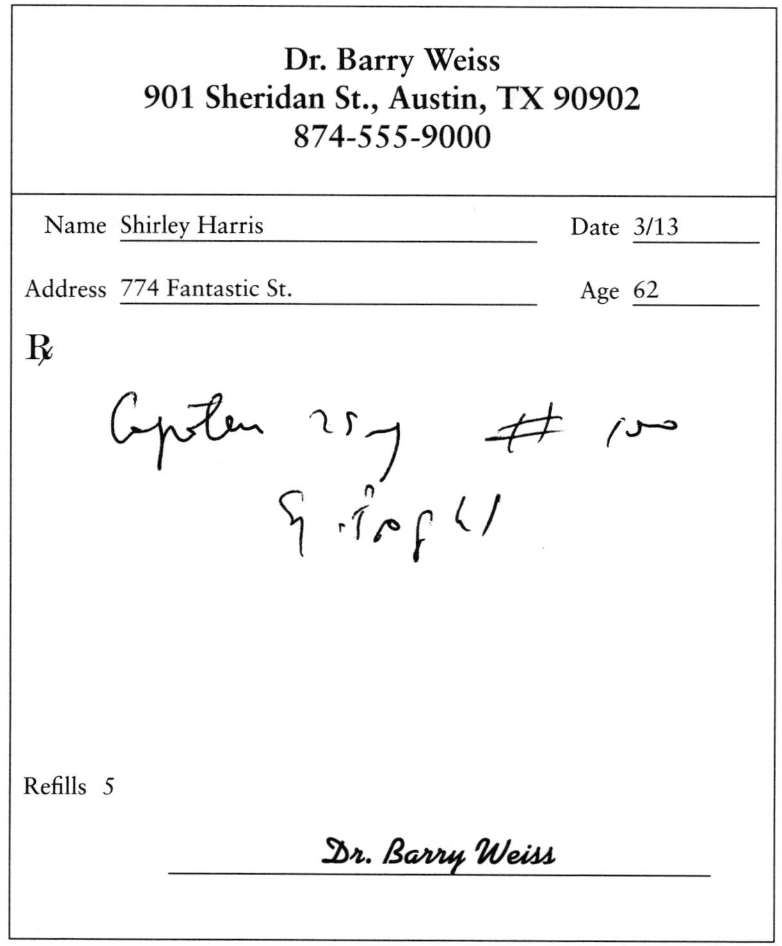
Dr. Barry Weiss
901 Sheridan St., Austin, TX 90902
874-555-9000

Name Shirley Harris Date 3/13

Address 774 Fantastic St. Age 62

℞

Capoten 25 mg #100

[illegible]

Refills 5

Dr. Barry Weiss

2.13b

2.14 PT. NAME: **KURT THOMAS** AGE: **71** GENDER: **M** DX: **HTN, CHF, BPH, INFECTION** ADDRESS: **522 ELEPHANT DR.** ALLERGY: **SULFA** WEIGHT: **170** HEIGHT: **5′ 8″**

MEDICATION	SIG.	PRESCRIBER	ORIG. DATE	REFILL DATE	REFILL DATE	REFILL DATE	REFILL DATE
Digoxin 0.25 mg #90	1 q am	Robins	4/9	7/12			
Keflex 250 mg #28	1 qid × 7 d	Robins	3/20				

Dr. Calvin Robins
7823 Tea Rose Trail, Miami, FL 44718
463-555-8000

Name Kurt Thomas Date 7/14

Address 522 Elephant Dr. Age 71

℞

Hytrin
Aj 1.0mg po QHS
#30

Refills 1

Dr. Calvin Robins

2.14a

Dr. Calvin Robins
7823 Tea Rose Trail, Miami, FL 44718
463-555-8000

Name Kurt Thomas Date 7/14

Address 522 Elephant Dr. Age 71

℞

1) Lasix 40mg — #100
1 tab ~~qd~~

2) Lanoxin 0.25mg #100
1 tab qd.

3) Capoten 12.5mg
#100
1 tab bid

Refills 1

Dr. Calvin Robins

2.14b

2.15

PT. NAME: **ARNOLD JOHNSON**	GENDER: **M**	ADDRESS: **333 DEXTER AVE.**	WEIGHT: **139**	HEIGHT: **5′ 3″**
AGE: **72**	DX: **HTN, A-FIB, OA PAIN**	ALLERGY: **NKA**	HX: **SEDENTARY, DOES NOT WANT TO WALK**	

MEDICATION	SIG.	PRESCRIBER	ORIG. DATE	REFILL DATE	REFILL DATE	REFILL DATE	REFILL DATE
Coumadin 5 mg #30	I q am	Thomas	8/5				
Tylenol No. 3 #50	I q 4–6 h prn	Thomas	7/20				
Furosemide 40 mg #60	I bid	Thomas	8/5				
Digoxin 0.25 mg #30	I q am	Thomas	8/5				

Dr. Erin Thomas
988 North Ridge, New York, NY 88364
813-555-7554

Name Arnold Johnson Date 8/16

Address 333 Dexter Ave. Age 72

℞

Vaseretic 10/25
#30
Sig i QAM.

Refills 4

Dr. Erin Thomas

2.15a

Dr. Erin Thomas
988 North Ridge, New York, NY 88364
813-555-7554

Name Arnold Johnson Date 8/16

Address 333 Dexter Ave. Age 72

℞

Coumadin 2.5 mg
#100
sig: i QD

Refills 4

Dr. Erin Thomas

2.15b

2.16

PT. NAME: **ART HARRIS**	GENDER: **M**	ADDRESS: **71 CAPITOL AVE.**	WEIGHT: **151**	HEIGHT: **5′ 4″**
AGE: **61**	DX: **HTN, BPH, TYPE 2 DM, OA, GOUT**	ALLERGY: **PCN**	HX: **HIGH SCHOOL PRINCIPAL**	

MEDICATION	SIG.	PRESCRIBER	ORIG. DATE	REFILL DATE	REFILL DATE	REFILL DATE	REFILL DATE
Colchicine 0.6 mg #90	1 daily	Griffin	12/8	3/8			
Tylenol No. 3 #50	1 q 4–6 h prn	Griffin	12/8				
Glyburide 2.5 mg #90	1 qd in am	Griffin	11/8				

Dr. Doug Griffin
7611 147th Terrace, Monterey, CA 38411
705-555-6644

Name Art Harris Date 3/18

Address 71 Capitol Ave Age 61

℞

Capoten 12.5 mg
Sig: 1 p.o. q 8°
Disp: #90

Refills 2

Dr. Doug Griffin

2.16a

Dr. Doug Griffin
7611 147th Terrace, Monterey, CA 38411
705-555-6644

Name Art Harris Date 3/18

Address 71 Capitol Ave Age 61

℞

Hytrin 5 #30

Sig: T q hs - for prostate

Refills

Dr. Doug Griffin

2.16b

2.17

PT. NAME: **MARTIN EDWARDS** GENDER: **M** ADDRESS: **555 BUNION WAY** WEIGHT: **150** HEIGHT: **5′ 10″**
AGE: **80** DX: **CHF, FE^{2+} DEFICIENCY, ANGINA, ARRHYTHMIA, BPH** ALLERGY: **PCN** HX: **HAPPILY MARRIED, TRAVELS, PLAYS GOLF, SOCIAL DRINKER**

MEDICATION	SIG.	PRESCRIBER	ORIG. DATE	REFILL DATE	REFILL DATE	REFILL DATE	REFILL DATE
$FeSO_4$ 325 mg #C	I tid	Sauls	1/10				
NTG 1/150 gr (0.4 mg) #C	I sl prn	Sauls	1/10				
Digoxin 0.25 mg #30	I q am	Sauls	1/10				
Hytrin 2 mg #30	I hs	Sauls	1/10				

Dr. Alfred Sauls
151212 S. High Rd., Chicago, IL 23875
954-555-1300

Name Martin Edwards Date 2/1

Address 555 Bunion Way Age 80

℞

Hytrin 5mg
Disp #100
Sig: i hs.

Refills 3

Dr. Alfred Sauls

2.17a

Dr. Alfred Sauls
151212 S. High Rd., Chicago, IL 23875
954-555-1300

Name Martin Edwards Date 2/1

Address 555 Bunion Way Age 80

℞

Adalat 60u #100
i qd

ī Rythmol 150 #60
B.I.D.

Refills NR

Dr. Alfred Sauls

2.17b

2.18

PT. NAME: **ARNOLD CAPLAN**	GENDER: **M**	ADDRESS: **224 ALBERTY CIR.**	WEIGHT: **178**	HEIGHT: **5′ 6″**
AGE: **82**	DX: **HTN, CHF**	ALLERGY: **NKA**	HX: **SOCIAL DRINKER, SMOKES 3 TIMES A DAY**	

MEDICATION	SIG.	PRESCRIBER	ORIG. DATE	REFILL DATE	REFILL DATE	REFILL DATE	REFILL DATE
Lasix 40 mg #30	1 bid	Weiss	4/3				
Lanoxin 0.125 mg #30	1 qd	Weiss	4/3				

Dr. Barry Weiss
901 Sheridan St., Austin, TX 90902
874-555-9000

Name Arnold Caplan Date 5/2

Address 224 Alberty Cir. Age 82

℞

[illegible] 10

#30 [illegible]

Refills 4

Dr. Barry Weiss

2.18a

Dr. Barry Weiss
901 Sheridan St., Austin, TX 90902
874-555-9000

Name Arnold Caplan Date 5/2

Address 224 Alberty Cir. Age 82

℞

Lanoxin 0.125mg
100

Sig: tab T daily

Refills NR

Dr. Barry Weiss

2.18b

2.19

PT. NAME: **BEN SMITH**	GENDER: **M**	ADDRESS: **14 HALL ST.**	WEIGHT: **179**	BMI: **28**
AGE: **58**	DX: **HTN, SUGAR (FBS: 123 mg%)**	ALLERGY: **ASA**	HX: **DIVORCED, POOR FOOD SELECTION, UNEMPLOYED**	

MEDICATION	SIG.	PRESCRIBER	ORIG. DATE	REFILL DATE	REFILL DATE	REFILL DATE	REFILL DATE
Cardizem CD 120 mg #30	1 q am	Robins	2/1	3/20	5/10	7/1	

Dr. Calvin Robins
7823 Tea Rose Trail, Miami, FL 44718
463-555-8000

Name Ben Smith Date 7/15

Address 14 Hall Street Age 58

℞

Lasix 40 mg
#60
1 BID

Refills 1

Dr. Calvin Robins

2.19a

Dr. Calvin Robins
7823 Tea Rose Trail, Miami, FL 44718
463-555-8000

Name Ben Smith Date 7/15

Address 14 Hall Street Age 58

℞

Altace 5 mg
i qd
#100

Refills 1

Dr. Calvin Robins

2.19b

2.20

PT. NAME: **WILLIAM GREEN** GENDER: **M** ADDRESS: **2688 UNIVERSITY ST.** WEIGHT: **150** HEIGHT: **5′ 4″**

AGE: **69** DX: **HTN, ANGINA, INSOMNIA** ALLERGY: **NKA** HX: **NERVOUS, CRITICAL, COMPLAINS FREQUENTLY**

MEDICATION	SIG.	PRESCRIBER	ORIG. DATE	REFILL DATE	REFILL DATE	REFILL DATE	REFILL DATE
Furosemide 20 mg #90	1 q am	Thomas	6/4	9/6			
Ambien 5 mg #60	1–2 hs prn	Thomas	4/3	6/8			
Nitro-Dur 0.2 mg/hr #30	1 qd	Thomas	6/4	7/3	8/4	9/2	

Dr. Erin Thomas
988 North Ridge, New York, NY 88364
813-555-7554

Name William Green Date 9/8

Address 2688 University St. Age 69

℞

Prinivil 5

#30

i q AM

Refills 0

Dr. Erin Thomas

2.20a

Dr. Erin Thomas
988 North Ridge, New York, NY 88364
813-555-7554

Name William Green Date 9/8

Address 2688 University St. Age 69

℞

Tenormin 50 mg

Sig: 1/2 p.o. q day

Disp: # 100

Refills 0

Dr. Erin Thomas

2.20b

2.21

PT. NAME: **MARK BLACK**	GENDER: **M**	ADDRESS: **474 HURRICANE ALLEY**	WEIGHT: **175**	BMI: **28**
AGE: **68**	DX: **HTN, ANGINA, BACTERIAL INFECTION, RASH**	ALLERGY: **PCN**	HX: **STORE CLERK, GAMBLER, DRINKS FREQUENTLY**	

MEDICATION	SIG.	PRESCRIBER	ORIG. DATE	REFILL DATE	REFILL DATE	REFILL DATE	REFILL DATE
Erythromycin 250 mg #28	1 qid × 7 d	Griffin	6/4				
Robitussin Syr 120 mL	5 mL q 4–6 h prn cough	Griffin	6/4				
Lanoxin 0.25 mg #30	1 qd	Griffin	7/10				
Lotrisone Cr. 15 g	Apply prn rash ud	Griffin	5/9				

Dr. Doug Griffin
7611 147th Terrace, Monterey, CA 38411
705-555-6644

Name Mark Black Date 7/11

Address 474 Hurricane Alley Age 68

℞

Clonidine
TTS #2
1 box
Use wkly

Refills 5

Dr. Doug Griffin

2.21a

Dr. Doug Griffin
7611 147th Terrace, Monterey, CA 38411
705-555-6644

Name Mark Black Date 7/11

Address 474 Hurricane Alley Age 68

℞

Imdur 60,
1 – P.O. day
#30

Refills 0

Dr. Doug Griffin

2.21b

2.22

PT. NAME: **ALAN JOHNSON** GENDER: **M** ADDRESS: **92 IBIS LANE** WEIGHT: **173** HEIGHT: **5′ 6″**

AGE: **69** DX: **HTN, ANGINA, TYPE 2 DM, CHF** ALLERGY: **NKA** HX: **SMOKER FOR 20 YEARS; SMOKES 1 PACK/DAY**

MEDICATION	SIG.	PRESCRIBER	ORIG. DATE	REFILL DATE	REFILL DATE	REFILL DATE	REFILL DATE
DiaBeta 5 mg #90	1 q am	Sauls	4/3	7/6			
NTG 1/150 gr (0.4 mg) #25	1 sl prn	Sauls	4/3	7/1			
Humulin N 10 mL	24 U am & 12 U pm	Sauls	7/1	7/6			

Dr. Alfred Sauls
151212 S. High Rd., Chicago, IL 23875
954-555-1300

Name Alan Johnson Date 7/14

Address 92 Ibis Lane Age 69

℞

Altace 2.5 mg

#30

1 cap daily

Refills 0

Dr. Alfred Sauls

2.22a

Dr. Alfred Sauls
151212 S. High Rd., Chicago, IL 23875
954-555-1300

Name Alan Johnson Date 7/14

Address 92 Ibis Lane Age 69

℞

Lanoxin 0.25

#100

1 tab q day po

Refills

Dr. Alfred Sauls

2.22b

2.23	PT. NAME: **FRED LEWEY**	GENDER: **M**	ADDRESS: **9 EAGLE RUN**	WEIGHT: **ABOUT 130**
	AGE: **80**	DX: **HTN, DEMENTIA, EDEMA, ANGINA, OA PAIN**	ALLERGY: **NKA**	HX: **FORMER SALESMAN, QUIET LIFESTYLE**

MEDICATION	SIG.	PRESCRIBER	ORIG. DATE	REFILL DATE	REFILL DATE	REFILL DATE	REFILL DATE
HCTZ 25 mg #50	1 q am	Weiss	9/2				
K-Dur 10 mEq #50	1 bid	Weiss	9/2				
Robitussin Syr 4 oz	5 mL tid	Weiss	8/3	9/12	11/5		
Tylenol No. 3 #21	1 q 4–6 h prn	Weiss	8/6	10/1			

Dr. Barry Weiss
901 Sheridan St., Austin, TX 90902
874-555-9000

Name Fred Lewey Date 11/9

Address 9 Eagle Run Age 80

℞

Clonidine .1 mg
1 po tid

☑ Label

Refill ______ times (PRN) NR

Dr. Barry Weiss

2.23a

Dr. Barry Weiss
901 Sheridan St., Austin, TX 90902
874-555-9000

Name Fred Lewey Date 11/9

Address 9 Eagle Run Age 80

℞

Nitropatch 0.2 mg/hr #30
Sig: Apply q AM, may remove q HS

Refills 6

Dr. Barry Weiss

2.23b

2.24	PT. NAME: **GEORGE BAKER** AGE: **72**	GENDER: **M** DX: **HTN, ANGINA, P.U.D.**	ADDRESS: **3975 BLACK DR.** ALLERGY: **PCN**	WEIGHT: **155** HX: **ACTIVE IN CHURCH ACTIVITIES, SOCIAL DRINKER**	BMI: **27**

MEDICATION	SIG.	PRESCRIBER	ORIG. DATE	REFILL DATE	REFILL DATE	REFILL DATE	REFILL DATE
Lasix 40 mg #30	1 q am	Robins	7/1	8/2			
Digoxin 0.125 mg #30	1 q am	Robins	7/1	8/2			
K-Dur 20 mEq #30	1 q am	Robins	7/1	10/4			
Nitro-Dur 0.2 mg/hr #30	Apply 1 on 12 hrs, off 12 hrs	Robins	7/1	8/2			

Dr. Calvin Robins
7823 Tea Rose Trail, Miami, FL 44718
463-555-8000

Name George Baker Date 10/15

Address 3975 Black Dr. Age 72

℞

Capoten 25 mg

#100 T BID

Refills 1

Dr. Calvin Robins

2.24a

Dr. Calvin Robins
7823 Tea Rose Trail, Miami, FL 44718
463-555-8000

Name George Baker Date 10/15

Address 3975 Black Dr. Age 72

℞

Zantac 150 mg

#100

T BID AC (B&D)

Refills 1

Dr. Calvin Robins

2.24b

2.25	PT. NAME: **ANDREW PHILLIPS** AGE: **82**	GENDER: **M** DX: **CHF, TYPE 2 DM, HTN**	ADDRESS: **61 GREEN ST.** ALLERGY: **NKA**	WEIGHT: **244** HX: **ON A DIET, BUYS CANDY**	BMI: **36**

MEDICATION	SIG.	PRESCRIBER	ORIG. DATE	REFILL DATE	REFILL DATE	REFILL DATE	REFILL DATE
Lanoxin 0.125 mg #90	1 q am	Thomas	2/1	5/3			
OTC 81 mg ASA #36	1 q am	Thomas	2/1	3/8			
Glucotrol 10 mg #90	1 bid ac	Thomas	1/5	2/21	4/8		
HCTZ 25 mg #50	1 q am	Thomas	2/1	3/20			

Dr. Erin Thomas
988 North Ridge, New York, NY 88364
813-555-7554

Name Andrew Phillips Date 5/25

Address 61 Green St. Age 82

℞

Capoten 50 mg tab
Sig: ½ tab PO BID
#/a

Refills 3

Dr. Erin Thomas

2.25a

Dr. Erin Thomas
988 North Ridge, New York, NY 88364
813-555-7554

Name Andrew Phillips Date 5/25

Address 61 Green St. Age 82

℞

Catapres TTS-1
patch #4
ue ī q wk

Refills 3

Dr. Erin Thomas

2.25b

2.26

PT. NAME: **JACK DAVIS** AGE: **72** GENDER: **M** DX: **HTN, PSVT** ADDRESS: **500 SE 2 ST.** ALLERGY: **NKA** WEIGHT: **277** HX: **FORMER SMOKER, SEDENTARY** BMI: **32**

MEDICATION	SIG.	PRESCRIBER	ORIG. DATE	REFILL DATE	REFILL DATE	REFILL DATE	REFILL DATE
HCTZ 25 mg #90	1 q am	Robins	6/4				
Prinivil 10 mg #90	1 q am	Robins	6/4				
Avapro 150 mg #90	1 q am	Robins	6/4				

Dr. Calvin Robins
7823 Tea Rose Trail, Miami, FL 44718
463-555-8000

Name Jack Davis Date 7/15

Address 500 SE 2 St. Age 72

℞

Tambocor 50g #100

1 BID

Refills 3

Dr. Calvin Robins

2.26a

Dr. Calvin Robins
7823 Tea Rose Trail, Miami, FL 44718
463-555-8000

Name Jack Davis Date 7/15

Address 500 SE 2 St. Age 72

℞

Slow K

#50

Sig: i tid

Refills

Dr. Calvin Robins

2.26b

2.27

PT. NAME: **ANTHONY JOHNSON** GENDER: **M** ADDRESS: **654 IBIS CT.** WEIGHT: **229** BMI: **36**
AGE: **70** DX: **HTN, OA, BACTERIAL INFECTION** ALLERGY: **NKA** HX: **SMOKER**

MEDICATION	SIG.	PRESCRIBER	ORIG. DATE	REFILL DATE	REFILL DATE	REFILL DATE	REFILL DATE
Tenormin 25 mg #30	I q am	Thomas	10/3	10/31			
Lasix 20 mg #30	I q am	Thomas	10/3	10/31			
Ultram 50 mg #24	I tid prn	Thomas	8/5				
Doxycycline 100 mg #10	I qd	Thomas	6/30				

Dr. Barry Weiss
901 Sheridan St., Austin, TX 90902
874-555-9000

Name Anthony Johnson Date 11/5

Address 654 Ibis Court Age 70

℞

Vasotec 5mg
1 each am
Send 60

Refills 2

Dr. Barry Weiss

2.27a

Dr. Barry Weiss
901 Sheridan St., Austin, TX 90902
874-555-9000

Name Anthony Johnson Date 11/5

Address 654 Ibis Court Age 70

℞

Calan SR 240
Sig: i po QAM

Refills 2

Dr. Barry Weiss

2.27b

2.28

PT. NAME: **JOHN ADAMS**	GENDER: **M**	ADDRESS: **555 W. 123RD AVE.**	WEIGHT: **182**	HEIGHT: **5′ 5″**
AGE: **73**	DX: **HTN, ANEMIA, HIGH TRIGLYCERIDES, DEPRESSED**	ALLERGY: **NKA**	HX: **ALWAYS WORRIES**	

MEDICATION	SIG.	PRESCRIBER	ORIG. DATE	REFILL DATE	REFILL DATE	REFILL DATE	REFILL DATE
Folic acid 1 mg #C	1 qd	Weiss	3/5	6/10			
Prozac 20 mg #30	1 q am	Weiss	2/5	3/10			

Dr. Barry Weiss
901 Sheridan St., Austin, TX 90902
874-555-9000

Name John Adams Date 7/20

Address 555 W. 123 Ave. Age 73

℞

Cozaar 50, # 60
S 1 PO daily

Refills 0

Dr. Barry Weiss

2.28a

Dr. Barry Weiss
901 Sheridan St., Austin, TX 90902
874-555-9000

Name John Adams Date 7/20

Address 555 W. 123 Ave. Age 73

℞

Fenofibrate 200
30 Thirty
i po qd

Refills 0

Dr. Barry Weiss

2.28b

2.29 PT. NAME: **BRIAN BLACK** AGE: **73** GENDER: **M** DX: **HTN, NERVES, DIZZINESS, JOCK ITCH** ADDRESS: **7584 GREEN AVE.** ALLERGY: **NKA** WEIGHT: **188** HX: **SMOKER** BMI: **33**

MEDICATION	SIG.	PRESCRIBER	ORIG. DATE	REFILL DATE	REFILL DATE	REFILL DATE	REFILL DATE
Xanax 0.25 mg #50	I bid prn itch	Thomas	6/3	7/20			
HCTZ 25 mg #90	I q am	Thomas	5/12	8/25			
Antivert 12.5 mg #30	I prn dizziness	Thomas	5/12				

Dr. Calvin Robins
7823 Tea Rose Trail, Miami, FL 44718
463-555-8000

Name Brian Black Date 8/30

Address 7584 Green Ave. Age 73

℞

Vasotec 10 mg #100
Take ÷ tab po qAm
Vasotec 5 mg #100
Take ÷ tab po qPm

Refills 4

Dr. Calvin Robins

2.29a

Dr. Calvin Robins
7823 Tea Rose Trail, Miami, FL 44718
463-555-8000

Name Brian Black Date 8/30

Address 7584 Green Ave. Age 73

℞

Lotrisone Cream
30 gm
Apply BID to affected area

☐ Label

Refill ______ times

Dr. Calvin Robins

2.29b

2.30

PT. NAME: **HENRY SMITH**	GENDER: **M**	ADDRESS: **54417 SW 197TH AVE.**	WEIGHT: **235**	BMI: **32**
AGE: **73**	DX: **HTN, DIABETES TYPE 2, LDL-C: 150 mg/dL**	ALLERGY: **NKA**	HX: **ALWAYS OBESE, BAD FOOD SELECTION**	

MEDICATION	SIG.	PRESCRIBER	ORIG. DATE	REFILL DATE	REFILL DATE	REFILL DATE	REFILL DATE
Glucophage 850 mg #60	I qd	Sauls	7/25	9/5	10/16		
Glucotrol XL 10 mg #60	I bid	Sauls	7/10	8/17	10/16		
Lotensin 40 mg #90	I bid	Sauls	6/13	9/8			
OTC-Imodium A-D #24	I bid	Sauls	8/4	9/20			

Dr. Alfred Sauls
151212 S. High Rd., Chicago, IL 23875
954-555-1300

Name Henry Smith Date 10/20

Address 54417 SW 197th Ave. Age 73

℞

Hctz 25 mg #100

Sig: 1 daily

Refills 1

Dr. Alfred Sauls

2.30a

Dr. Alfred Sauls
151212 S. High Rd., Chicago, IL 23875
954-555-1300

Name Henry Smith Date 10/20

Address 54417 SW 197th Ave. Age 73

℞

Lipitor 10 mg

#90

i day

Refills 1

Dr. Alfred Sauls

2.30b

2.31

PT. NAME: **MARJORIE JONES** GENDER: **F** ADDRESS: **154 ORIOLE AVE.** WEIGHT: **187** BMI: **29**
AGE: **71** DX: **HTN, TYPE 2 DM, "BAD BACK," LDL-C: 160 mg/dL** ALLERGY: **NKA** HX: **ALWAYS ON A DIET**

MEDICATION	SIG.	PRESCRIBER	ORIG. DATE	REFILL DATE	REFILL DATE	REFILL DATE	REFILL DATE
Tylenol No. 3 #30	I q 4–6 h prn pain	Thomas	10/25				
Accupril 40 mg #60	I bid	Thomas	9/29				
Medrol Dosepak 4 mg #1	Follow instructions on Dosepack	Thomas	9/13				
Amaryl 4 mg #30	I qd	Thomas	9/6				

Dr. Erin Thomas
988 North Ridge, New York, NY 88364
813-555-7554

Name Marjorie Jones Date 10/28

Address 154 Oriole Ave. Age 71

℞

Lipitor 10 mg
#60
Sig: i PO daily

Refills 2

Dr. Erin Thomas

2.31a

Dr. Erin Thomas
988 North Ridge, New York, NY 88364
813-555-7554

Name Marjorie Jones Date 10/28

Address 154 Oriole Ave. Age 71

℞

Relafan 500 g
dis: #20
sig: ii p.o. QD

Refill (0) 1 - 2 - 3 - 4 - PRN

Dr. Erin Thomas

2.31b

2.32	PT. NAME: **MARION BLACK**	GENDER: **F**	ADDRESS: **7053 130TH AVE.**	WEIGHT: **150**	BMI: **24**
	AGE: **82**	DX: **HTN, CHF, IBS, ANGINA**	ALLERGY: **NKA**	HX: **SEDENTARY, DYSPEPTIC**	

MEDICATION	SIG.	PRESCRIBER	ORIG. DATE	REFILL DATE	REFILL DATE	REFILL DATE	REFILL DATE
Digoxin 0.125 mg #60	1 qd	Thomas	2/5	4/18			
Furosemide 40 mg #60	1 qd	Thomas	2/5	4/18			
Levbid ER tabs #30	1 q am & 1 hs prn	Thomas	1/15	1/30	2/20		

Dr. Erin Thomas
988 North Ridge, New York, NY 88364
813-555-7554

Name Marion Black Date 4/30

Address 7053 130th Ave. Age 82

℞

10% KCl pint no sugar
1
ʒi T Tablespoon BID

Refills 3

Dr. Erin Thomas

2.32a

Dr. Erin Thomas
988 North Ridge, New York, NY 88364
813-555-7554

Name Marion Black Date 4/30

Address 7053 130th Ave. Age 82

℞

N.T.G. 1/150 #100
Sig 1 tab S.L. p.r.n.
for chest pain.

Refills 3

Dr. Erin Thomas

2.32b

2.33

PT. NAME: **RODNEY DESIR** AGE: **58** GENDER: **M** DX: **HTN, CHOLESTEROL, GUM ABSCESS** ADDRESS: **443 SOUTH AVE.** ALLERGY: **MILK** WEIGHT: **204** HX: **TAXI DRIVER, VERY ACTIVE** BMI: **31**

MEDICATION	SIG.	PRESCRIBER	ORIG. DATE	REFILL DATE	REFILL DATE	REFILL DATE	REFILL DATE
Hyzaar 50-12.5 mg #30	1 qd	Curvelo	5/6	7/1	8/10	9/14	
Vitamin D 1000 IU #30	1 q am	Curvelo	5/6	6/4	7/2	8/9	9/2
Toprol XL 25 mg #30	1 qd	Curvelo	7/1	9/3	9/15		
Norvasc 10 mg #30	1 qd	Curvelo	7/5	8/3	9/1		

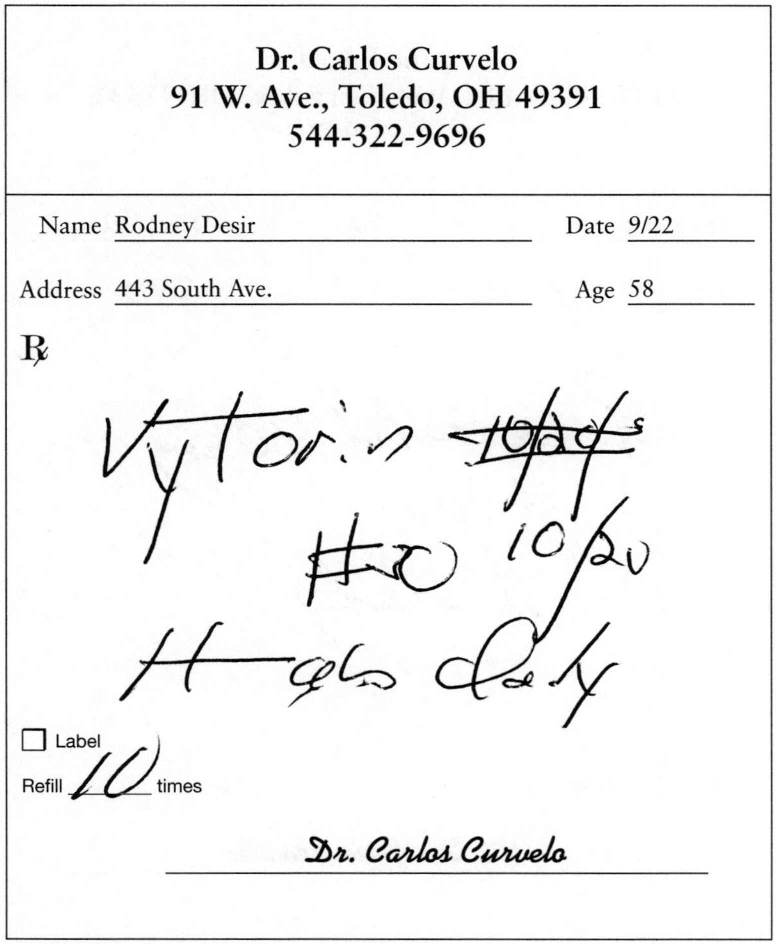

Dr. Carlos Curvelo
91 W. Ave., Toledo, OH 49391
544-322-9696

Name Rodney Desir Date 9/22
Address 443 South Ave. Age 58

℞
Vytorin #30 10/20
1 qhs daily

☐ Label
Refill 10 times

Dr. Carlos Curvelo

2.33a

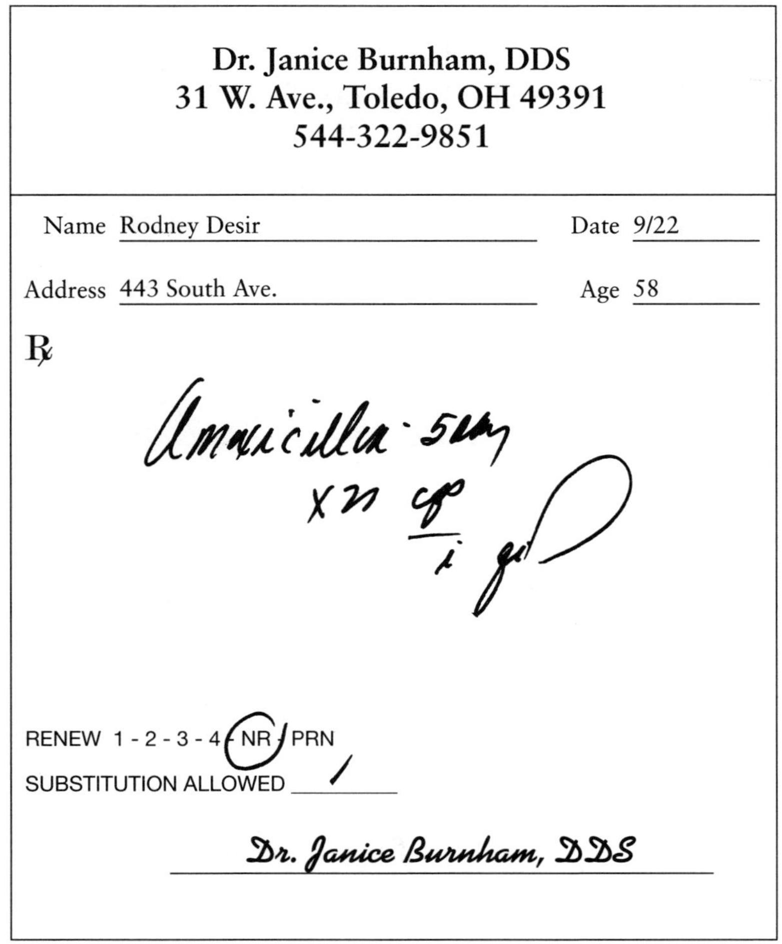

Dr. Janice Burnham, DDS
31 W. Ave., Toledo, OH 49391
544-322-9851

Name Rodney Desir Date 9/22
Address 443 South Ave. Age 58

℞
Amoxicillin 500 mg
x21 cp
i qd

RENEW 1 - 2 - 3 - 4 - NR - PRN
SUBSTITUTION ALLOWED ✓

Dr. Janice Burnham, DDS

2.33b

2.34

PT. NAME: **JEFF SCOTT** GENDER: **M** ADDRESS: **99 CORVALLIS AVE.** WEIGHT: **153** BMI: **27**
AGE: **65** DX: **HTN, HIGH CHOLESTEROL, OA, HERNIATED DISK** ALLERGY: **ERYTHROMYCIN, BIAXIN**

MEDICATION	SIG.	PRESCRIBER	ORIG. DATE	REFILL DATE	REFILL DATE	REFILL DATE	REFILL DATE
Zetia 10 mg #30	1 qd	Blasberg	11/5	12/6			
Oxycodone ER 80 mg #60	1 bid	Blasberg	11/30				
Peri-Colace #30	1 qd	OTC	12/2				

Dr. Jane Bearden
44 No Corvallis Ave., Corvallis, OR 97331
222-666-9876

Name Jeff Scott Date 12/20

Address 99 Corvallis Ave. Age 65

℞

lisinopril HCT 20/12.5

#30

1 q AM

☐ LABEL

REFILL prn TIMES PRN NR

Dr. Jane Bearden

2.34a

Dr. Jane Bearden
44 No Corvallis Ave., Corvallis, OR 97331
222-666-9876

Name Jeff Scott Date 12/20

Address 99 Corvallis Ave. Age 65

℞

Pravachol 40 mg

#100

i daily

Refill 3 times

Dr. Jane Bearden

2.34b

2.35

PT. NAME: **ROZ BARRON** GENDER: **F** ADDRESS: **22 SOUTH 3000 EAST** WEIGHT: **133** HEIGHT: **5′ 1″**
AGE: **65** DX: **HTN, HYPOTHYROID, BAD BACK, GLAUCOMA** ALLERGY: **PCN, ASA** HX: **ACTIVE, GOLFER, SMOKES**

MEDICATION	SIG.	PRESCRIBER	ORIG. DATE	REFILL DATE	REFILL DATE	REFILL DATE	REFILL DATE
Synthroid 125 mcg #30	1 qd	Cassidy	10/20	11/19			
Lorazepam 1 mg #30	1 bid prn	Cassidy	10/20				
Clarinex 5 mg #30	1 qd prn	Cassidy	6/7	8/9			
Xalatan 0.005% 2.5 mL	1 gtt ou qd	Bascomb	6/16	7/24			

Dr. Annette Cassidy
88 South 6000 East
Salt Lake City, UT 84112
801-543-2828

Name Roz Barron Date 12/3

Address 22 South 3000 East Age 65

℞

Diovan 80mg
#30
1 in AM - 10AM + 1 at 10PM

2x Refs

Dr. Annette Cassidy

2.35a

Dr. Omar Viscarando
34 South 500 East
Salt Lake City, UT 84112
801-543-1236

Name Roz Barron Date 12/3

Address 22 South 3000 East Age 65

℞

Soma Compd
#XXX
Sig: i tid

REFILL ______ TIMES

Dr. Omar Viscarando

2.35b

2.36

PT. NAME: **JOAN LOBATO** GENDER: **F** ADDRESS: **840 HUNTINGTON AVE.** WEIGHT: **122** BMI: **22**

AGE: **63** DX: **HTN, TYPE 2 DM, ARRHYTHMIA, INCONTINENCE, HIGH CHOLESTEROL, INSOMNIA** ALLERGY: **PCN** HX: **ETOH, OCCASIONAL SMOKER**

MEDICATION	SIG.	PRESCRIBER	ORIG. DATE	REFILL DATE	REFILL DATE	REFILL DATE	REFILL DATE
Insulin syringes U-100 #100	Use ud	Bernstein	10/1				
Humulin N 100 U/mL 10 mL	Use according to instructions	Bernstein	10/1				
Amitriptyline HCl 10 mg #30	1 hs	Bernstein	6/7	7/5	8/3	9/1	10/5
Sonata 5 mg caps #30	1 hs prn	Bernstein	9/27	10/29			

Dr. Roger Bernstein
999 Fenway Park Drive, Boston, MA 02115
617-554-9876

Name Joan Lobato Date 11/3

Address 8840 Huntington Ave. Age 63

℞

Zocor
40mg po qPM
disp 30

☐ LABEL

REFILL (3) TIMES PRN NR

Dr. Roger Bernstein

2.36a

Dr. Roger Bernstein
999 Fenway Park Drive, Boston, MA 02115
617-554-9876

Name Joan Lobato Date 11/3

Address 8840 Huntington Ave. Age 63

℞

Sotalol
80mg
po qAM & qPM
disp 60

☐ LABEL

REFILL (3) TIMES PRN

Dr. Roger Bernstein

2.36b

2.37

PT. NAME: **JASON GRAY**
AGE: **56**
GENDER: **M**
DX: **TYPE 2 DM, HTN, ANGINA, CHOLESTEROL**
ADDRESS: **5 SAUSALITO ST.**
ALLERGY: **NKA**
WEIGHT: **189**
HX: **TRUCK DRIVER**
BMI: **30**

MEDICATION	SIG.	PRESCRIBER	ORIG. DATE	REFILL DATE	REFILL DATE	REFILL DATE	REFILL DATE
Coreg 3.125 mg #60	1 bid	Babbit	8/31	9/29	10/11		
Coreg 6.25 mg #60	1 bid	Babbit	11/9	12/8			
Actos 15 mg #30	1 qd	Babbit	8/31	10/11			
Metformin 500 mg #60	1 bid	Babbit	8/31	9/2	10/5	11/28	
Ezetimibe 10 mg #60	1 qd	Babbit	10/30				

Dr. Leslie Babbit
112 Parnassus Ave., San Francisco, CA 94143
415-777-3456

Name Jason Gray Date 12/11

Address 5 Sausalito St. Age 56

℞

Altace 5 mg #50

Sig T po daily

REFILL 1 - 2 - 3 - NR - (PRN)

(LABEL WITH NAME OF MEDICATION DISPENSED)

Dr. Leslie Babbit

2.37a

Dr. Leslie Babbit
112 Parnassus Ave., San Francisco, CA 94143
415-777-3456

Name Jason Gray Date 12/11

Address 5 Sausalito St. Age 56

℞

Nitrolingual spray 1/150 #1.

as directed

REFILL 1 - 2 - (3) - NR - PRN

LABEL WITH NAME OF MEDICATION DISPENSED

Dr. Leslie Babbit

2.37b

2.38

PT. NAME: **LEIGH CRESPO**
AGE: **71**
GENDER: **F**
DX: **HTN, DEPRESSION, OSTEOPOROSIS**
ADDRESS: **55 WEST MARKHAM**
ALLERGY: **NKA**
WEIGHT: **102**
HX: **FORMER TEACHER, SEDENTARY LIFESTYLE**
BMI: **20**

MEDICATION	SIG.	PRESCRIBER	ORIG. DATE	REFILL DATE	REFILL DATE	REFILL DATE	REFILL DATE
Zoloft 50 mg #30	1 qd	Hopkins	10/1	11/2			
Lipitor 10 mg #30	1 qd	Hopkins	9/2	10/3	11/2	12/1	

Dr. Kim Hopkins
88 West Markham, Little Rock, AR
501-444-3469

Name Leigh Crespo Date 12/3
Address 55 West Markham Age 71

℞

ZESTORETIC 20/12.5
ONE q AM
#30

REPEAT 6 TIMES

Dr. Kim Hopkins

2.38a

Dr. Kim Hopkins
88 West Markham, Little Rock, AR
501-444-3469

Name Leigh Crespo Date 12/3
Address 55 West Markham Age 71

℞

Fosamax 70 mg
Sig i po q week
#4

12 Refills

Dr. Kim Hopkins

2.38b

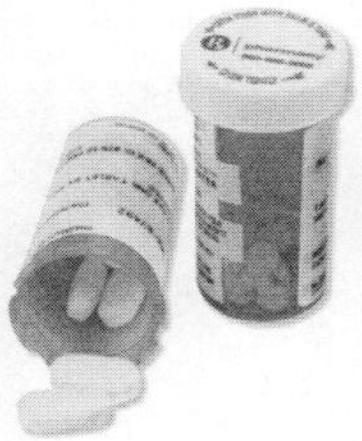

3 • GERIATRICS

UPON COMPLETION OF THIS CHAPTER, THE STUDENT WILL BE ABLE TO:

- describe the mechanism of action of Zyloprim and thereby understand the interaction with azathioprine and 6-mercaptopurine.
- understand the interaction between aspirin and uricosuric drugs.
- recognize and discuss the two uses of lactulose.
- instruct the patient regarding the importance of drinking adequate amounts of water when taking laxatives.
- counsel the patients on the correct methods for taking Fosamax and other oral bisphosphonates.
- give appropriate instructions for the application of scopolamine patches.
- instruct the person taking thyroid products about compliance.
- counsel the patient taking thyroid products that the medication should be taken on an empty stomach. Vitamins, minerals, antacids, and all other products should be taken later in the day.
- advise the patient who is taking colchicine that the dose should not be increased unless ordered by the prescriber.

DRUG LIST

Actonel
Allopurinol
Antivert
Boniva
Colchicine
Docusate
Estradiol
Fosamax
Lactulose
Premarin/Prempro
Probenecid
Propylthiouracil/Tapazole
Synthroid
Transderm Scop
Uloric

• DRUG **HOT POINTS**

Allopurinol
Inhibits xanthine oxidase, reduces uric acid formation
Interaction with azathioprine and 6-MP (6-mercaptopurine)
Compare to Uloric

Antivert
OTC & Rx (Bonine, meclizine)
Watch: additive anticholinergic effects

Docusate (sodium: Colace; calcium: Surfak)
Full glass of water with each dose
Do not take with mineral oil
Daily intake of fiber-containing foods

Fosamax
Tablets, liquid, and tablets with vitamin D
Take 30 minutes before breakfast on an empty stomach; no juice, coffee, milk, or food
Take with lots of water; sit upright for 30 minutes
5 mg/day (prevention) or 10 mg/day (treatment)
70 mg once-a-week tablet (35 mg also)
For men or women
Routine weight-bearing exercise
Adequate calcium & vitamin D intake, if needed
Treatment for Paget's disease (40 mg/day × 6 months)
Compare with Miacalcin
Compare with Boniva and Actonel

Lactulose
May be mixed with fruit juice or water
May cause abdominal discomfort
Don't take other laxatives
Counsel: increased gas production
Metabolized in colon to lactic, formic, and acetic acids
Uses:
- As laxative (osmosis)
- For portal-systemic encephalopathy (NH_3 trapped as NH_4^+ in the colon)

Premarin: oral and vaginal formulations
Derived from urine of pregnant mares
Intact uterus: Prempro or Premphase
Not intact uterus: Premarin (estrogen)
Vaginal formulation: external & internal
Estrace (estradiol)—compare with Premarin
Estrogen patch application advice
Evista: SERM—compare with Premarin
Caution: ankle swelling
Warnings about potential hazards

Probenecid
Mechanism: uricosuric (increases uric acid excretion)
Aspirin interaction
Dietary advice
Caution regarding dehydration
Compare with colchicine

Propylthiouracil (PTU)
Mechanism in treating hyperthyroidism
Use in pregnancy compared with Tapazole

Synthroid
qd in am on regular schedule
Interactions: iron products and other polyvalent cations
Dosage equivalents (approximate equivalent strength, based on clinical response): 50 mcg up to 100 mcg is equal to the effect of 60 mg (1 grain) of thyroid hormone
Thyroid lab test: TSH (elevated TSH: hypothyroid; depressed TSH: hyperthyroid)
Compare with Cytomel (liothyronine, triiodothyronine [T_3])

Transderm Scop
Apply behind ear every 3 days
Uses: travel, vertigo, hospice patients (to dry bronchial secretions)
Anticholinergic cautions

• QUESTIONS TO BE ANSWERED IN PREPARATION FOR CHAPTER 3 LAB

- Using receptors, how does meclizine work in the treatment of dizziness (vertigo)?
- What is the mechanism of action of Zyloprim?
- What is the usual adult dose for Zyloprim?
- How many grams of lactulose are contained in each 15 mL of lactulose syrup?
- Compare and contrast the two mechanisms of lactulose: one in the treatment of constipation and the other in the treatment of portal–systemic encephalopathy, including hepatic coma.
- What is the problem if a diabetic patient takes lactulose?
- Probenecid is a uricosuric agent. Define "uricosuric."
- Explain the reason why aspirin may block the uricosuric action of probenecid.
- Why is it important to take Synthroid on an empty stomach?
- Explain the interaction between certain vitamin–mineral products with Synthroid.
- What are some signs and symptoms of an overdose of a thyroid product?
- Explain the advantages of Synthroid over the crude thyroid hormone.
- Explain the milligram dosing conversion from Synthroid to crude thyroid products.
- What are important counseling points for the use of Miacalcin nasal spray?
- Explain the advantages of using Miacalcin nasal spray over Fosamax.
- Explain the advantages of using Fosamax over Miacalcin nasal spray.
- What are the important counseling points for Fosamax?
- What is the most common side effect with the use of Fosamax?
- What advantage does the 70 mg once-a-week dose of Fosamax offer?
- What is the difference between Premarin and Prempro?
- How does Prempro differ from Premphase?
- Which patients should use the estrogen product alone, and which should use the combination of estrogen and progestin?
- Compare the action of Estrace with that of Premarin.
- Why should the patient be warned not to smoke when taking estrogen products?
- Which estradiol patches are used once a week, and which are used twice a week?
- Which area of the body is the preferred site for estradiol patches?
- What is the mechanism of action of Evista?
- Which adverse effects of Evista should the patient be aware of?
- In the treatment of hyperthyroidism in a pregnant patient, which product is preferred, PTU or Tapazole? Explain the reason for your answer.
- What is the pharmacological effect of bisphosphonates on osteoclasts?
- Which bisphosphonates are available in a PO once-monthly tablet?

• GERIATRIC MEDICATION THERAPY MANAGEMENT QUESTIONS AND COMMENTS

- You are taking pills to help strengthen your bones. You mentioned that you swim and do yoga. These exercises are not as effective as long, brisk walks; stretching exercises in the standing position; or other activities that will cause the bones to be stronger. These are called "weight bearing." Would you like a list of these exercises to help build your bones?
- Did your doctor tell you how important it is for you to keep taking your thyroid pills indefinitely, even if you feel good?
- You are taking a medication for your bowels. Are you drinking at least four glasses of water daily, if approved by your doctor? Are you aware of foods that contain fiber that will help?
- Your medication is prescribed to control uric acid in your body. Would you like a list of foods and drinks that should be avoided?
- Your doctor has prescribed a medication that will help your body remove extra uric acid. Are you aware that any aspirin-containing product, even OTC or nonprescription medication, will decrease the action of the prescription medication?
- Did you know that this nasal spray to strengthen your bones should be used the following way: one spray in the right nostril on the first day, then one spray in the left nostril the next day, and so on?
- You are taking medications to strengthen your bones. Did the doctor tell you to take enough calcium products and foods to help the medications?
- Calcium citrate with vitamin D is very effective.
- I notice that the test we just did with your heel shows that your bones need more strength. Are you seeing a doctor?
- Your doctor has prescribed a pill to take for dizziness. Did you tell the doctor that you are taking other medications from another doctor that might cause side effects with the new medicine?
- Your thyroid medication has an important caution. It should be taken on an empty stomach with a full glass of water, first thing in the morning, with no foods or other vitamins or pills for about 1 hour. This will make it work better.
- Your medication to make your bones strong has an important caution. It should be taken on an empty stomach with a full glass of water, first thing in the morning, with no foods, other vitamins, or pills for about 1 hour. This will make it work better.
- I notice that you are using two prescribed laxatives, and you also purchase other laxatives without a prescription. Did your doctor advise you to limit the amount of laxatives to use?
- You are taking a female hormone. Please contact us or your doctor if you notice any aches or pains in your knee or in the back of the knee or other parts of your legs.
- I notice that you and your doctor have decided to stop the female hormone medications that you were taking. If you need something to help vaginal dryness, we carry very effective OTC products that can prevent this problem.
- Because you have mentioned that you are experiencing rapid heartbeats and you cannot sleep well, I recommend that you see your doctor soon to have a complete checkup and thyroid test.
- We can recommend a nutritionist, registered dietitian, as well as a local physical or occupational therapist. If you or your doctor would like, we can put you in contact.

3.1	PT. NAME: **ALICE SMITH**	GENDER: **F**	ADDRESS: **223 ORIOLE AVE.**	WEIGHT: **188**	BMI: **31**
	AGE: **65**	DX: **POSTMENOPAUSAL, HTN, CHF, NASAL ALLERGY, BRONCHIAL INFECTION**	ALLERGY: **NKA**	HX: **ETOH**	

MEDICATION	SIG.	PRESCRIBER	ORIG. DATE	REFILL DATE	REFILL DATE	REFILL DATE	REFILL DATE
Z-Pak	Take ud	Weiss	9/25				
Flonase nasal spray 16 g	Use ud	Weiss	7/3	8/28			
Lanoxin 0.125 mg #30	1 qd	Weiss	8/25	9/25			
Lasix 40 mg #30	1 qd	Weiss	9/25				

Dr. Barry Weiss
901 Sheridan St., Austin, TX 90902
874-555-9000

Name Alice Smith Date 9/29

Address 223 Oriole Ave. Age 65

℞

Estrace 1 mg Tab

Sig: i po qd

#100

Refills 2

Dr. Barry Weiss

3.1a

Dr. Barry Weiss
901 Sheridan St., Austin, TX 90902
874-555-9000

Name Alice Smith Date 9/29

Address 223 Oriole Ave. Age 65

℞

Aldactone 25 #30

Sig: i bid

Refills 2

Dr. Barry Weiss

3.1b

3.2	PT. NAME: **ANNA MYERS** AGE: **65**	GENDER: **F** DX: **NERVES, ANGINA, HTN, HYPOTHYROID, NASAL ALLERGIES**	ADDRESS: **822 WEST RD.** ALLERGY: **NKA**	WEIGHT: **226** HX: **ALWAYS ON A DIET**	BMI: **34**

MEDICATION	SIG.	PRESCRIBER	ORIG. DATE	REFILL DATE	REFILL DATE	REFILL DATE	REFILL DATE
Xanax 0.25 mg #30	1/2 tab bid	Hunter	8/1	9/4			
Nitrostat 1/150 gr (0.4 mg) #C	1 sl prn	Hunter	5/30				
Capoten 25 mg #60	1 bid	Hunter	6/29	8/3	9/12	9/29	
Claritin 10 mg #30	1 qd	Hunter	7/7	7/27			
Sudafed 30 mg #24	1 bid prn runny nose	OTC	2/22	5/12	8/29		

Dr. Calvin Hunter
4000 Lake Dr., New Orleans, LA 44718
463-555-0009

Name Anna Myers Date 9/30

Address 822 West Road Age 65

℞

Synthroid 0.1 mg #30
1 po qd

Refills PRN

Dr. Calvin Hunter

3.2a

Dr. Calvin Hunter
4000 Lake Dr., New Orleans, LA 44718
463-555-0009

Name Anna Myers Date 9/30

Address 822 West Road Age 65

℞

Norvasc 5 mg
#C
[illegible]

Refills PRN

Dr. Calvin Hunter

3.2b

3.3	PT. NAME: **JOYCE MURPHY** AGE: **58**	GENDER: **F** DX: **POSTMENOPAUSAL SX, HTN, HYPOTHYROID, HIGH CHOLESTEROL**	ADDRESS: **67 BLOOMINGDALE ST.** ALLERGY: **PCN**	WEIGHT: **218** HX: **RETIRED TEACHER; STRESSFUL LIFESTYLE; FREQUENT GAMBLER**	BMI: **35**

MEDICATION	SIG.	PRESCRIBER	ORIG. DATE	REFILL DATE	REFILL DATE	REFILL DATE	REFILL DATE
Detrol 1 mg #30	1 bid	Abrahamsson	6/27	8/4			
Lac-Hydrin 12% 225 mL	apply bid	Abrahamsson	8/24				
Prempro 0.625/2.5 mg #28	1 qd	Fine	7/13	8/4	9/1	10/4	
Lunesta 1 mg #30	1 hs	Fine	10/1				

Dr. Mark Fine
600 Beacon St., Boston, MA 48484
813-555-7555

Name Joyce Murphy Date 10/15

Address 67 Bloomingdale St. Age 58

℞

Premarin cream Apply
1/2 applicator
daily x 7 days, then
QOD ī large
tube

Refills 2

Dr. Mark Fine

3.3a

Dr. J.V. Abrahamsson
988 Beacon St., Boston, MA 48484
813-555-2222

Name Joyce Murphy Date 10/15

Address 67 Bloomingdale St. Age 58

℞

① Synthroid .025 #100
i qd

② Lasix 20 mg #100
i qd

③ Pravachol #100
20 mg

Refills 2

Dr. J.V. Abrahamsson

3.3b

3.4

PT. NAME: **KATE ANDERSON** | AGE: **81** | GENDER: **F** | DX: **ANXIETY, THYROID (ELEVATED TSH), GOUT, OA** | ADDRESS: **87 SOUTH ST.** | ALLERGY: **NKA** | WEIGHT: **132** | HX: **SOCIAL DRINKER** | BMI: **26**

MEDICATION	SIG.	PRESCRIBER	ORIG. DATE	REFILL DATE	REFILL DATE	REFILL DATE	REFILL DATE
BuSpar 5 mg #90	I tid	Griffin	9/8	10/13			
Synthroid 0.05 mg #30	I qd	Griffin	8/23	9/25	10/25		
Temazepam 15 mg #30	I hs prn sleep	Griffin	8/21	9/15	10/8		
Anacin tabs #C	I tid prn headaches	OTC	8/5	9/6	10/3		

Dr. Doug Griffin
7611 147th Terrace, Monterey, CA 38411
705-555-6644

Name Kate Anderson Date 10/28

Address 87 South St. Age 81

℞

lactulose [illegible]
16 oz
Sig: [illegible] bid

Refills 2

Dr. Doug Griffin

3.4a

Dr. Doug Griffin
7611 147th Terrace, Monterey, CA 38411
705-555-6644

Name Kate Anderson Date 10/28

Address 87 South St. Age 81

℞

Benemid 0.5 g
#100
T BID

Refills 2

Dr. Doug Griffin

3.4b

3.5

PT. NAME: **EDNA JOHNSON** GENDER: **F** ADDRESS: **500 CUMMINGS ST.** WEIGHT: **105** HEIGHT: **5′**

AGE: **79** DX: **HTN, TYPE 2 DM, THYROID, ANGINA** ALLERGY: **NKA** HX: **SMOKES 1/2 PACK/DAY**

MEDICATION	SIG.	PRESCRIBER	ORIG. DATE	REFILL DATE	REFILL DATE	REFILL DATE	REFILL DATE
Nitrostat 1/150 gr (0.4 mg) #C	1 sl ud	Crawford	5/2	6/13			
BD Ultra-Fine insulin syringes with needles 1/2 cc	Use ud	Crawford	3/16	4/30			
Toprol XL 50 mg #90	1 qd	Crawford	5/2				
Synthroid 0.05 mg #90	1 qd	Crawford	2/15	5/20			
Lopressor 50 mg #45	1/2 tab qd	Crawford	2/15				

Dr. Alfred Crawford
2100 Cummings St., Valdosta, GA 31601
954-555-1348

Name Edna Johnson Date 6/15

Address 500 Cummings St. Age 79

℞

NTG Spray
use for tightness
in chest

Refills 3

Dr. Alfred Crawford

3.5a

Dr. Alfred Crawford
2100 Cummings St., Valdosta, GA 31601
954-555-1348

Name Edna Johnson Date 6/15

Address 500 Cummings St. Age 79

℞

Armour Thyroid 60 mg
#30
sig: 1 daily in a.m.

Refills 3

Dr. Alfred Crawford

3.5b

3.6

PT. NAME: **CHARLES SCHMIDT** GENDER: **M** ADDRESS: **1002 WEST RD.** WEIGHT: **159** BMI: **26**
AGE: **62** DX: **HTN, HEMORRHOIDS ("PILES"), BACTERIAL EYE INFECTION, VERTIGO** ALLERGY: **PCN** HX: **SMOKER**

MEDICATION	SIG.	PRESCRIBER	ORIG. DATE	REFILL DATE	REFILL DATE	REFILL DATE	REFILL DATE
Zestril 20 mg #30	I qd	Weiss	8/5				
HCTZ 25 mg #30	I qd	Weiss	8/5				
Cipro 500 mg #6	I bid × 3 d	Weiss	6/1				
Ciloxan ophthalmic solution 5 mL	I gtt ou qid	Sanders	4/8				

Dr. Barry Weiss
901 Sheridan St., Austin, TX 90902
874-555-9000

Name Charles Schmidt Date 8/28

Address 1002 West Rd. Age 62

℞

Antivert 25
T qid prn
dizziness
#30

Refills 1

Dr. Barry Weiss

3.6a

Dr. Lynn Jacobson
4850 NW 10th St., Austin, TX 90902
874-555-8200

Name Charles Schmidt Date 8/28

Address 1002 West Rd. Age 62

℞

Anusol HC Supp (generic)
#14
T pr post BM daily

Refills 1

Lynn Jacobson

3.6b

3.7	PT. NAME: **ELIZABETH KELLY**	GENDER: **F**	ADDRESS: **5007 TALLAHASSEE CT.**	WEIGHT: **117**	BMI: **22**
	AGE: **63**	DX: **HTN, OSTEOPOROSIS, ANXIETY**	ALLERGY: **PCN**	HX: **ACTIVE IN BUSINESS; PARTICIPATES IN ATHLETIC HOBBIES**	

MEDICATION	SIG.	PRESCRIBER	ORIG. DATE	REFILL DATE	REFILL DATE	REFILL DATE	REFILL DATE
Adalat CC 30 mg #30	I qd	Sauls	4/10	5/8	6/4		
Lasix 40 mg #90	I qd	Sauls	4/10				
Xanax 0.25 mg #5	I qd prn anxiety	Sauls	5/10				

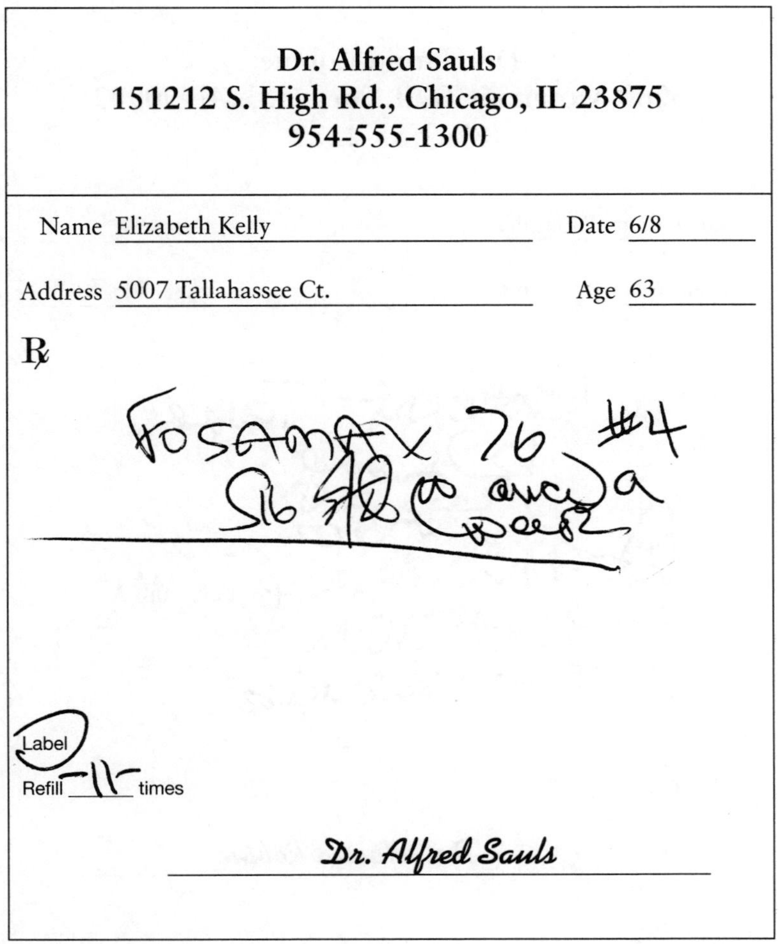

Dr. Alfred Sauls
151212 S. High Rd., Chicago, IL 23875
954-555-1300

Name Elizabeth Kelly Date 6/8

Address 5007 Tallahassee Ct. Age 63

℞

Fosamax 70 #4
[illegible]

Label
Refill —||— times

Dr. Alfred Sauls

3.7a

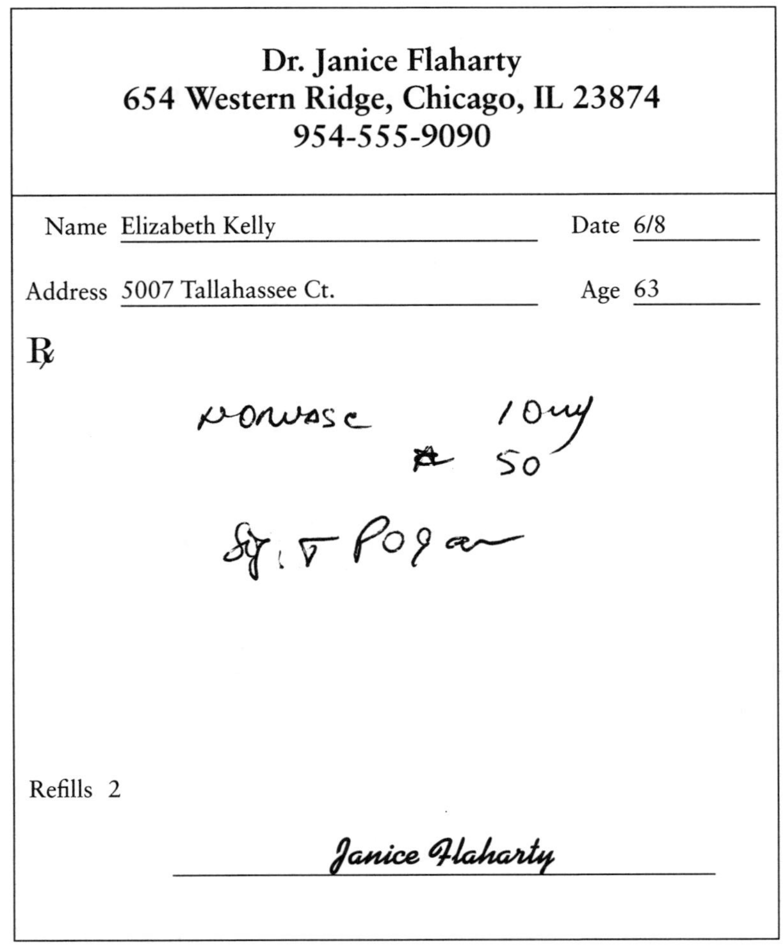

Dr. Janice Flaharty
654 Western Ridge, Chicago, IL 23874
954-555-9090

Name Elizabeth Kelly Date 6/8

Address 5007 Tallahassee Ct. Age 63

℞

Norvasc 10 mg
50

Sig: i T PO q am

Refills 2

Janice Flaharty

3.7b

3.8

PT. NAME: **EMMA GONZALEZ**	GENDER: **F**	ADDRESS: **6 SKI TRAIL LANE**	WEIGHT: **179**	BMI: **31**
AGE: **72**	DX: **TYPE 2 DM, HTN, VERTIGO, CONSTIPATION**	ALLERGY: **NKA**	HX: **SEDENTARY LIFESTYLE**	

MEDICATION	SIG.	PRESCRIBER	ORIG. DATE	REFILL DATE	REFILL DATE	REFILL DATE	REFILL DATE
Lopressor 50 mg #30	1/2 tab bid	Robine	4/12	5/10			
Elocon lotion 30 mL	Apply to scalp bid	Robine	6/1				
Glyburide 2.5 mg #90	1 bid	Robine	1/5	4/8			
Dramamine tabs #36	1 tab prn dizziness	OTC	3/3	5/14			

Dr. Bart Knee
777 High St., Portland, ME 90902
874-555-8888

Name Emma Gonzalez Date 6/4

Address 6 Ski Trail Lane Age 72

℞

LACTULOSE SYRUP

SIG: 1 TBSP AS NEEDED
B.ID

DISP: 1 LG TUBE

Refills 6

Dr. Bart Knee

3.8a

Dr. Harold Robine
6060 Mountain Trail, Portland, ME 90902
874-555-2222

Name Emma Gonzalez Date 6/3

Address 6 Ski Trail Lane Age 72

℞

Antivert Tabs
12½ mg
#50
Sig: i for walking in day;
i at 3PM
i at bedtime

Refills 6

Dr. Harold Robine

3.8b

3.9

PT. NAME: ETHEL PETERSON	GENDER: F	ADDRESS: 564 CAPITOL AVE.	WEIGHT: 116	HEIGHT: 5′ 2″
AGE: 50	DX: IBS, OSTEOPOROSIS, POSTNASAL DRIP, DIZZINESS	ALLERGY: NKA	HX: FAMILY HISTORY OF OSTEOPOROSIS; YEARS OF GI UPSET (SINCE CHILDHOOD)	

MEDICATION	SIG.	PRESCRIBER	ORIG. DATE	REFILL DATE	REFILL DATE	REFILL DATE	REFILL DATE
Librax #50	1 tid ac	Thomas	6/4	6/28	7/17	8/1	
Allegra D 12-h 60 mg #30	1 bid	Thomas	7/12				
Benadryl 25 mg #48	1 bid for sinus	OTC	2/27	3/30	4/15	5/30	

Dr. Erin Thomas
988 North Ridge, New York, NY 88364
813-555-7554

Name Ethel Peterson Date 8/5

Address 564 Capitol Ave. Age 50

℞

Meclizine 12.5 mg bid po

#60

Refills 2

Dr. Erin Thomas

3.9a

Dr. John Samuels
411 North Ridge, New York, NY 88364
813-555-9876

Name Ethel Peterson Date 8/5

Address 564 Capitol Ave. Age 50

℞

Prevacid 30mg qd

Fosamax

70 mg

once a week

wait 1 hr for breakfast

Refills 2

Dr. John Samuels

3.9b

3.10 PT. NAME: **MAMIE WILLIAMS** AGE: **63** GENDER: **F** DX: **CHF, ANXIETY, SKIN INFECTION, HEART RHYTHM DISTURBANCE, CONSTIPATION** ADDRESS: **321 WEST RD.** ALLERGY: **NKA** WEIGHT: **148** HX: **SMOKER FOR 40 YEARS** BMI: **30**

MEDICATION	SIG.	PRESCRIBER	ORIG. DATE	REFILL DATE	REFILL DATE	REFILL DATE	REFILL DATE
BuSpar 5 mg #90	I tid	Griffin	2/5	3/8	4/6		
Lanoxin 0.125 mg #30	I qd	Griffin	3/10				
Bactroban Cream 15 g	Apply bid	Griffin	1/15				
Betapace 80 mg #30	I bid	Griffin	5/12				
Lasix 40 mg #50	I bid	Griffin	3/10				
KCl 10% liq. 473 mL	I tbs bid	Griffin	3/10	4/8	5/4	5/19	

Dr. Doug Griffin
7611 147th Terrace, Monterey, CA 38411
705-555-6644

Name Mamie Williams Date 5/20

Address 321 West Rd. Age 63

℞

Lactulose Syrup
8 ℥
SIG: T teaspoon
TID

Refills 6

Dr. Doug Griffin

3.10a

Dr. Doug Griffin
7611 147th Terrace, Monterey, CA 38411
705-555-6644

Name Mamie Williams Date 5/20

Address 321 West Rd. Age 63

℞

Plavix 75,
#30
T qd n x6

Dr. Doug Griffin

3.10b

3.11

PT. NAME: **FLORENCE WILSON** GENDER: **F** ADDRESS: **566 EAST CT.** WEIGHT: **122** HEIGHT: **5′ 3″**
AGE: **69** DX: **HTN, OSTEOPOROSIS, OA, TENSION HEADACHES** ALLERGY: **NKA** HX: **SMOKES 1 PACK/DAY**

MEDICATION	SIG.	PRESCRIBER	ORIG. DATE	REFILL DATE	REFILL DATE	REFILL DATE	REFILL DATE
Tenormin 50 mg #30	1 qd	Weiss	11/3	12/4			
Tylenol No. 4 #30	1–2 q 4–6 h prn	Weiss	11/2				
Fioricet #12	1–2 ud	Sauls	11/10				
Percocet 5 mg/325 mg #6	1 q 6 h prn pain	Sauls	10/12				
Ibuprofen 600 mg #30	1 bid, alternate Tylenol	Weiss	11/4				
Acetaminophen 500 mg #C	1–2 q 4 h prn pain	OTC	7/6	8/7	9/1	10/16	11/20

Dr. Barry Weiss
901 Sheridan St., Austin, TX 90902
874-555-9000

Name Florence Wilson Date 12/15
Address 566 East Ct. Age 69

℞

Miacalcin inh
i spray qd

Ag (2)

Refills 3

Dr. Barry Weiss

3.11a

Dr. Lynn Jacobson
4850 NW 10th St., Austin, TX 90902
874-555-8200

Name Florence Wilson Date 12/15
Address 566 East Ct. Age 69

℞

Esgic
#100

Sig: i tab i or ii q 6 h
prn cephalgia

Refills 3

Lynn Jacobson

3.11b

3.12

PT. NAME: **GEORGE HOFFMAN** GENDER: **M** ADDRESS: **23 SOUTH ST.** WEIGHT: **176** HEIGHT: **5′ 3″**

AGE: **72** DX: **HTN, HIGH CHOLESTEROL, GERD, BACK PAIN, VERTIGO, ANGINA** ALLERGY: **NKA** HX: **ACTIVE LIFESTYLE, DRINKS SOCIALLY**

MEDICATION	SIG.	PRESCRIBER	ORIG. DATE	REFILL DATE	REFILL DATE	REFILL DATE	REFILL DATE
Simvastatin 10 mg #30	I qd	Robins	4/12				
Procardia XL 60 mg #30	I qd	Robins	4/12				
Prilosec 20 mg #30	I bid	Robins	3/10	3/25			
Bufferin tabs #C	I tid for pain	OTC	5/1	5/29			
Bengay ultra 4 oz	Apply tid for muscle pain	OTC	5/1	5/29			

Dr. Calvin Robins
7823 Tea Rose Trail, Miami, FL 44718
463-555-8000

Name George Hoffman Date 5/30

Address 23 South St. Age 72

℞

Antivert 25 mg

#100 i PO tid prn

Refills 3

Dr. Calvin Robins

3.12a

Dr. Paul Gunion
3999 Tea Rose Trail, Miami, FL 44718
463-555-9543

Name George Hoffman Date 5/30

Address 23 South St. Age 72

℞

1) NTG 0.4mg one bottle
i SL q5′ x3 prn for chest pains

2) ECASA #30 i qd

Refills 3

Dr. Paul Gunion

3.12b

3.13

PT. NAME: **WILLIE MAE MILLER** AGE: **66**
GENDER: **F**
DX: **HTN, HYPERURICEMIA, GOUT PAIN, OA PAIN, EYE IRRITATION**
ADDRESS: **1 EAGLE RUN**
ALLERGY: **PCN**
WEIGHT: **155**
HX: **ETOH**
BMI: **26**

MEDICATION	SIG.	PRESCRIBER	ORIG. DATE	REFILL DATE	REFILL DATE	REFILL DATE	REFILL DATE
Procardia XL 60 mg #90	I q am	Wallace	4/12	7/10	10/24		
Pred Forte ophthalmic drops 5 mL	I gtt ou qid	Tenzel	2/24				
Tylenol No. 3 #30	I bid prn	Wallace	2/20				

Dr. Barry Wallace
977 Sheridan St., Austin, TX 90902
874-555-9099

Name Willie Mae Miller Date 10/25

Address 1 Eagle Run Age 66

℞

Colchicine 0.6mg #30
S: ī qd.

Refills 6

Dr. Barry Wallace

3.13a

Dr. Lynn Jacobson
4850 NW 10th St., Austin, TX 90902
874-555-8200

Name Willie Mae Miller Date 10/25

Address 1 Eagle Run Age 66

℞

Allopurinol 100g #30
ī po QD

Refills 6

Lynn Jacobson

3.13b

3.14

PT. NAME: **HENRIETTA GARCIA** GENDER: **F** ADDRESS: **92 IBIS LANE** WEIGHT: **180** BMI: **35**
AGE: **79** DX: **HTN, OSTEOPOROSIS, HYPOTHYROID (ELEVATED TSH), INSOMNIA** ALLERGY: **CHOCOLATE, MSG IN CHINESE FOOD** HX: **SMOKER FOR 50 YEARS**

MEDICATION	SIG.	PRESCRIBER	ORIG. DATE	REFILL DATE	REFILL DATE	REFILL DATE	REFILL DATE
Tenoretic 50/25 mg #30	I qd	Lippman	4/12				
K-Dur 20 mEq #30	I bid	Lippman	4/12				
Citracal +D #60	I tid	Lippman	2/15				
Restoril 30 mg #30	I hs prn	Lippman	1/20	2/18	3/16	4/18	

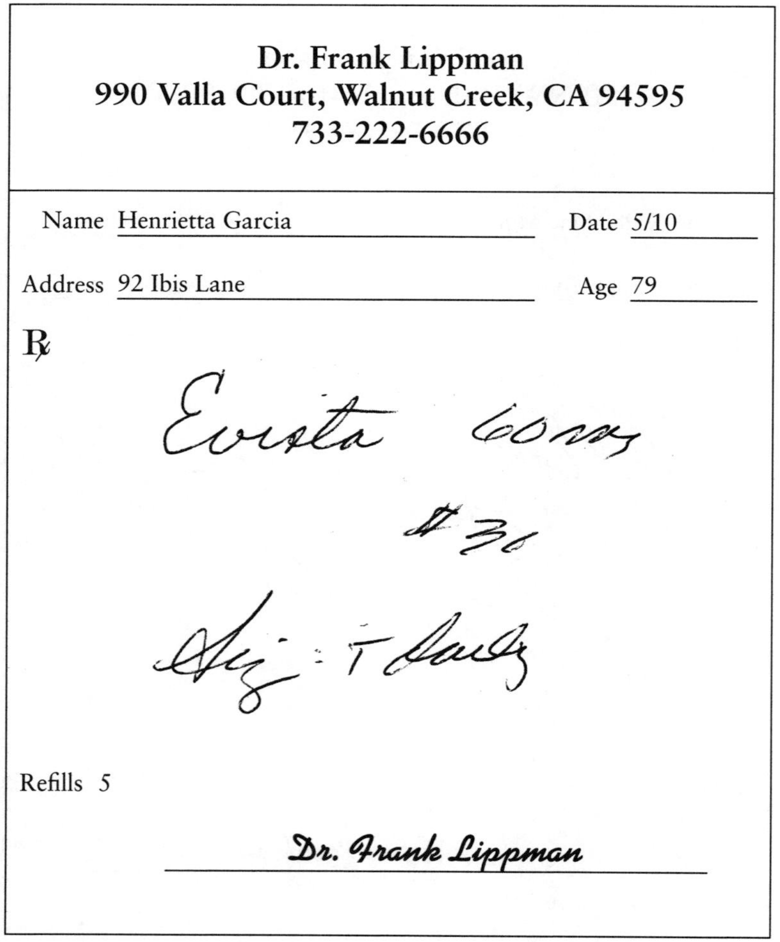

Dr. Frank Lippman
990 Valla Court, Walnut Creek, CA 94595
733-222-6666

Name Henrietta Garcia Date 5/10
Address 92 Ibis Lane Age 79
℞
Evista 60mg
#30
Sig: i daily

Refills 5
Dr. Frank Lippman

3.14a

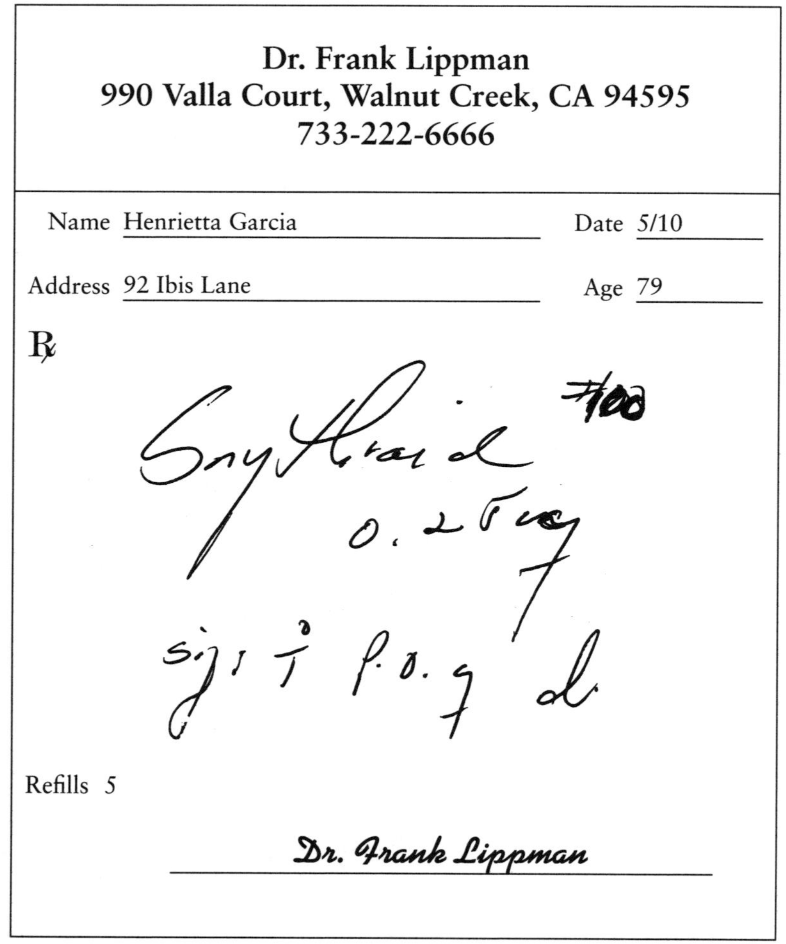

Dr. Frank Lippman
990 Valla Court, Walnut Creek, CA 94595
733-222-6666

Name Henrietta Garcia Date 5/10
Address 92 Ibis Lane Age 79
℞
Synthroid #100
0.25mg
sig: i p.o. q d

Refills 5
Dr. Frank Lippman

3.14b

3.15

PT. NAME: **GRACE NELSON**	GENDER: **F**	ADDRESS: **900 81ST ST.**	WEIGHT: **129**	HEIGHT: **5′**
AGE: **72**	DX: **GERD, OA, EDEMA, LEG CRAMPS WHILE WALKING, CONSTIPATION, SKIN FUNGUS, POSTMENOPAUSAL SX**		ALLERGY: **NKA**	HX: **SOCIAL DRINKER**

MEDICATION	SIG.	PRESCRIBER	ORIG. DATE	REFILL DATE	REFILL DATE	REFILL DATE	REFILL DATE
Lotrisone cream 15 g	Apply ud prn	Melnick	5/12				
Cilostazol 50 mg #60	1 bid	Melnick	3/15	4/12	5/15	6/15	
Senokot-S # 60	1 hs prn	Melnick	6/10				
Prilosec 20 mg #30	1 q am	Melnick	7/20				

Dr. Ralph Kaufman
600 N. Alfred, Los Angeles, CA 44718
181-555-8000

Name Grace Nelson Date 8/17

Address 900 81st St. Age 72

℞

Prempro 0.45/1.5
1 daily

Refills 0

Dr. Ralph Kaufman

3.15a

Dr. Alfred Melnick
400 Santa Monica Blvd., Santa Monica, CA 44718
181-555-5000

Name Grace Nelson Date 8/17

Address 900 81st St. Age 72

℞

Dyazide
#50
Sig: i tiw

Refills ad lib

Dr. Alfred Melnick

3.15b

3.16

PT. NAME: **HAROLD BROWN**	GENDER: **M**	ADDRESS: **3975 BLACK DR.**	WEIGHT: **225**	BMI: **36**
AGE: **72**	DX: **OA, HTN, ANGINA, COPD, LOW BONE DENSITY**	ALLERGY: **NKA**	HX: **SMOKED 2 PACKS/DAY FOR 15 YEARS; STILL SMOKES 2 OR 3 CIGARETTES DAILY; HAS TAKEN PREDNISONE FOR YEARS**	

MEDICATION	SIG.	PRESCRIBER	ORIG. DATE	REFILL DATE	REFILL DATE	REFILL DATE	REFILL DATE
Nitro Patch 0.4 mg/hr #30	Apply 1 qd	Griffin	1/15	2/13	3/12		
Corgard 40 mg #30	1 qd	Griffin	2/3	3/1	4/1		
Demadex 20 mg #30	1 qd	Griffin	1/15	3/12			
Prednisone 5 mg #C	1 q am	Griffin	1/3				
Advair Diskus 250/50 mcg #60	Use bid	Griffin	1/3	2/2	4/2		

Dr. Doug Griffin
7611 147th Terrace, Monterey, CA 38411
705-555-6644

Name Harold Brown Date 4/20

Address 3975 Black Dr. Age 72

℞

—Fosamax 5 mg po q-d
½ hour before meal c̄ full
glass of water
remain sit for ½ hour
after taking) #30

Refills 1

Dr. Doug Griffin

3.16a

Dr. Doug Griffin
7611 147th Terrace, Monterey, CA 38411
705-555-6644

Name Harold Brown Date 4/20

Address 3975 Black Dr. Age 72

℞

— ASA 81 mg po q-d #30
— Celebrex 200 mg
po q-d c̄ food
#30

Refills 1

Dr. Doug Griffin

3.16b

3.17

PT. NAME: **LILLIAN WAGNER** GENDER: **F** ADDRESS: **61 GREEN ST.** WEIGHT: **126** HEIGHT: **5′ 5″**

AGE: **64** DX: **HTN, OA, TENSION HEADACHE, HYPOTHYROID, DYSPEPSIA, OSTEOPOROSIS** ALLERGY: **CATS** HX: **SMOKER; SEDENTARY LIFESTYLE**

MEDICATION	SIG.	PRESCRIBER	ORIG. DATE	REFILL DATE	REFILL DATE	REFILL DATE	REFILL DATE
Mobic 7.5 mg #30	1 qd	Sauls	5/12	5/21	5/30		
Fioricet #50	1–2 ud	Sauls	6/20				
Synthroid 0.1 mg #90	1 q am	Sauls	3/10	6/20			
Surfak 240 mg #C	1 qd	OTC	2/4	4/9	6/17		
Nexium 40 mg #30	1 q am 30 min ac	Sauls	3/22	4/28	5/30	6/19	

Dr. Alfred Sauls
151212 S. High Rd., Chicago, IL 23875
954-555-1300

Name Lillian Wagner Date 6/22

Address 61 Green St. Age 64

℞

Miacalcin Nasal Inhaler
1 month's supply
Sig T per nostril qd

Refills 5

Dr. Alfred Sauls

3.17a

Dr. Alfred Sauls
151212 S. High Rd., Chicago, IL 23875
954-555-1300

Name Lillian Wagner Date 6/22

Address 61 Green St. Age 64

℞

Levothroid 100mcg
Sig: i po daily
#30.

Refills 5

Dr. Alfred Sauls

3.17b

3.18

PT. NAME: **MABEL LOPEZ**	GENDER: **F**	ADDRESS: **654 IBIS CT.**	WEIGHT: **121**	BMI: **21**
AGE: **63**	DX: **HTN, EPILEPSY, POSTMENOPAUSAL**	ALLERGY: **NKA**	HX: **FAMILY HISTORY OF OSTEOPOROSIS**	

MEDICATION	SIG.	PRESCRIBER	ORIG. DATE	REFILL DATE	REFILL DATE	REFILL DATE	REFILL DATE
Tenormin 25 mg #90	1 q am	Robins	3/12				
Fosamax 70 mg #4	1 q wk	Robins	2/12				
Dilantin 100 mg #90	3 qd	Robins	1/15	2/16	3/14		

Dr. Calvin Robins
7823 Tea Rose Trail, Miami, FL 44718
463-555-8000

Name Mabel Lopez Date 4/15

Address 654 Ibis Ct. Age 63

℞

Prempro
2.5 mg
i po qd
#3 cycles

Refills 3

Dr. Calvin Robins

3.18a

Dr. Calvin Robins
7823 Tea Rose Trail, Miami, FL 44718
463-555-8000

Name Mabel Lopez Date 4/15

Address 654 Ibis Ct. Age 63

℞

Lasix
20
#30
i BIW
1 hr water

Refills 3

Dr. Calvin Robins

3.18b

3.19

PT. NAME: **JOHN SMITH**	GENDER: **M**	ADDRESS: **977 IBIS LANE**	WEIGHT: **205**	BMI: **31**
AGE: **68**	DX: **GOUT, HTN, CHF**	ALLERGY: **NKA**	HX: **ETOH**	

MEDICATION	SIG.	PRESCRIBER	ORIG. DATE	REFILL DATE	REFILL DATE	REFILL DATE	REFILL DATE
Lanoxin 0.125 mg #90	1 q am	Thomas	2/3	6/1			
Lasix 40 mg #180	1 bid	Thomas	2/3	5/4			
Vasotec 10 mg #90	1 q am	Thomas	2/3	6/1			
Colchicine 0.6 mg #90	1 qd	Thomas	5/19				

Dr. Erin Thomas
988 North Ridge, New York, NY 88364
813-555-7554

Name John Smith Date 6/2

Address 977 Ibis Lane Age 68

℞

Allopurinol

#50 300 mg

Sig 1/2 tablet qd.

a. breakfast

Refills 3

Dr. Erin Thomas

3.19a

Dr. Erin Thomas
988 North Ridge, New York, NY 88364
813-555-7554

Name John Smith Date 6/2

Address 977 Ibis Lane Age 68

℞

COLCHICINE

0.6 mg PO QD

100

Refills 3

Dr. Erin Thomas

3.19b

3.20	PT. NAME: **MARGARET JONES**	GENDER: **F**	ADDRESS: **684 HURRICANE ALLEY**	WEIGHT: **107**	BMI: **20**
	AGE: **63**	DX: **COPD, OSTEOPOROSIS, HTN**	ALLERGY: **SULFA**	HX: **SMOKES 1 PACK/DAY**	

MEDICATION	SIG.	PRESCRIBER	ORIG. DATE	REFILL DATE	REFILL DATE	REFILL DATE	REFILL DATE
Theophylline SR 200 mg #90	1 bid pc	Shaw	3/5	4/30			
Ativan 1 mg #30	1 hs prn sleep	Shaw	3/7	4/15			
Serevent Diskus #60	1 puff bid	Shaw	1/4	3/5			
Flovent HFA 110 mcg/inh 12 g	2 puffs bid	Shaw	1/4	3/5			
Prednisone 1 mg #90	2 qd	Shaw	1/4	2/19			

Dr. G. Donald Shaw
333 Hedgehog St., Palm Desert, CA 22999
399-333-6666

Name Margaret Jones Date 5/23

Address 684 Hurricane Alley Age 63

℞

Fosamax 70mg
#30

1 weekly in AM
as directed
Cobal

Refills 2

Dr. G.D. Shaw

3.20a

Dr. G. Donald Shaw
333 Hedgehog St., Palm Desert, CA 22999
399-333-6666

Name Margaret Jones Date 5/23

Address 684 Hurricane Alley Age 63

℞

Actonel 5, #60
S, i d

Refills 5

Dr. G.D. Shaw

3.20b

3.21

PT. NAME: **MARIE MEYER** GENDER: **F** ADDRESS: **1984 GREEN ST.** WEIGHT: **155** HEIGHT: **5′ 6″**
AGE: **63** DX: **INSOMNIA, HYPOTHYROID, ELEVATED CHOLESTEROL, SKIN INFECTION** ALLERGY: **ASA** HX: **SOCIAL DRINKER**

MEDICATION	SIG.	PRESCRIBER	ORIG. DATE	REFILL DATE	REFILL DATE	REFILL DATE	REFILL DATE
Keflex 250 mg #30	1 qid × 7 d	Sauls	6/10				
Bactroban Ung. 15 g	Apply qd ud	Sauls	6/10				
Restoril 15 mg #30	1 hs	Sauls	4/6	5/8	6/12	7/13	

Dr. Alfred Sauls
151212 S. High Rd., Chicago, IL 23875
954-555-1300

Name Marie Meyer Date 7/20

Address 1984 Green St. Age 63

℞

Syn Thyroid .15
#100
Sig: i q am

Refills 3

Dr. Alfred Sauls

3.21a

Dr. Janice Flaharty
654 Western Ridge, Chicago, IL 23874
954-555-9090

Name Marie Meyer Date 7/20

Address 1984 Green St. Age 63

℞

Questran (4gm)
disp 50
packets
one po bid
in 6oz water

Refills 3

Janice Flaharty

3.21b

3.22

PT. NAME: **MARIE BRYANT** AGE: **70**
GENDER: **F** DX: **INTERMITTENT CLAUDICATION, NASAL ALLERGY, HYPOTHYROID, HTN, GERD**
ADDRESS: **774 DUBLIN LANE** ALLERGY: **SULFA**
WEIGHT: **167** HX: **SMOKER**
HEIGHT: **5′ 8″**

MEDICATION	SIG.	PRESCRIBER	ORIG. DATE	REFILL DATE	REFILL DATE	REFILL DATE	REFILL DATE
Claritin 10 mg #30	1 qd for allergy	Geary	2/5	3/10	4/15		
Norvasc 5 mg #30	1 qd	Geary	1/15	2/25	3/30	4/29	5/16
Prevacid 30 mg #30	1 q am	Geary	1/25	2/20	3/10	4/1	4/30
Synthroid 100 mcg #90	1 q am	Geary	1/3	4/9			

Dr. Tom Geary
66 Victory Place, E. Brunswick, NJ 33399
585-868-9998

Name Marie Bryant Date 5/18

Address 774 Dublin Lane Age 70

℞

Synthroid 0.025mg

Sig: i po QD with 0.1mg

Dr. Tom Geary

3.22a

Dr. Tom Geary
66 Victory Place, E. Brunswick, NJ 33399
585-868-9998

Name Marie Bryant Date 5/18

Address 774 Dublin Lane Age 70

℞

Trental 400mg

#90

i TID c meals

Refills PRN

Dr. Tom Geary

3.22b

3.23 PT. NAME: **SAMANTHA RIVERA** AGE: **61** GENDER: **F** DX: **OA, TYPE 2 DM, POSTMENOPAUSAL, DIZZINESS** ADDRESS: **522 ELEPHANT DR.** ALLERGY: **NKA** WEIGHT: **118** HX: **SMOKER**

MEDICATION	SIG.	PRESCRIBER	ORIG. DATE	REFILL DATE	REFILL DATE	REFILL DATE	REFILL DATE
Glipizide 5 mg #30	1 bid ac	Thomas	2/20				
Celebrex 200 mg #30	1 bid	Thomas	2/20				
Mycolog cream 15 g	Apply bid prn	Thomas	2/28				

Dr. Erin Thomas
988 North Ridge, New York, NY 88364
813-555-7554

Name Samantha Rivera Date 3/1

Address 522 Elephant Dr. Age 61

℞

Estraderm 0.05 mg #24

Sig as directed (twice a week)

Refills PRN

Dr. Erin Thomas

3.23a

Dr. Erin Thomas
988 North Ridge, New York, NY 88364
813-555-7554

Name Samantha Rivera Date 3/1

Address 522 Elephant Dr. Age 61

℞

Antivert 12½ #30

i q 8 h prn vertigo

Refills PRN

Dr. Erin Thomas

3.23b

3.24

PT. NAME: **BETTY RAMIREZ** AGE: **65** | GENDER: **F** | DX: **HTN, OSTEOPOROSIS, ANXIETY, VERTIGO** | ADDRESS: **494 WEST GROVE ST.** | ALLERGY: **PCN, ASA** | WEIGHT: **111** | HX: **SMOKES HALF PACK/DAY; HISTORY OF 1 PACK/DAY FOR 10 YEARS** | BMI: **21**

MEDICATION	SIG.	PRESCRIBER	ORIG. DATE	REFILL DATE	REFILL DATE	REFILL DATE	REFILL DATE
Lorazepam 1 mg #60	1 bid	Botwin	8/16	10/18			
Buspirone 10 mg #60	1 bid	Botwin	11/16	12/19			
Lisinopril-HCTZ 20/12.5 mg #30	1 qd	Botwin	9/5	10/4	11/4	12/6	
Altace 2.5 mg #30	1 cap qd	Botwin	9/5	10/4	11/4	12/6	

Dr. Sharon Botwin
3 Sheridan St., Austin, TX 90902
874-555-9493

Name Betty Ramirez Date 12/20

Address 494 W. Grove St. Age 65

℞

Evista 60mg #30
ī po qd

LABEL ALL PRESCRIPTIONS

REFILL .....6..... TIMES

Dr. Sharon Botwin

3.24a

Dr. Sharon Botwin
3 Sheridan St., Austin, TX 90902
874-555-9493

Name Betty Ramirez Date 12/20

Address 494 W. Grove St. Age 65

℞

Antivert/25
#30
Sig: ī tid TIW)

Dr. Sharon Botwin

3.24b

3.25 PT. NAME: **ANITA KAMOROV** AGE: **54** GENDER: **F** DX: **HTN, VAGINAL DRYNESS, DEPRESSION, URI, SINUS DRIP** ADDRESS: **1623 38TH ST.** ALLERGY: **PENICILLIN, TETRACYCLINE** WEIGHT: **189** HX: **ALWAYS ON A DIET** HEIGHT: **5′ 6″**

MEDICATION	SIG.	PRESCRIBER	ORIG. DATE	REFILL DATE	REFILL DATE	REFILL DATE	REFILL DATE
Zoloft 50 mg #30	1 qd in am	Boros	11/28	12/26			
Toprol XL 50 mg #30	1 qd	Boros	8/2	9/2	10/3	11/4	12/1
Z-Pak	Take ud	Boros	6/4				

Dr. Shelby Boros
22 Valla Court, Walnut Creek, CA 94595
733-222-9394

Name Anita Kamorov Date 12/29

Address 1623 38th St. Age 54

℞ Premarin Vag Cream
no Plunger
apply bid x 1mo

Ref PRN

Dr. Shelby Boros

3.25a

Dr. Shelby Boros
22 Valla Court, Walnut Creek, CA 94595
733-222-9394

Name Anita Kamorov Date 12/29

Address 1623 38th St. Age 54

℞ Claritin 10 #15

Sig T daily

Ref PRN

Dr. Shelby Boros

3.25b

3.26

PT. NAME: **ANNE HALL** GENDER: **F** ADDRESS: **77 BLOOMINGDALE ST.** WEIGHT: **112** BMI: **21**

AGE: **66** DX: **POSTMENOPAUSAL SX, HTN, DENTAL INFECTION, OSTEOPOROSIS, HYPERLIPIDEMIA, OA, GERD** ALLERGY: **PCN** HX: **LICENSED NURSE PRACTITIONER**

MEDICATION	SIG.	PRESCRIBER	ORIG. DATE	REFILL DATE	REFILL DATE	REFILL DATE	REFILL DATE
Ambien CR 12.5 mg #30	1 hs	Damon	11/5	12/4			
Lipitor 10 mg #90	1 qd	Damon	9/30				
Mobic 15 mg #50	1 qd for arthritis	Damon	10/7	11/22			
Prevacid 24HR #28	1 qd	OTC	11/24	12/20			

Dr. James Damon
800 Fenway Place, Boston, MA 48484
813-555-0001

Name Anne Hall Date 12/28

Address 77 Bloomingdale St. Age 66

℞ Boniva 150 mg
#3 Tablets
i̊ q monthly

☐ Label

Refill - 0 - 1 - 2 - 3 - 4 - PRN (circled)

Dr. James Damon

3.26a

Dr. Jerome Fink, DDS
33 Beacon St., Boston, MA 48484
813-555-1634

Name Anne Hall Date 12/29

Address 77 Bloomingdale St. Age 66

℞ Cipro - 750 mg tabs.
Dispense 14 tabs.
T tab B.i.D. until finished

Dr. Jerome Fink, DDS

3.26b

3.27

PT. NAME: **ANNE TAYLOR** GENDER: **F** ADDRESS: **8809 WEST AVE.** WEIGHT: **120** HEIGHT: **5′ 4″**

AGE: **81** DX: **ANXIETY, ANGINA, HTN, HYPERTHYROID (VERY LOW TSH)** ALLERGY: **ASA** HX: **SOCIAL DRINKER, SMOKES 3 CIGARETTES DAILY**

MEDICATION	SIG.	PRESCRIBER	ORIG. DATE	REFILL DATE	REFILL DATE	REFILL DATE	REFILL DATE
NTG SL 0.4 mg #C	I sl prn chest pain	Hilton	9/12				
Lisinopril 10 mg #50	I qd	Hilton	9/1	10/18	12/9		
Clonazepam 0.5 mg #12	I hs	Hilton	9/1				
Clonazepam 0.5 mg #50	I hs	Hilton	9/10	10/28	12/10		
Lomotil #30	I tid	Hilton	9/1	10/3	11/2	12/6	
Furosemide 20 mg #30	I qd	Hilton	9/1	10/1	10/28	11/30	

Dr. Ray Hilton
12 NE 4 Terrace, Monterey, CA 38411
705-555-9994

Name Anne Taylor Date 12/11

Address 8809 West Ave. Age 81

℞

Tapazole 10 mg

#100

i daily

☑ Label

Refill 3 times PRN NR

Dr. Ray Hilton

3.27a

Dr. Ray Hilton
12 NE 4 Terrace, Monterey, CA 38411
705-555-9994

Name Anne Taylor Date 12/11

Address 8809 West Ave. Age 81

℞

Inderal 40 mg

i daily

#100

Refills 2

Dr. Ray Hilton

3.27b

3.28

PT. NAME: **GRETA HOFFMAN** GENDER: **F** ADDRESS: **99 SOUTH ELM** WEIGHT: **129** HEIGHT: **5′ 4″**

AGE: **62** DX: **OSTEOPOROSIS, LUMBAR PAIN, DEPRESSION, BACTERIAL SKIN INFECTION** ALLERGY: **NKA** HX: **SMOKER; SEDENTARY LIFESTYLE; LOW CALCIUM INTAKE**

MEDICATION	SIG.	PRESCRIBER	ORIG. DATE	REFILL DATE	REFILL DATE	REFILL DATE	REFILL DATE
Bactroban 2% cream 15 g	Apply to AA tid	Parrish	7/15				
Z-Pak	Take ud	Parrish	7/15				
Hydroxyzine HCl 25 mg #30	1 qd for itch	Parrish	7/15	9/2			
Wellbutrin XL 150 mg #30	1 qd in am	Gray	5/3	6/2	7/7	8/9	9/4

Dr. Kurt Steinsnyder
221 Sheridan St., Austin, TX 90902
874-555-0302

Name Greta Hoffman Date 9/12

Address 99 South Elm Age 62

℞ Actonel 35 mg
#4
Sig T tab weekly

☐ LABEL

REFILL 2 TIMES

Dr. Kurt Steinsnyder

3.28a

Dr. Kurt Steinsnyder
221 Sheridan St., Austin, TX 90902
874-555-0302

Name Greta Hoffman Date 9/12

Address 99 South Elm Age 62

℞ Celebrex 200 mg
#30
Sig T tab QD

☐ LABEL

REFILL 12 TIMES

Dr. Kurt Steinsnyder

3.28b

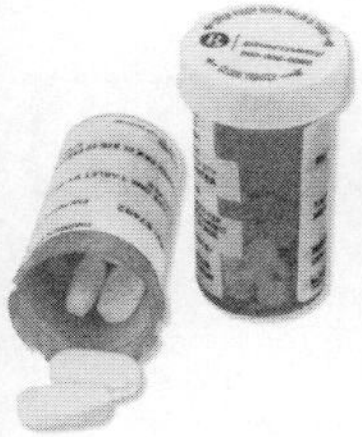

4 • PAIN AND CONTROLLED DRUGS

UPON COMPLETION OF THIS CHAPTER, THE STUDENT WILL BE ABLE TO:

- accurately fill out the appropriate forms for ordering Schedule II controlled drugs.
- identify the legal implications regarding narcotics. In particular, the student shall demonstrate knowledge of laws pertaining to emergency fills and partial fills of Schedule II controlled substances.
- describe the differences in the formulas of certain pain medications that contain aspirin and acetaminophen.
- discuss chronic pain caused by cancer, particularly the role of "by-the-clock" and "PRN" dosing in the instructions.
- describe the equivalent analgesic doses of narcotics.
- understand important safety procedures in case of narcotic robbery and theft.
- advise the patient or caregiver regarding the appropriate techniques for administering and disposing of fentanyl patches.

DRUG LIST

Buprenorphine
Demerol
Dilaudid
Duragesic patch
Fiorinal/Fioricet
Marinol
Methadone
Morphine
Nucynta
Oxycodone
Paregoric
Percocet
Percodan
Suboxone
Subutex
Tincture of opium
Tylenol #3
Ultram/Ultracet
Vicodin

• DRUG HOT POINTS

Buprenorphine
Buprenex injectable for relief of moderate-to-severe pain
Sublingual tabs and film for treatment of opioid dependence
Transdermal patch (Butrans) for moderate-to-severe pain requiring continous around-the-clock treatment for an extended period

Demerol
Uses and misuses (elderly)
Interaction with MAOIs
75 mg IM = 300 mg PO
Metabolite may accumulate
Warnings: be careful in driving, etc.

Dilaudid
Drug abuse problems
Safety of personnel
High doses in terminal cancer patients
Narcotic laws
Relative potencies against other narcotics

Duragesic patch
Strengths (mcg/hr)
Application (q 72 h)
Disposal procedure (not in regular trash)

Fiorinal/Fioricet
Differences, warnings

Marinol
Controlled drug
Appetite stimulant, for nausea or glaucoma

Methadone
Long-acting opioid agonist for pain
For detoxification and maintenance therapy of opioid dependence

Morphine
Inexpensive, predictable, various forms
MS-Contin, Oramorph SR, Kadian, and Avinza
Also solutions (20:1, etc.) and other forms (suppositories, tabs, injections)
Potential for constipation
Do not crush long-acting tablets
Alcohol caution: ER products may release early
Cancer pain: dose by the clock with breakthrough doses of short-acting MS
Form 222 for ordering narcotics
Equianalgesic dosing
Pain management

Oxycodone
Schedule II
Immediate release-IR
Long-acting—OxyContin (abuse potential)
Concentrated solutions

Paregoric
Camphorated tincture of opium
C-III controlled drug
For diarrhea
Morphine content: 2 mg/5 mL

Percocet
Color differences—different strengths
Compare oxycodone with morphine potency
Acetaminophen: watch overuse (Rx & OTC)
No alcohol, take with food or milk

Percodan
Contains aspirin
Monitor for ASA sensitivity; ask questions
Watch color of tablet
Take with food or milk, no alcohol
Monitor other Rxs: Coumadin, probenecid

Suboxone
For treatment of opioid dependence
Contains naloxone
SL tablet and film

Subutex
For treatment of opioid dependence

Tincture of opium
C-II controlled drug
Morphine content: 10 mg/mL

• DRUG HOT POINTS (*continued*)

Tylenol #3
Maximum APAP 4 g/day total
Take with food or milk
No alcohol, caution driving, etc.
Strengths (mg per dose compared with #)
Tablets are C-III
Potential for abuse
Actions of both ingredients

Ultram
Mechanism: SNRI & mild opioid agonist
Maximum dose—400 mg/day (adjust dose in elderly)
Overdose—potential seizures
Counseling, compliance
Caution—MAOI interaction
Ultracet—combination with acetaminophen
Compare with Nucynta

Vicodin
Abuse potential
Contains APAP
Many forms (ES, HP); new warnings: 325 mg APAP/tab will be implemented
Other similar drugs (Lorcet)
Compare with Vicoprofen

• QUESTIONS TO BE ANSWERED IN PREPARATION FOR CHAPTER 4 LAB

- How many milligrams of hydrocodone are contained in each Vicodin tablet?
- What is the milligram strength of the other analgesic product in Vicodin?
- What is the quantity of barbiturate in each Fiorinal tablet?
- Identify the differences in ingredients and controlled drug class between Fiorinal tablets and Fioricet tablets.
- What is the brand name for a long-acting form of morphine tablets?
- Identify the ingredients in Vicoprofen.
- What is the equipotent PO strength, in milligrams, of hydromorphone to a 100-mg PO dose of meperidine?
- A prescription is written for Duragesic 75. Explain what the 75 means in terms of metric quantity and time in which that quantity is released.
- What is the name of the active metabolite of Demerol and its route of excretion?
- Explain why Demerol may not be an ideal analgesic for the elderly person. (Note: It is in the Beers List.)
- What is the generic name of Dilaudid?
- Explain some security measures that a pharmacy should exercise when stocking Dilaudid.
- What is the number of the form that is used to order Schedule II controlled drugs?
- What is the generic name of Duragesic patches?
- What is the smallest size milligram tablet of Demerol?
- How would you fill and label a prescription for Demerol 25-mg tabs PO q 4 to 6 h PRN pain?
- How many milligrams of codeine are contained in each tablet of Tylenol #2, #3, and #4?
- What is the advantage of the use of sublingual buprenorphine tablets in the office-based treatment of opioid dependence?
- How many milligrams of Demerol PO is equipotent to 7.5 mg of Dilaudid PO?
- Explain the correct disposal method of Duragesic patches after they have been used and removed by the patient.
- What is the generic name of Marinol?
- What are the two mechanisms involved in the therapeutic action of Ultram?
- What is the maximum amount of Ultram tablets that can be taken daily?
- Which adverse effect is most possible with higher than usual doses of Ultram?
- Identify the various strengths of Percocet.
- What interaction could occur when combining meperidine and phenelzine (an MAOI)?
- What interaction could occur when combining Demerol and Eldepryl?
- What is the brand name of a long-acting product containing oxycodone?
- Which adverse effect is most common among terminally ill patients who chronically take opioids?
- What is the difference between an opioid and an opiate?
- Explain the theory of the mechanism of analgesia produced by opiates and opioids.
- If a person took 10 Vicoprofen tablets per day plus Restoril and alcohol, what serious adverse effect is he or she at risk for?
- Which classes of antidepressants should be avoided in patients who are taking tramadol?
- How does the dose of Paregoric compare with that of tincture of opium?
- Compare Ultram to Nucynta (mechanism and DEA category)
- What is the purpose of naloxone in Suboxone?

• PAIN AND CONTROLLED DRUGS MEDICATION THERAPY MANAGEMENT QUESTIONS AND COMMENTS

- Has your doctor mentioned that alcohol should not be taken with your pain medications?
- If using buprenorphine tablet for use under the tongue is difficult for you, many doctors recommend that it be placed between the cheek and tongue to dissolve. I would like to congratulate you for staying with the buprenorphine program that your doctor and you have created. Keep up the good work. We are always here to help you with whatever medication information you need.
- Your pain pill has a direction that says, "Take as needed." Did your doctor tell you exactly when to take it?
- You mentioned that your pain is not helped by the new pain medication. Could you tell me a number from 1 to 10 to describe the pain before and now with the new medication? Here is a list with pictures for you to describe the number.
- Your pain patch has an important caution. Please place it on skin with no hair. Use it only every 3 days or as the doctor prescribed. Also, do not use a heating pad, or use lotion or alcohol on the area before you apply the patch. The old patch must be taken off when the new patch is applied in 3 days. Even if the pain is on your foot or knee, the patch goes on the chest, not on the other areas. When you are disposing the pain patch, it must not be placed in the regular trash unless it is thoroughly mixed with kitty litter or sand from your garden. This is the safest way to put it in the trash.
- Did the doctor mention that an OTC laxative called Senna with docusate sodium (many brands and generics) would be helpful to prevent or treat constipation from your pain pills?
- Your prescription is for a liquid called opium tincture to treat your diarrhea. The medication must be taken by mouth only by drops placed in a glass of water and swallowed according to the instructions on the prescription.
- I notice that your doctor is in another state. Would you mind letting me know the circumstances behind the need for this pain medication?
- Your doctor has prescribed Fioricet. I would like to mention that it is prescribed "as needed for headache." It would be good for you to limit the amount of this medication because it contains a barbiturate that could impair your movements and driving ability. Also, remember not to take OTC Tylenol products with this because the prescription medication of these products contains the same medication.
- Because you are the caregiver for your patient on the hospice program, make sure that there is enough ventilation in the room so it will not be too stuffy. A small fan near the bed would be helpful. The nurse is placing an eye drop called atropine sulfate under the patient's tongue. This is to dry the lung fluid that has been causing difficult breathing.
- Because there is acetaminophen combined in many of your medications, please remember to totally avoid alcohol, and do not take any additional products that contain acetaminophen.

4.1 PT. NAME: **DONALD DAVIS** AGE: **42** GENDER: **M** DX: **BACK AND NECK PAIN, OA** ADDRESS: **61 GREEN ST.** ALLERGY: **ASA** WEIGHT: **168** HX: **SPORTS-RELATED INJURIES** BMI: **24**

MEDICATION	SIG.	PRESCRIBER	ORIG. DATE	REFILL DATE	REFILL DATE	REFILL DATE	REFILL DATE
Restoril 30 mg #30	1 hs	Johns	8/2	9/15			
Klonopin 1 mg #60	1 bid	Johns	5/6	6/5	7/1	7/20	8/25
Tylenol 500 mg #C	1–2 qid for pain	OTC	6/1	6/19	7/5	7/30	8/12

Dr. Donna Johns
7000 SW 1st Ave., Santa Fe, NM 54545
766-555-9097

Name Donald Davis Date 9/20

Address 61 Green St. Age 42

℞

Fioricet #60

Sig T or TT q 4h prn Headache

Refills 0

Dr. Donna Johns

4.1a

Dr. Mathew Xavier
5456 Southern Trail, Santa Fe, NM 54545
766-555-6600

Name Donald Davis Date 9/20

Address 61 Green St. Age 42

℞

Vicodin

1 Q4H PRN

pain

#180 (One hundred & Eighty)

☒ ~~DO~~ NOT REFILL

☐ REFILL _______ TIMES

Dr. Mathew Xavier

DEA# AM1234563

4.1b

4.2

PT. NAME: **FRANK SCHNEIDER** | AGE: **42** | GENDER: **M** | DX: **PAIN, SPASMS** | ADDRESS: **500 SE 2ND ST.** | ALLERGY: **ASA** | WEIGHT: **155** | HX: **ETOH** | HEIGHT: **5′ 4″**

MEDICATION	SIG.	PRESCRIBER	ORIG. DATE	REFILL DATE	REFILL DATE	REFILL DATE	REFILL DATE
Soma 350 mg #100	I tid	Griffin	10/31				
Xanax 2 mg #60	I bid	Griffin	10/31				

Dr. Doug Griffin
7611 147th Terrace, Monterey, CA 38411
705-555-6644

Name Frank Schneider Date 11/5

Address 500 SE 2nd St. Age 42

℞

Vicodin

#30 (thirty)

i po q 3 hrs prn severe pain

Refills 0

Dr. Doug Griffin

DEA# AG1234563

4.2a

Dr. Doug Griffin
7611 147th Terrace, Monterey, CA 38411
705-555-6644

Name Frank Schneider Date 11/5

Address 500 SE 2nd St. Age 42

℞

Fiorinal Tabs

100 -

Sig i q 4-6 h
prn cough

Not Valid for Class II Drugs

☑ Label

Refill NR times PRN (NR)

Dr. Doug Griffin

4.2b

4.3 PT. NAME: **FRANK HERNANDEZ** AGE: **79** GENDER: **M** DX: **PROSTATE CA, HTN, A-FIB, ANXIETY, GERD** ADDRESS: **555 W. 123RD AVE.** ALLERGY: **NKA** WEIGHT: **145** HX: **SMOKER** HEIGHT: **5′ 6″**

MEDICATION	SIG.	PRESCRIBER	ORIG. DATE	REFILL DATE	REFILL DATE	REFILL DATE	REFILL DATE
Coumadin 5 mg #90	I qd	Halloway	2/15	5/20	8/25		
Pepcid 20 mg #60	I bid	Halloway	3/30	4/25	5/30	6/29	
Alprazolam 0.25 mg #30	I bid	Halloway	6/1	7/30			
Lanoxin 0.25 mg #90	I q am	Halloway	2/15	5/20	8/25		
Lasix 20 mg #90	I q am	Halloway	2/15	5/20	8/25		

Dr. Janet Halloway
4414 W. Bridge Rd., San Francisco, CA 40001
154-555-8558

Name Frank Hernandez Date 8/29

Address 555 W 123rd Ave. Age 79

℞

Percodan
① as directed

#30

Refills 0

Dr. Janet Halloway

DEA# AH1234563

4.3a

Dr. Janet Halloway
4414 W. Bridge Rd., San Francisco, CA 40001
154-555-8558

Name Frank Hernandez Date 8/29

Address 555 W 123rd Ave. Age 79

℞

Casodex 50 mg
Disp # 14
Sig: Take ① PO QD

Label

Refill 3 times

Dr. Janet Halloway

4.3b

4.4

PT. NAME: **HANK CARLSON**	GENDER: **M**	ADDRESS: **7584 GREEN AVE.**	WEIGHT: **140**	BMI: **26**
AGE: **72**	DX: **HTN, CHF, OA, VENOUS THROMBOSIS**	ALLERGY: **SULFA, PCN**	HX: **GOLFER, TENNIS PLAYER**	

MEDICATION	SIG.	PRESCRIBER	ORIG. DATE	REFILL DATE	REFILL DATE	REFILL DATE	REFILL DATE
Coumadin 5 mg #90	I qd ud	Isaacs	8/7				
Coreg 3.125 mg #30	I bid, 8 am & 8 pm	Isaacs	4/20	5/16	6/18	7/17	
Celebrex 100 mg #60	I bid prn pain	Isaacs	5/20	5/30	6/12		
K-Dur 20 mEq #90	I tab/day	Isaacs	4/20	7/25			
Bumex I mg #90	I tab/day	Isaacs	4/20	8/18			

Dr. Howard Isaacs
1115 Turnaround Lane, Detroit, MI 64789
343-555-7000

Name Hank Carlson Date 8/20

Address 7584 Green Ave. Age 72

℞

Vicoprofen
i po q6h prn pn
#40

Refills 0

Dr. Howard Isaacs

DEA# AI1234563

4.4a

Dr. Howard Isaacs
1115 Turnaround Lane, Detroit, MI 64789
343-555-7000

Name Hank Carlson Date 8/20

Address 7584 Green Ave. Age 72

℞

Slow-K 20mg
#50
2 T/d

Refills PRN

Dr. Howard Isaacs

4.4b

4.5

PT. NAME: **JANET MARTIN** GENDER: **F** ADDRESS: **6 PENNSYLVANIA AVE. NW** WEIGHT: **153** HEIGHT: **5′ 8″**
AGE: **48** DX: **SEVERE BACK PAIN, DYSPEPSIA, DEPRESSION, BACTERIAL INFECTION** ALLERGY: **PCN** HX: **SMOKER, ETOH**

MEDICATION	SIG.	PRESCRIBER	ORIG. DATE	REFILL DATE	REFILL DATE	REFILL DATE	REFILL DATE
Amitriptyline 25 mg #60	1 q 12 h	Keller	9/12	10/11			
Levaquin 250 mg #11	2 today then 1 qd × 9 days	Keller	9/20				
Prilosec 10 mg #30	1 qd	Keller	6/20	7/18	8/18	9/30	
Ecotrin 325 mg #C	1 tab bid	OTC	5/1	6/12	7/26	9/10	

Dr. Daniel Keller
5007 Turtle Drive, Miami, FL 98887
247-555-9876

Name Janet Martin Date 10/30

Address 6 Pensylvania Ave. NW Age 48

℞

Tylenol #4

i q4h p pain

#30

Refills 0

Dr. Daniel Keller

DEA# AK1234563

4.5a

Dr. Daniel Keller
5007 Turtle Drive, Miami, FL 98887
247-555-9876

Name Janet Martin Date 10/30

Address 6 Pensylvania Ave. NW Age 48

℞

Ultram 50 mg

i q4h p pain

#50

Refills 0

Dr. Daniel Keller

4.5b

4.6 PT. NAME: **MARK JOHNSON** AGE: **58** GENDER: **M** DX: **BACK PAIN, CHRONIC RHINORRHEA, BACTERIAL INFECTION** ADDRESS: **564 CAPITOL AVE.** ALLERGY: **NKA** WEIGHT: **179** HEIGHT: **5′ 7″**

MEDICATION	SIG.	PRESCRIBER	ORIG. DATE	REFILL DATE	REFILL DATE	REFILL DATE	REFILL DATE
Claritin 10 mg #20	1 qd	Halloway	5/6	6/9	7/18		
Z-Pak	Take ud	Halloway	5/6				
Nizoral shampoo 2% 120 mL	Use ud for dandruff	Halloway	2/15	7/30			

Dr. Janet Halloway
4414 W. Bridge Rd., San Francisco, CA 40001
154-555-8558

Name Mark Johnson Date 8/20
Address 564 Capitol Ave. Age 58

℞

Percocet 7.5mg
#30 (XXX)
i - ii po q4-6h prn pain

Refills 1

Dr. Janet Halloway

4.6a

Dr. Janet Halloway
4414 W. Bridge Rd., San Francisco, CA 40001
154-555-8558

Name Mark Johnson Date 8/20
Address 564 Capitol Ave. Age 58

℞

Atarax 10mg
#30
T po bid

Refills 1

Dr. Janet Halloway

4.6b

4.7

PT. NAME: **JOSEPHINE MARTINS** GENDER: **F** ADDRESS: **321 WEST ROAD** WEIGHT: **133** BMI: **21**
AGE: **63** DX: **CA, NERVES, BACK PAIN** ALLERGY: **ASA**

MEDICATION	SIG.	PRESCRIBER	ORIG. DATE	REFILL DATE	REFILL DATE	REFILL DATE	REFILL DATE
Neurontin 300 mg #100	1 qid × 7 d	Keller	5/21	6/30			
Evista 60 mg #30	1 qd	Keller	3/4	3/31	4/25		
Remeron 30 mg #60	2 hs	Keller	2/15	3/10	4/9	5/9	6/8
Celexa 20 mg #30	1 qd	Keller	6/5				

Dr. Daniel Keller
5007 Turtle Drive, Miami, FL 98887
247-555-9876

Name Josephine Martins Date 7/1

Address 321 West Rd. Age 63

℞

Oxy IR 5mg
#30 (Thirty)
Sig: i tab PO QD prn breakthrough pain

Refills 0

Dr. Daniel Keller
DEA# AK1234563

4.7a

Dr. Daniel Keller
5007 Turtle Drive, Miami, FL 98887
247-555-9876

Name Josephine Martins Date 7/1

Address 321 West Rd. Age 63

℞

Oxycontin 10mg
#60 (sixty)
Sig: i tab PO Q12°

Refills 0

Dr. Daniel Keller
DEA# AK1234563

4.7b

4.8

PT. NAME: **MATHEW ZIMMERMAN** | GENDER: **M** | ADDRESS: **566 EAST CT.** | WEIGHT: **144** | BMI: **28**

AGE: **73** | DX: **CA, HTN, HIGH CHOLESTEROL, HEARTBURN** | ALLERGY: **NKA**

MEDICATION	SIG.	PRESCRIBER	ORIG. DATE	REFILL DATE	REFILL DATE	REFILL DATE	REFILL DATE
Duragesic 25 mcg/hr #5	I q 72 h	Griffin	4/12				
Percocet 5/325 #100	I q 6 h	Griffin	3/15				
Pravachol 20 mg #90	I hs	Strozier	2/28	6/15			
Duragesic 50 mcg/hr #10	I q 72 h	Griffin	8/20				
Lasix 40 mg #180	I bid	Strozier	2/28	6/15			

Dr. Doug Griffin
7611 147th Terrace, Monterey, CA 38411
705-555-6644

Name Mathew Zimmerman Date 9/25

Address 566 East Ct. Age 73

℞

#30 (thirty)

Duragesic 75 mg/hour
1 patch q 72 hours

Refills 0

Dr. Doug Griffin

DEA# AG1234563

4.8a

Dr. Doug Griffin
7611 147th Terrace, Monterey, CA 38411
705-555-6644

Name Mathew Zimmerman Date 9/25

Address 566 East Ct. Age 73

℞

Zantac 150 mg
#50

Sig: i ½ hr ac breakfast;
i HS.

Refills 3

Dr. Doug Griffin

4.8b

4.9

PT. NAME: **RUTH LARSON**	GENDER: **F**	ADDRESS: **92 IBIS LANE**	WEIGHT: **130**	BMI: **21**
AGE: **58**	DX: **OA, GERD, SEVERE HEADACHES, BACTERIAL INFECTION**	ALLERGY: **ASA**	HX: **SOCIAL DRINKER**	

MEDICATION	SIG.	PRESCRIBER	ORIG. DATE	REFILL DATE	REFILL DATE	REFILL DATE	REFILL DATE
Prevacid 30 mg #60	1 qd	Keller	2/7	3/30	4/29	5/18	
Keflex 500 mg #14	1 q 6 h	Keller	5/20				
Tylenol Arthritis Strength #C	1 bid	OTC	1/12	2/20	3/10	4/15	5/20

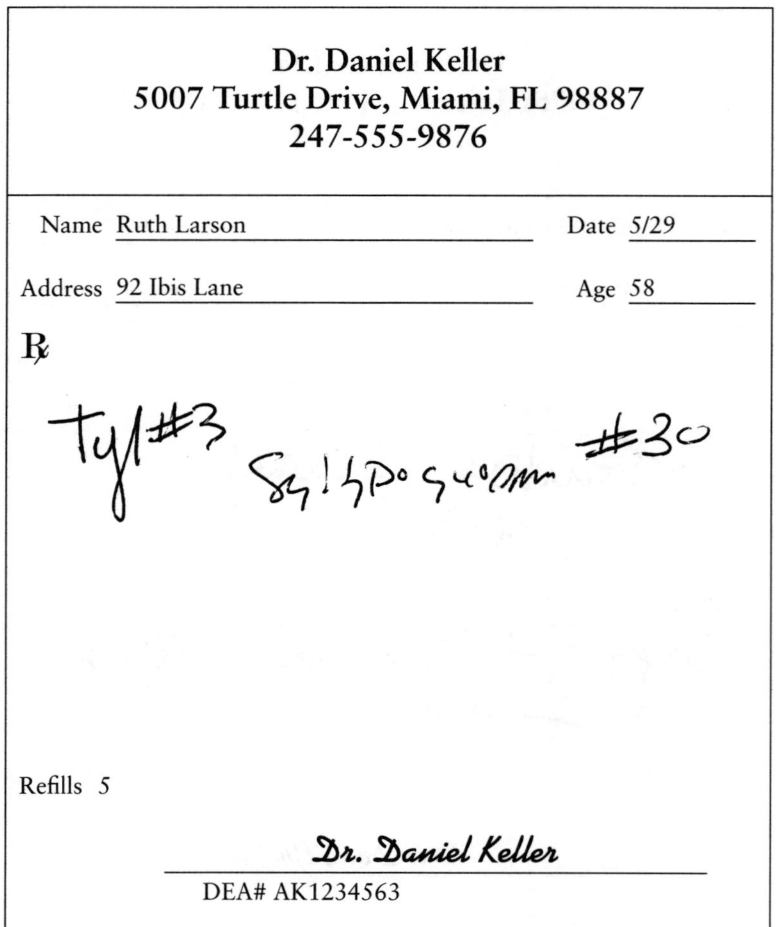

Dr. Daniel Keller
5007 Turtle Drive, Miami, FL 98887
247-555-9876

Name Ruth Larson Date 5/29

Address 92 Ibis Lane Age 58

℞

Tyl #3 Sig: 1 po q4h prn #30

Refills 5

Dr. Daniel Keller

DEA# AK1234563

4.9a

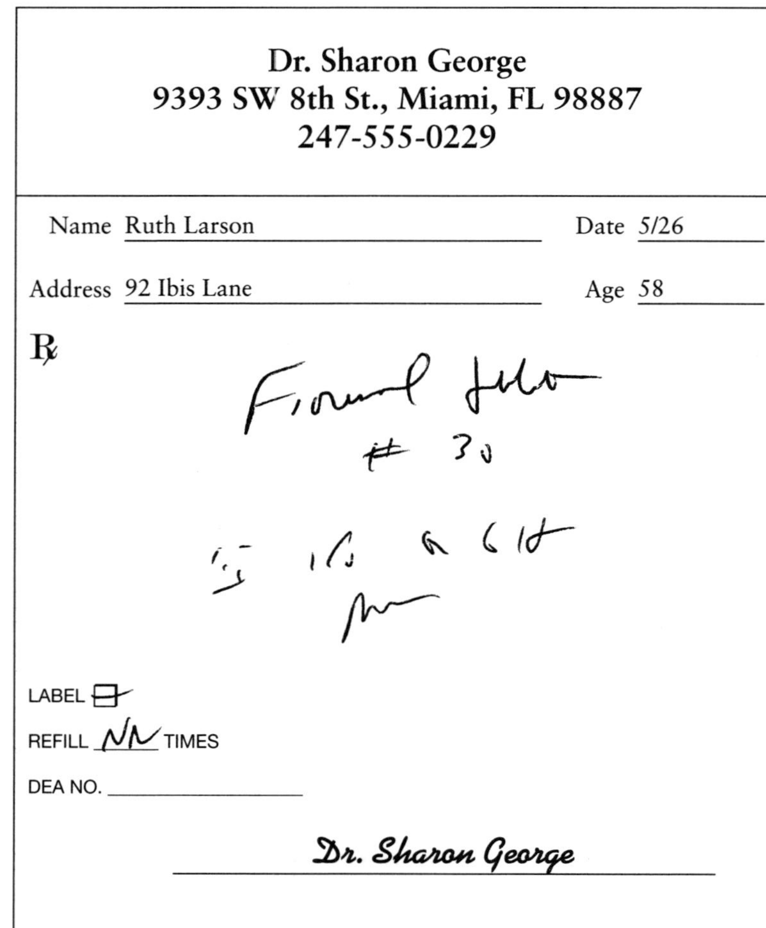

Dr. Sharon George
9393 SW 8th St., Miami, FL 98887
247-555-0229

Name Ruth Larson Date 5/26

Address 92 Ibis Lane Age 58

℞

Fiorinal tabs
#30
Sig: 1-2 q 6h
prn

LABEL ☑

REFILL NR TIMES

DEA NO. ______________

Dr. Sharon George

4.9b

4.10

PT. NAME: **SHIRLEY ANDERSON**
AGE: **62**
GENDER: **F**
DX: **NERVES, DIARRHEA, OA, GUM INFECTION**
ADDRESS: **9 EAGLE RUN**
ALLERGY: **NKA**
WEIGHT: **198**
BMI: **29**

MEDICATION	SIG.	PRESCRIBER	ORIG. DATE	REFILL DATE	REFILL DATE	REFILL DATE	REFILL DATE
Trazodone 50 mg #30	1 hs	Isaacs	6/29	7/28	9/18	10/19	
Celebrex 200 mg #30	1 qd	Isaacs	3/14	5/26	6/29		

Dr. Howard Isaacs
1115 Turnaround Lane, Detroit, MI 64789
343-555-7000

Name Shirley Anderson Date 10/21

Address 9 Eagle Run Age 62

℞ Codeine 30 mg tabs
1 tid for loose
diarrhea
Disp 20

Refills 0

Dr. Howard Isaacs

DEA# AI1234563

4.10a

Sean Smith, DDS
30 NE 5th St., Detroit, MI 64789
343-821-1100

Name Shirley Anderson Date 10/21

Address 9 Eagle Run Age 62

℞ cephalexin /500
Disp 28
Sig: i q6h

☑ Label

Refill ________ times PRN (NR)

Sean Smith, DDS

4.10b

4.11

PT. NAME: **CAROL SMITH** GENDER: **F** ADDRESS: **145 NORTH AVE.** WEIGHT: **AVERAGE (NOT AVAILABLE)**
AGE: **48** DX: **BACK TRAUMA, SEVERE BACK PAIN, NERVES** ALLERGY: **PCN, ASA**

MEDICATION	SIG.	PRESCRIBER	ORIG. DATE	REFILL DATE	REFILL DATE	REFILL DATE	REFILL DATE
Ultram 50 mg #40	2 qid	Griffin	3/20	3/24	3/28		
Atarax 25 mg #30	1 hs	Griffin	3/20				
Ambien 5 mg #30	1 hs	Griffin	3/20				
Alprazolam 0.5 mg #100	1 q 4 h or prn	Griffin	2/15				

Dr. Doug Griffin
7611 147th Terrace, Monterey, CA 38411
705-555-6644

Name Carol Smith Date 4/5

Address 145 North Ave. Age 48

℞

Ultram 50 mg
T po q 4 H prn
#30

Refills 1

Dr. Doug Griffin

4.11a

Dr. Doug Griffin
7611 147th Terrace, Monterey, CA 38411
705-555-6644

Name Carol Smith Date 4/5

Address 145 North Ave. Age 48

℞

MS Contin 30 mg
Sig: 1 p.o. Q 12 H
Disp: # 60

Refills 1

Dr. Doug Griffin
DEA# AG1234563

4.11b

4.12	PT. NAME: **ANN RILEY**	GENDER: **F**	ADDRESS: **500 SE 2ND ST.**	WEIGHT: **198**	HEIGHT: **6′**
	AGE: **48**	DX: **BACK PAIN, IBS, GOUT, ACNE VULGARIS**	ALLERGY: **ASA**	HX: **ETOH**	

MEDICATION	SIG.	PRESCRIBER	ORIG. DATE	REFILL DATE	REFILL DATE	REFILL DATE	REFILL DATE
Prilosec 20 mg #30	1 qd	Johns	9/1				
Retin-A 0.025% cream 20 g	Apply ud	Johns	7/10	8/30	9/23		
Zyloprim 100 mg #30	1 qd	Johns	7/10	8/9	9/1		
Donnatal tabs #120	1 ac & hs	Johns	8/22	9/20			

Dr. Donna Johns
7000 SW 1st Ave., Santa Fe, NM 54545
766-555-9097

Name Ann Riley Date 9/25

Address 500 SE 2nd St. Age 48

℞

Tylenol #4
#50

Sig: [illegible]

Refills 0

Dr. Donna Johns

DEA# AJ1234563

4.12a

Dr. Donna Johns
7000 SW 1st Ave., Santa Fe, NM 54545
766-555-9097

Name Ann Riley Date 9/25

Address 500 SE 2nd St. Age 48

℞

Soma
#100

Sig: [illegible]

Refills 0

Dr. Donna Johns

4.12b

4.13

PT. NAME: **JONAS WILLIAMS**
AGE: **38**
GENDER: **M**
DX: **SICKLE CELL**
ADDRESS: **654 IBIS CT.**
ALLERGY: **NKA**
WEIGHT: **168**
HX: **HAS USED DURAGESIC PATCH FOR MONTHS**
BMI: **29**

MEDICATION	SIG.	PRESCRIBER	ORIG. DATE	REFILL DATE	REFILL DATE	REFILL DATE	REFILL DATE
Tylenol No. 4 #50	1 q 4 h prn	Griffin	6/5	6/29			
Hydrea 500 mg #30	2 qd	Griffin	7/12				
Duragesic 75 mcg/hr #30	Apply 1 patch q 72 h	Griffin	7/12				

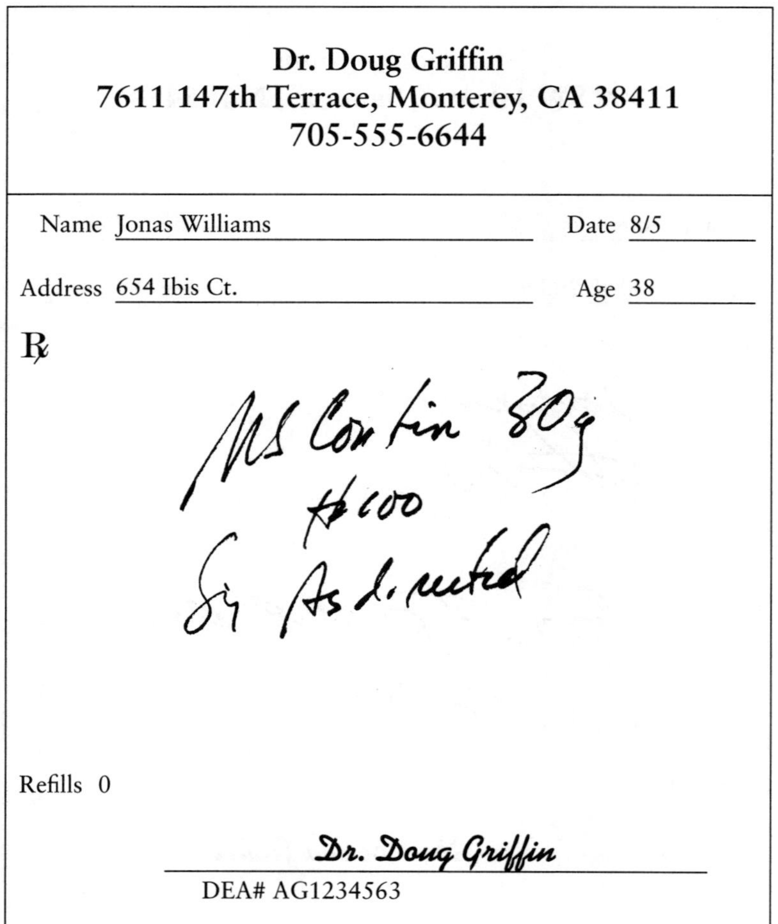

Dr. Doug Griffin
7611 147th Terrace, Monterey, CA 38411
705-555-6644

Name Jonas Williams Date 8/5

Address 654 Ibis Ct. Age 38

℞

MS Contin 80 mg
#100
Sig As directed

Refills 0

Dr. Doug Griffin

DEA# AG1234563

4.13a

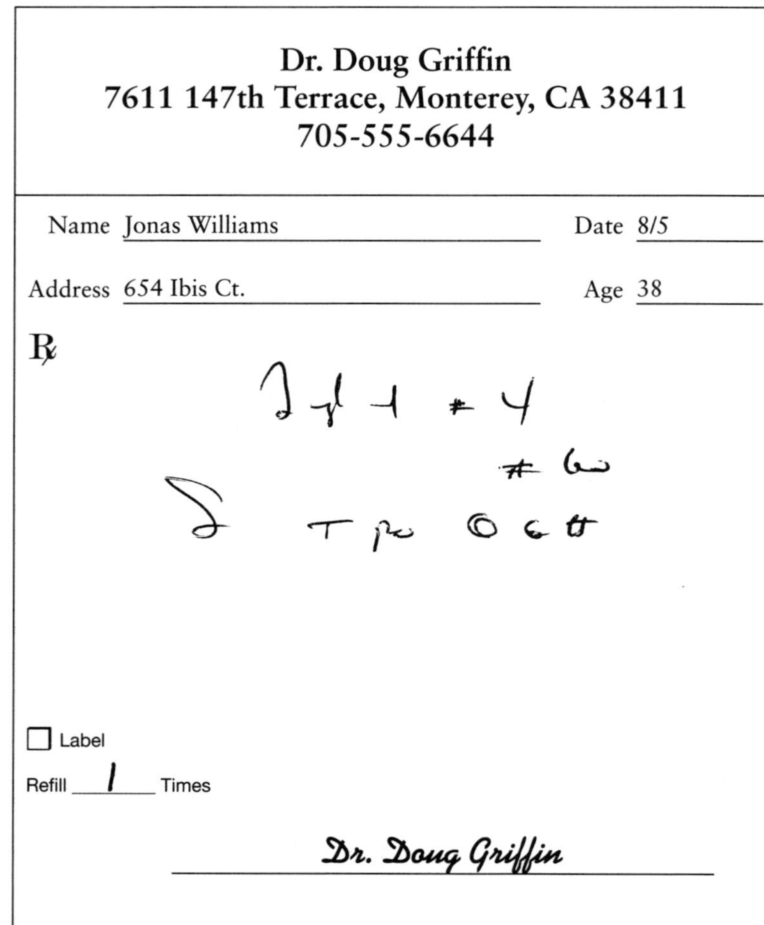

Dr. Doug Griffin
7611 147th Terrace, Monterey, CA 38411
705-555-6644

Name Jonas Williams Date 8/5

Address 654 Ibis Ct. Age 38

℞

Tyl #4
#60
S T po Q 6 h

☐ Label

Refill 1 Times

Dr. Doug Griffin

4.13b

4.14	PT. NAME: BARBARA ERICKSON	GENDER: F	ADDRESS: 854 GREEN ST.	WEIGHT: NA (UNWILLING TO DISCUSS)
	AGE: 31	DX: MULTIPLE SCLEROSIS, PAIN, INSOMNIA, DEPRESSION	ALLERGY: PCN	HX: SMOKER FOR LIFE

MEDICATION	SIG.	PRESCRIBER	ORIG. DATE	REFILL DATE	REFILL DATE	REFILL DATE	REFILL DATE
Elavil 50 mg #30	1 hs	Isaacs	10/7				
Amoxicillin 500 mg #15	1 bid	Isaacs	8/29				

Dr. Howard Isaacs
1115 Turnaround Lane, Detroit, MI 64789
343-555-7000

Name Barbara Erickson Date 10/15

Address 854 Green St. Age 31

℞

Oxycodone c̄ APAP
#60
i PO q6° PRN

Refills 0

Dr. Howard Isaacs

DEA# AI1234563

4.14a

Dr. Marilyn Zoeller
45 Alabama Place, Detroit, MI 64789
343-555-7771

Name Barbara Erickson Date 10/10

Address 854 Green St. Age 31

℞

Relafen 750
Sig ii PO QD

#30

☒ Label

Refill 1 times PRN NR

Dr. Marilyn Zoeller

4.14b

4.15

PT. NAME: **JAMES WILSON** | GENDER: **M** | ADDRESS: **53 IRIS BLVD.** | WEIGHT: **122** | HEIGHT: **5′ 7″** | BMI: **19**

AGE: **55** | DX: **CA, NAUSEA, WEIGHT LOSS, MOUTH SORES (THRUSH)** | ALLERGY: **NKA** | HX: **SMOKER**

MEDICATION	SIG.	PRESCRIBER	ORIG. DATE	REFILL DATE	REFILL DATE	REFILL DATE	REFILL DATE
Megace 40 mg/mL susp. 240 mL	2 tsp hs	Johns	9/19	10/9	10/28		
Diflucan 100 mg #12	1 qd	Johns	7/7	7/19			
Xylocaine Viscous 2% 100 mL	1 tbs swish & swallow prn	Johns	6/9				
Compazine tab 10 mg #7	1 q 4 h	Johns	6/9	6/12	6/22		

Dr. Donna Johns
7000 SW 1st Ave., Santa Fe, NM 54545
766-555-9097

Name James Wilson Date 11/5

Address 53 Iris Blvd. Age 55

℞

Percocet 5/325
Disp: #120
Sig: i tab po q 4-6° prn

Refills 0

Dr. Donna Johns

DEA# AJ1234563

4.15a

Dr. Donna Johns
7000 SW 1st Ave., Santa Fe, NM 54545
766-555-9097

Name James Wilson Date 11/5

Address 53 Iris Blvd. Age 55

℞

Compazine Suppos 25 mg
#12
i q6° prn severe nausea

Dr. Donna Johns

4.15b

4.16 PT. NAME: **CATHERINE KLINE** AGE: **37** GENDER: **F** DX: **MIGRAINES, HYPOTHYROID, NAUSEA** ADDRESS: **5577 BLACK DR.** ALLERGY: **NKA** WEIGHT: **128** BMI: **23**

MEDICATION	SIG.	PRESCRIBER	ORIG. DATE	REFILL DATE	REFILL DATE	REFILL DATE	REFILL DATE
Imitrex 50 mg tab #45	Use ud	Keller	6/20	9/6	9/18	10/24	
Diazepam 5 mg #30	1/2 to 1 bid	Keller	9/6	9/28	10/24		
Synthroid 0.125 mg #30	1 qd	Keller	10/30				
Phenergan suppository 50 mg #6	Use PR prn	Keller	11/6				

Dr. Daniel Keller
5007 Turtle Drive, Miami, FL 98887
247-555-9876

Name Catherine Kline Date 11/24

Address 5577 Black Dr. Age 37

℞ Vicodin

#40 (Forty)

sig i tab po q4–6h prn pain

Refills 0

Dr. Daniel Keller

DEA# AK1234563

4.16a

Dr. Daniel Keller
5007 Turtle Drive, Miami, FL 98887
247-555-9876

Name Catherine Kline Date 11/24

Address 5577 Black Dr. Age 37

℞ Fioricet tabs

#50

S i–ii po tab q 4–6 h for severe headache

Refills 0

Dr. Daniel Keller

4.16b

4.17

PT. NAME: **JOAN O'BRIEN**	GENDER: **F**	ADDRESS: **23 SOUTH ST.**	WEIGHT: **168**	BMI: **30**
AGE: **64**	DX: **HTN, HA, CHOLESTEROL, POSTMENOPAUSAL**	ALLERGY: **ASA**	HX: **SMOKER; 20 PACK-YEARS**	

MEDICATION	SIG.	PRESCRIBER	ORIG. DATE	REFILL DATE	REFILL DATE	REFILL DATE	REFILL DATE
Lipitor 10 mg #30	1 hs	Griffin	11/2				
Lopressor 50 mg #60	1 bid	Griffin	11/2				
Prempro 0.45/2.5 mg #28	1 qd	Griffin	10/15	11/1			

Dr. Doug Griffin
7611 147th Terrace, Monterey, CA 38411
705-555-6644

Name Joan O'Brien Date 11/10

Address 23 South St. Age 64

℞

Fioricet #100
Sig: as directed

Refills 0

Dr. Doug Griffin

4.17a

Dr. Doug Griffin
7611 147th Terrace, Monterey, CA 38411
705-555-6644

Name Joan O'Brien Date 11/10

Address 23 South St. Age 64

℞

Tylenol #3
Sig: 1 p.o. q 12
prn for severe HA
Disp: #40 (forty)

Refills 0

Dr. Doug Griffin

DEA# AG1234563

4.17b

4.18

PT. NAME: **BRITTNEY JOHNSON** GENDER: **F** ADDRESS: **23 SOUTH ST.** WEIGHT: **85**

AGE: **13** DX: **ATTENTION DEFICIT HYPERACTIVITY DISORDER (ADHD), URTICARIA, SKIN INFECTION** ALLERGY: **ASA** HX: **BEHAVIOR PROBLEMS IN SCHOOL**

MEDICATION	SIG.	PRESCRIBER	ORIG. DATE	REFILL DATE	REFILL DATE	REFILL DATE	REFILL DATE
Ritalin 5 mg #50	1 am & 1/2 pm	Lambert	6/1				
Claritin 10 mg #30	1 tab/day	Lambert	2/6	3/10	4/2	5/12	
Augmentin susp. 400-57 100 mL	1 tsp bid × 10 d	Lambert	1/29				
Bactroban Ointment 15 g	Apply tid to AA	Lambert	2/27				

Dr. Daniel Lambert
5007 Turtle Drive, Miami, FL 98887
247-555-9876

Name Brittney Johnson Date 7/1

Address 23 South St. Age 13

℞

Ritalin 5mg / tablet
TI am
T noon

#90

Refills 0

Dr. Daniel Lambert

4.18a

Dr. Albert Kaplan
3 SW. Dade Blvd., Miami, FL 98887
247-555-1235

Name Brittney Johnson Date 7/18

Address 23 South St. Age 13

℞

Triamcinolone
Cr.
0.1%
80 gm
in SARNA QS
240 gm

☐ Label

Refill 2 times PRN NR

Dr Albert Kaplan

4.18b

4.19

PT. NAME: **NICOLE DAVIS** AGE: **50** GENDER: **F** DX: **GERD, INSOMNIA, SEVERE BACK PAIN** ADDRESS: **66 NORTH DRIVE** ALLERGY: **PCN** WEIGHT: **154** HX: **REAL ESTATE AGENT, SMOKES, SOCIAL DRINKER** HEIGHT: **5′ 4″**

MEDICATION	SIG.	PRESCRIBER	ORIG. DATE	REFILL DATE	REFILL DATE	REFILL DATE	REFILL DATE
Metoclopramide 5 mg #90	1 tid ac	Tumaneng	9/2	10/1	11/3	12/5	
Ambien 10 mg #30	1 hs prn	Tumaneng	5/9	6/11	7/15		
Lunesta 2 mg #30	1 hs prn	Tumaneng	8/9	9/22	10/29	11/29	
Oxycodone 30 mg #30	1 tab tid prn pain	Tumaneng	10/22				
Oxycodone 30 mg #30	1 tab tid prn pain	Tumaneng	11/28				

Dr. Howard Tumaneng
90 East Drive, Santa Fe, NM 54545
766-555-9390

Name Nicole Davis Date 12/10

Address 66 North Drive Age 50

℞

Duragesic 25 mcg
#1 PO Q72hrs
#10

Refills 0

Dr. Howard Tumaneng

DEA# AT1234563

4.19a

Dr. Howard Tumaneng
90 East Drive, Santa Fe, NM 54545
766-555-9390

Name Nicole Davis Date 12/10

Address 66 North Drive Age 50

℞

Zantac 150 # xiv
ʒ i BID

Refills
PRN

Dr. Howard Tumaneng

4.19b

4.20

PT. NAME: **MEGAN HARRIS**	GENDER: **F**	ADDRESS: **19523 NE 21ST AVE.**	WEIGHT: **132**	BMI: **25**
AGE: **42**	DX: **PAIN, SPASMS, URI, NAUSEA**	ALLERGY: **CIPRO, PCN**	HX: **ETOH, SMOKING, DIVORCED, UNEMPLOYED**	

MEDICATION	SIG.	PRESCRIBER	ORIG. DATE	REFILL DATE	REFILL DATE	REFILL DATE	REFILL DATE
Soma 350 mg #100	I tid	Parlato	10/31	11/27			
Xanax 2 mg #60	I bid	Parlato	10/31	11/27			
Z-Pak	Take ud	Parlato	10/31				
Phenergan 25 mg tabs #30	I tid	Parlato	10/31	11/8	12/3	12/17	

Dr. Jessica Hartmann
55 1st Terrace, Monterey, CA 38411
705-555-5180

Name Megan Harris Date 12/19

Address 19523 NE 21 Ave. Age 42

℞

Ultracet c̄ (24)

sig i q4-6h prn pain

NR

Dr. Jessica Hartmann

4.20a

Dr. Waldo Terranova
9052 188 Terrace, Monterey, CA 38411
705-555-0001

Name Megan Harris Date 12/18

Address 19523 NE 21 Ave. Age 42

℞

Soma 350 mg

50 (fifty)

i tid as directed

☐ Label

Refill 1X times

Dr. Waldo Terranova

4.20b

4.21 PT. NAME: **MARK SPENCER** AGE: **47** GENDER: **M** DX: **NERVES, URI, OPIOID DEPENDENCE** ADDRESS: **12 GROVE AVE.** ALLERGY: **NKA** WEIGHT: **135** HX: **DRUG ABUSE** BMI: **22**

MEDICATION	SIG.	PRESCRIBER	ORIG. DATE	REFILL DATE	REFILL DATE	REFILL DATE	REFILL DATE
Vicodin #C	I q 6 h prn	Jarvis	3/7	5/7	6/8	7/9	8/30
Z-Pak	Take ud	Young	6/5				
Cipro 500 mg #12	I bid	Young	9/2				
Subutex 8 mg #10	I qd	Young	11/20				

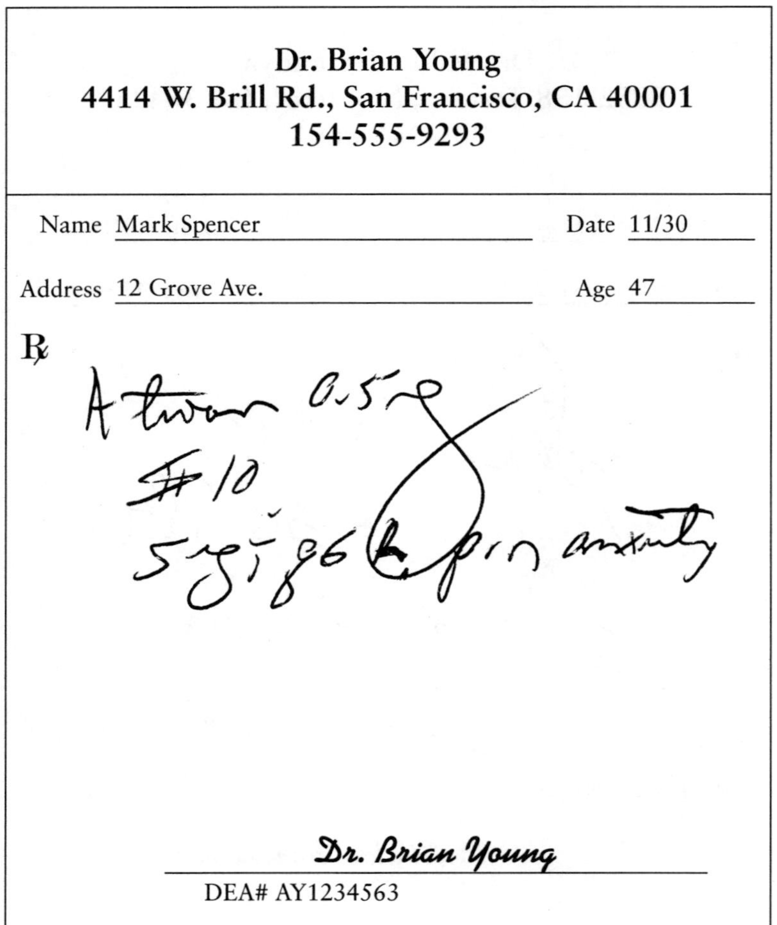

Dr. Brian Young
4414 W. Brill Rd., San Francisco, CA 40001
154-555-9293

Name Mark Spencer Date 11/30
Address 12 Grove Ave. Age 47

℞
Ativan 0.5 mg
#10
Sig i q6h prn anxiety

Dr. Brian Young
DEA# AY1234563

4.21a

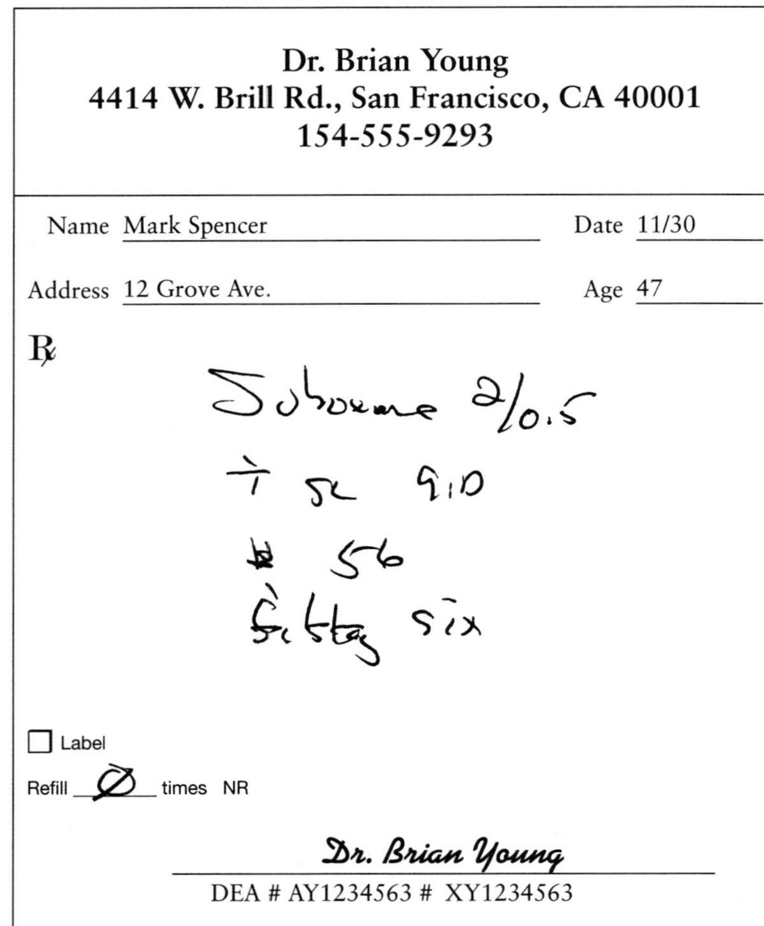

Dr. Brian Young
4414 W. Brill Rd., San Francisco, CA 40001
154-555-9293

Name Mark Spencer Date 11/30
Address 12 Grove Ave. Age 47

℞
Suboxone 2/0.5
i SL QID
56
fifty six

☐ Label
Refill Ø times NR

Dr. Brian Young
DEA # AY1234563 # XY1234563

4.21b

4.22 PT. NAME: **MICHAEL FELIX** AGE: **38** GENDER: **M** DX: **OPIOID DEPENDENCE, ED** ADDRESS: **44 GRAY ST.** ALLERGY: **ASA, PCN** WEIGHT: **120** HX: **DRUG ABUSE** HEIGHT: **5′ 7″**

MEDICATION	SIG.	PRESCRIBER	ORIG. DATE	REFILL DATE	REFILL DATE	REFILL DATE	REFILL DATE
Viagra 100 mg #5	Use ud	Boyles	4/22				
Valium 10 mg #50	1 bid prn	Boyles	4/22	5/30	8/3	8/30	
Subutex 8 mg #10	1 qd	Chappell	10/30	11/30			

Dr. John Chappell
28 St. Lawrence Ave., Detroit, MI 64789
343-555-5959

Name Michael Felix Date 12/5

Address 44 Gray St. Age 38

℞

Suboxone (8) #21
1/2 tab TID SL
twenty one

☐ Label

Refill 0 times NR

Dr. John Chappell
DEA# BC1234563 XC1234563

4.22a

Dr. John Chappell
28 St. Lawrence Ave., Detroit, MI 64789
343-555-5959

Name Michael Felix Date 12/5

Address 44 Gray St. Age 38

℞

Valium 10mg
i po BID
28
Twenty eight

☐ Label

Refill 0 times NR

Dr. John Chappell
DEA# BC1234563

4.22b

4.23 PT. NAME: **PAMELA RICHARDS** AGE: **48** GENDER: **F** DX: **INSOMNIA, BACK PAIN, DRUG DEPENDENCE** ADDRESS: **3 HOWARD LANE** ALLERGY: **PCN** WEIGHT: **113** HX: **SMOKER, ETOH, DRUGS** BMI: **20**

MEDICATION	SIG.	PRESCRIBER	ORIG. DATE	REFILL DATE	REFILL DATE	REFILL DATE	REFILL DATE
Oxycontin 80 mg #100	1 tid prn	Gold	10/19				
Valium 5 mg #90	1 tid prn	Gold	3/5	4/7	6/7	8/12	10/19
Ultram 50 mg #100	1–2 tid prn pain	Harris	6/22	8/30			
Clonazepam 1 mg #30	1/2 tab prn sleep	Midkiff	9/15	10/4	10/20		
Gabapentin 300 mg #90	1 tid	Midkiff	9/15	10/4	10/20		

Dr. Ray Lopez
40 Green Road, Tampa, FL 49857
786-555-5657

Name Pamela Richards Date 11/4

Address 3 Howard Lane Age 48

℞

SUBUTEX 8mg
#10 (TEN)

SIG i qd

Label

Refill NR times

Dr. Ray Lopez

DEA# BL1234563 XL1234563

4.23a

Dr. Ray Lopez
40 Green Road, Tampa, FL 49857
786-555-5657

Name Pamela Richards Date 11/4

Address 3 Howard Lane Age 48

℞

Flexeril 10mg tbs
i tab po qhs prn
#30

No Refills

Dr. Ray Lopez

4.23b

4.24

PT. NAME: **JOANNIE FRANCIS** AGE: **68** GENDER: **F** DX: **HTN, DIARRHEA, IBS, DEPRESSION, BACK PAIN** ADDRESS: **88 BRUNSWICK AVE.** ALLERGY: **NKA** WEIGHT: **139** BMI: **22**

MEDICATION	SIG.	PRESCRIBER	ORIG. DATE	REFILL DATE	REFILL DATE	REFILL DATE	REFILL DATE
Norvasc 5 mg #30	I qd	Daley	2/4	3/6	4/3	5/2	6/30
Carisoprodol 350 mg #30	I tid prn	Daley	3/2				
Carisoprodol 350 mg #120	I tid prn	Daley	3/20	4/21	6/28	8/15	9/12
Dicyclomine 20 mg #30	I bid prn cramps	Daley	5/6	8/9			
Fluoxetine 20 mg #30	I qd am	Daley	9/3	10/5			

Dr. Aaron Daley
7 Harbor Drive, San Francisco, CA 40001
959-555-3211

Name Joannie Francis Date 10/8

Address 88 Brunswick Ave. Age 68

℞

Tincture of Opium
5gtts q 20' ac
#8oz

Label

Refill Ø times

Dr. Aaron Daley

DEA# AD1234563

4.24a

Dr. Aaron Daley
7 Harbor Drive, San Francisco, CA 40001
959-555-3211

Name Joannie Francis Date 10/8

Address 88 Brunswick Ave. Age 68

℞

Tyl #4
#30
Sig: i-ii po q4° prn

Refills 0

Dr. Aaron Daley

DEA# AD1234563

4.24b

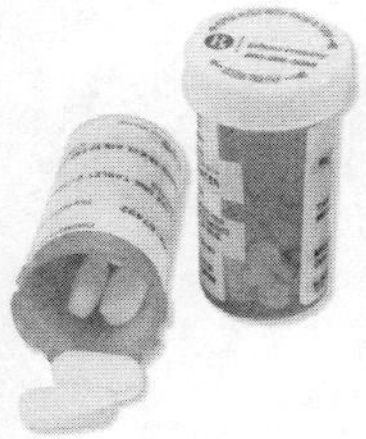

5 • DRUGS FOR NEOPLASTIC DISORDERS AND IMMUNOSUPPRESSANTS

UPON COMPLETION OF THIS CHAPTER, THE STUDENT WILL BE ABLE TO:

- counsel patients on the potency of antineoplastic agents and the importance of taking them exactly as prescribed.
- counsel patients on the special dietary and fluid requirements associated with cancer chemotherapy.
- demonstrate the proper application of 5-FU topical preparations.
- discuss the benefit of Lupron combination therapy.
- calculate the dose reduction of Imuran if allopurinol is added to the drug regimen.
- counsel the patients on compliance with drugs that are necessary to take along with other chemotherapy drugs.
- caution patients about OTC products, which may have important drug interactions with prescription drugs.
- discuss the various glucocorticoids and compare their glucocorticoid and mineralocorticoid potencies.

DRUG LIST

5-FU (topical forms)
Arimidex
Aromasin
Casodex
CellCept
Cytoxan
Femara
Imuran
Leucovorin Calcium
Leukeran
Lupron
Megace
Methotrexate
Nystatin
Prednisone
Tamoxifen

• DRUG HOT POINTS

5-FU
Antimetabolite
1% cream: Fluoroplex for topical use
5% cream: Efudex
Cream: proper application
Correct period of administration
Compliance: avoid exposure to sun, avoid the eyes
Used IV for CA of the colon, rectum, breast, stomach, and pancreas

Casodex
Prostate CA treatment
Antiandrogen at target tissue
Possible warfarin interaction
Role of Lupron
Both agents should be started together
Do not D/C without consulting prescriber
Compare with Eulexin

Cytoxan
Alkylating agent: cross-links DNA
Take with water (2 to 3 L/day)
Adverse effect: hemorrhagic cystitis
MESNA: detoxifying agent to inhibit hemorrhagic cystitis
Compare with Leukeran

Imuran
Immunosuppressive
Allopurinol interaction: (↓ dose of Imuran by 3/4 to 1/4 of original dose)
Report sore throat
No live vaccines
AZT/azathioprine confusion
Many uses: kidney transplant rejection, lupus, RA, Crohn's disease, myasthenia gravis
Compare with Purinethol (6-MP)
Compare with CellCept (MMF) as an inhibitor of IMP dehydrogenase

Leucovorin Calcium
Folinic acid, **not** folic acid
The active form
Leucovorin rescue after high-dose MTX
PO use with folic acid antagonists

Lupron
LHRH agonist
Continuous use results in decrease in LH & FSH
Estrogen & testosterone production are decreased
Indicated for endometriosis & prostate CA
Comply with appointments for injection

Megace
Two different uses
Tablets
Liquid (40 mg/mL)
Dose: 800 mg/day for appetite stimulant
Concentrated formulation: Megace ES

Methotrexate (MTX)
Resembles folic acid; antagonist
Different indications/dosage ranges
CA, psoriasis, RA
PO taken once a week, at 12-hour intervals, or taken all at one time
Drug interactions (OTC & Rx): avoid salicylates & NSAIDs
Caution: sulfonylureas
Avoid sunlight
Compliance with blood tests
Checkup for liver tests

Nolvadex (Tamoxifen)
Breast CA, women or men
Potent antiestrogen
Take with food
Check history for other Rxs containing estrogen products (interaction)
Potential for hot flashes
Compare with Arimidex, Femara, Aromasin

Nystatin (oral, topical, and vaginal)
Oral: S-S (swish and swallow or spit): thrush
Shake, then place liquid in buccal areas of both sides of mouth
Retain in mouth as long as possible
Continue for 2 days postasymptomatic
Commonly included in various "magic mouthwash" formulas

Prednisone
Glucocorticoid with some mineralocorticoid activity
Take with food or milk
Compliance with scheduled doses
High doses should be tapered down
Compare potency with other glucocorticoids
Compare PO mineralocorticoid activity with other glucocorticoids (methylprednisolone, dexamethasone, triamcinolone)
Potential for hyperglycemia
Potential for osteoporosis (long-term use)

• QUESTIONS TO BE ANSWERED IN PREPARATION FOR CHAPTER 5 LAB

- What is the mechanism of action of Lupron?
- In a community pharmacy, how should the label be typed for the following prescription? Megace Suspension Sig: 800 mg qd
- A patient takes 1 tablespoonful of Megace suspension daily. How many milligrams of active ingredient is the patient taking on a daily basis?
- If a physician prescribes 5-FU cream to be used on the skin, which product would you dispense?
- What is the equipotent dose of dexamethasone PO to prednisone 20 mg PO?
- If a doctor wanted to switch a patient from 10 mg of prednisone a day to methylprednisolone, what would the dose be for the methylprednisolone?
- How many milligrams of active drug are contained in each tablet of methotrexate?
- A prescription is written for MTX 7.5 mg PO weekly. How would you advise the patient concerning the dosing intervals?
- Explain the counseling for the administration of nystatin suspension for the treatment of oral candidiasis (thrush).
- Explain the problem if a person abruptly stops taking oral prednisone after long-term administration of 10 mg PO daily.
- What is the significance of the H-P-A axis in the preceding problem?
- Compare the action of azathioprine (Imuran) with that of CellCept.
- How many milligrams of active drug are contained in each Eulexin capsule?
- What is the advantage of Casodex over Eulexin?
- A patient is taking four Imuran 50 mg tablets daily. The physician adds a new product, Zyloprim, 300 mg once daily. What should be the new Imuran dose?
- What is the difference between azathioprine and Purinethol (6-MP)?
- A person taking Premarin is given a new prescription for tamoxifen. What is the outcome if they are taken concurrently?
- Why would folic acid not be appropriate for use as "leucovorin rescue" therapy with high-dose MTX therapy?
- What is the pharmacologic difference between folic acid and folinic acid?
- Your client is taking PO Cytoxan. He is at risk for which adverse effect? How much water should he drink each day to minimize the risk of the adverse effect?
- How does Megace suspension differ from Megace ES suspension?
- Explain the role of MESNA when used in a patient who has taken cyclophosphamide.

• DRUGS FOR NEOPLASTIC DISORDERS AND IMMUNOSUPPRESSIVE MEDICATION THERAPY MANAGEMENT QUESTIONS AND COMMENTS

- Did your doctor mention the correct manner of applying the cream for your skin condition? Also, were you informed to stay out of the sun during the 2-week period that you are using this cream? It is very important to avoid contact of the skin cream with your eyes. The cream is called 5-FU. It will cause some irritation in a few days. That shows that the cream is doing its job. Your doctor advises that you use a soothing cream during the day to reduce the irritation, which will go away in 2 weeks.
- You are taking a powerful medication. Do you have it on your calendar to visit the doctor for the blood tests that are needed?
- Your prescription for MTX, or methotrexate, has instructions to take six tablets per week. Please remember that the tablets should be taken as follows: all six tablets at once with water, or in three doses, at 12-hour intervals over 2 days. They must **never** be taken every day over a 6-day period.
- Are you aware that prednisone is a form of cortisone? This medicine should be taken with food or milk, not on an empty stomach. If necessary, when this medicine is stopped, it must be slowly stopped, according to the doctor's instructions.
- Are you seeing your doctor for the Lupron injections to go with your Casodex?
- Megace, or Megestrol liquid, should be shaken well before using. In addition, did the doctor tell you to increase your food intake to help you gain weight?
- Your medication is called Cytoxan or cyclophosphamide. Please remember to drink at least eight glasses of water (if allowed) each day to avoid problems with this medication.
- Your arthritis doctor has prescribed azathioprine. You are also seeing another doctor for your gout, for which you take allopurinol. We will have to call both doctors to calculate the correct dose of the azathioprine.
- Nystatin suspension is prescribed for the rash in your mouth, which has occurred because of your other medications. Please remember to shake the suspension well each time, and then swish it in the mouth, making sure that both sides and all tissues are exposed to the medication. Keep it in the mouth for 5 minutes if possible and then spit it out or swallow it, as the doctor ordered.
- Your doctor has prescribed a strong, effective medication called Leukeran. Because this medication is dosed by body weight, I would like to know your weight so I can verify that the dose on the prescription is correct. I know that you do not feel well and you are not happy to tell us your weight; however, my professional obligation is to make sure that the medications are correctly dosed and that you take them correctly to avoid problems while ensuring that they help you.
- I strongly recommend that you take absolutely no OTC herbal supplements while taking your prescription medication, unless the doctor recommends one. If one is recommended, it is very important for you to let me know so I can verify that it is safe or effective, and this must be documented on your profile in our computer.
- If you cannot afford your medication, let's contact the manufacturer to see if there is a coupon that is available to help you decrease the cost.
- Because you are taking a medication for your muscle weakness condition, which you mentioned and is called myasthenia gravis, it is very important to avoid any OTC medication unless you call us first. Cold, allergy, and sleep pills could make your condition worse.

5.1

PT. NAME: **CYNTHIA SMITH** GENDER: **F** ADDRESS: **894 WEST RD.** WEIGHT: **140** HEIGHT: **5′ 8″**
AGE: **59** DX: **HTN, IBS, RA, VERTIGO, EYE INFLAMMATION, CONSTIPATION** ALLERGY: **PCN**

MEDICATION	SIG.	PRESCRIBER	ORIG. DATE	REFILL DATE	REFILL DATE	REFILL DATE	REFILL DATE
Bentyl 20 mg #90	1 qid for abdominal pain	Thomas	8/3	8/30	9/28		
Antivert 12.5 mg #40	1 qid prn dizziness	Thomas	8/29				
Lasix 40 mg #60	1 bid	Thomas	9/7				
Ex-Lax Chocolate #48	1–2 hs	OTC	8/5	9/3	10/5		
Hypotears 15 mL	2 drops qid to ou	OTC	8/5	8/29	9/28		

Dr. Erin Thomas
988 North Ridge, New York, NY 88364
813-555-7554

Name Cynthia Smith Date 10/5

Address 894 West Rd. Age 59

℞

Prednisone 50

Sig 1 Tab daily PC Breakfast

Refills 3

Dr. Erin Thomas

5.1a

Dr. Erin Thomas
988 North Ridge, New York, NY 88364
813-555-7554

Name Cynthia Smith Date 10/5

Address 894 West Rd. Age 59

℞

Inflamase Forte 1%

10cc

gtts i OD Bid

Refills 3

Dr. Erin Thomas

5.1b

5.2

PT. NAME: **MICHAEL MURPHY**	GENDER: **M**	ADDRESS: **2 TALLAHASSEE CT.**	WEIGHT: **154**	BMI: **26**
AGE: **67**	DX: **PROSTATE CA, NASAL CONGESTION, DEPRESSION**	ALLERGY: **NKA**	HX: **SMOKER: 50 PACK-YEAR HISTORY**	

MEDICATION	SIG.	PRESCRIBER	ORIG. DATE	REFILL DATE	REFILL DATE	REFILL DATE	REFILL DATE
Claritin-D 24 Hr #15	I qd	Griffin	8/8				
St. John's wort 300 mg #50	I tid	OTC	7/2	7/20	8/6		

Dr. Doug Griffin
7611 147th Terrace, Monterey, CA 38411
705-555-6644

Name Michael Murphy Date 8/10

Address 2 Tallahassee Ct. Age 67

℞

Flutamide 125mg
ii P.O. TID
#100

Refills 2

Dr. Doug Griffin

5.2a

Dr. Doug Griffin
7611 147th Terrace, Monterey, CA 38411
705-555-6644

Name Michael Murphy Date 8/10

Address 2 Tallahassee Ct. Age 67

℞

Tylenol c̄ Codeine Elixer
20 cc p.o. q4° PRN
Disp: i pint.

REFILL ∅ TIMES

Dr. Doug Griffin

5.2b

5.3 PT. NAME: **DIANE MYERS** AGE: **46** GENDER: **F** DX: **TYPE 2 DM, BREAST CA, DEPRESSION** ADDRESS: **6 PENNSYLVANIA AVE. NW** ALLERGY: **NKA** WEIGHT: **138** BMI: **26**

MEDICATION	SIG.	PRESCRIBER	ORIG. DATE	REFILL DATE	REFILL DATE	REFILL DATE	REFILL DATE
Lorazepam 1 mg #90	1 hs	Stage	8/10				
Amoxicillin 500 mg #4	4 caps 1 h before appt.	Ely, DDS	1/6				
Glyburide 2.5 mg #90	1 qd	Stage	3/5	6/8	10/24		

Dr. Howard Isaacs
1115 Turnaround Lane, Detroit, MI 64789
343-555-7000

Name Diane Myers Date 11/5

Address 6 Pennsylvania Ave. NW Age 46

℞

Tamoxifen 10 mgm bid po
3 months supply

Refills 0

Dr. Howard Isaacs

5.3a

Dr. Marilyn Zoeller
45 Alabama Place, Detroit, MI 64789
343-555-7771

Name Diane Myers Date 11/5

Address 6 Pennsylvania Ave. NW Age 46

℞

Paxil, 20 mg
#30
sig: ½ qhs x 4 days,
then 1 qhs

REFILL ..∅..... TIMES

Dr. Marilyn Zoeller

5.3b

5.4

PT. NAME: **PATRICIA ANDERSON** GENDER: **F** ADDRESS: **564 CAPITOL AVE.** WEIGHT: **130** BMI: **24**

AGE: **69** DX: **HTN, HRT, DYSPAREUNIA, NEWLY DIAGNOSED BREAST CA** ALLERGY: **NKA** HX: **SMOKER FOR 40 YEARS**

MEDICATION	SIG.	PRESCRIBER	ORIG. DATE	REFILL DATE	REFILL DATE	REFILL DATE	REFILL DATE
HCTZ 25 #90	1 q am	Robins	4/12	5/15			
Premarin 0.625 #90	1 qd	Robins	5/10				
Replens vaginal moisturizer 35 g	As needed	OTC	3/1	5/10	7/15		

Dr. David Knowles
555 Tea Rose Trail, Miami, FL 44718
463-555-0098

Name Patricia Anderson Date 7/20

Address 564 Capitol Ave. Age 69

℞

Tamoxifen 10mg
1 PO BID
#100
Refill #3

Dr. David Knowles

5.4a

Dr. Calvin Robins
7823 Tea Rose Trail, Miami, FL 44718
463-555-8000

Name Patricia Anderson Date 7/20

Address 564 Capitol Ave. Age 69

℞

Avapro 150mg
1 PO qd
#30

☐ LABEL

REFILL 5 TIMES PRN

Dr. Calvin Robins

5.4b

5.5	PT. NAME: **JOHN JOHNSON**	GENDER: **M**	ADDRESS: **321 WEST RD.**	WEIGHT: **166**	HEIGHT: **5′ 10″**
	AGE: **68**	DX: **ACTINIC KERATOSIS, BACTERIAL INFECTION (COMMUNITY-ACQUIRED PNEUMONIA), COUGH**	ALLERGY: **SULFA**		

MEDICATION	SIG.	PRESCRIBER	ORIG. DATE	REFILL DATE	REFILL DATE	REFILL DATE	REFILL DATE
Levaquin 500 #7	1 qd × 7 d	Thomas	10/2				
Tessalon Perles 100 mg #15	1 qid	Thomas	10/2				

Dr. Erin Thomas
988 North Ridge, New York, NY 88364
813-555-7554

Name John Johnson Date 10/12

Address 321 West Rd. Age 68

℞

Efudex 5% cream

Disp: 25 gm

Sig: [illegible] BID × 2 wk

as [illegible] me

Refills 0

Dr. Erin Thomas

5.5a

Dr. Erin Thomas
988 North Ridge, New York, NY 88364
813-555-7554

Name John Johnson Date 10/12

Address 321 West Rd. Age 68

℞

TRIAMCINOLONE ACETONIDE

0.5% HP cream

15 gm

[illegible] BID

Refills 0

Dr. Erin Thomas

5.5b

5.6

PT. NAME: **MARY SCHMIDT** GENDER: **F** ADDRESS: **566 EAST CT.** WEIGHT: **118** BMI: **20**

AGE: **72** DX: **CA, HTN, MUSCLE PAIN, CACHEXIA (GENERAL WEIGHT LOSS)** ALLERGY: **NKA** HX: **SMOKER FOR 35 YEARS**

MEDICATION	SIG.	PRESCRIBER	ORIG. DATE	REFILL DATE	REFILL DATE	REFILL DATE	REFILL DATE
Percocet 5/325 #C	2 q 4 h	Griffin	8/21				
Soma 350 mg #90	1 hs	Griffin	6/23				

Dr. Doug Griffin
7611 147th Terrace, Monterey, CA 38411
705-555-6644

Name Mary Schmidt Date 8/30

Address 566 East Ct. Age 72

℞

Megace 1 Pint
(20mg/5cc)

Sig. 20ml
BID

Refills 0

Dr. Doug Griffin

5.6a

Dr. Jay Mack
52 West Drive, Monterey, CA 38411
705-555-3321

Name Mary Schmidt Date 8/29

Address 566 East Ct. Age 72

℞

HCTZ 25mg
Sig: i tab PO qd
#30

Label

Refill 3 times

Dr. Jay Mack

5.6b

5.7

PT. NAME: **LESTER KELLY** | GENDER: **M** | ADDRESS: **23 SOUTH ST.** | WEIGHT: **215** | BMI: **27**
AGE: **55** | DX: **GOUT, CROHN'S DISEASE** | ALLERGY: **NKA** | HX: **ENTERITIS**

MEDICATION	SIG.	PRESCRIBER	ORIG. DATE	REFILL DATE	REFILL DATE	REFILL DATE	REFILL DATE
Zyloprim 300 mg #90	I q am	Blank	4/12	7/20			
Xanax 0.25 #60	I q hs	Blank	6/18				

Dr. Alfred Sauls
151212 S. High Rd., Chicago, IL 23875
954-555-1300

Name Lester Kelly Date 7/30

Address 23 South St. Age 55

℞

Imuran 50mg
#30
T PO bid

Refills 0

Dr. Alfred Sauls

5.7a

Dr. Neil Blank
201 Baker St., Chicago, IL 23875
954-555-0001

Name Lester Kelly Date 7/31

Address 23 South St. Age 55

℞

Indocin 25mg
#15
Sig: 1 tid
for 5 days

REFILL 3 TIMES

Dr. Blank

5.7b

5.8

PT. NAME: **BENJAMIN MEYER**	GENDER: **M**	ADDRESS: **145 NORTH AVE.**	WEIGHT: **144**	HEIGHT: **5′ 7″**
AGE: **79**	DX: **OA, HTN, CHF, RESPIRATORY INFECTION**	ALLERGY: **NKA**		

MEDICATION	SIG.	PRESCRIBER	ORIG. DATE	REFILL DATE	REFILL DATE	REFILL DATE	REFILL DATE
Antivert 25 mg #90	I tid	Johns	9/29				
Cipro 500 mg #14	I bid	Johns	8/12				
Lanoxin 0.25 #30	I q am	Johns	8/30	9/30			

Dr. Donna Johns
7000 SW 1st Ave., Santa Fe, NM 54545
766-555-9097

Name Benjamin Meyer Date 10/25

Address 145 North Ave. Age 79

℞

Verapamil 80mg po tid
Dyazide i po qd
Digoxin 0.125mg po qd
Advil 400mg po qhs
Prednisone 5mg po bid

Refills 0

Dr. Donna Johns

5.8a

Dr. Donna Johns
7000 SW 1st Ave., Santa Fe, NM 54545
766-555-9097

Name Benjamin Meyer Date 10/25

Address 145 North Ave. Age 79

℞

Cipro 750 mg
i BID
#10

N.R.

Dr. Donna Johns

5.8b

5.9	PT. NAME: **LYNDON PETERSON**	GENDER: **M**	ADDRESS: **325 IRIS BLVD.**	WEIGHT: **198**	HEIGHT: **6′ 1″**
	AGE: **57**	DX: **ANEMIA, SUNSPOTS ON FOREHEAD AND CHEEK**	ALLERGY: **ASA**	HX: **RETIRED, FISHES, PLAYS GOLF**	

MEDICATION	SIG.	PRESCRIBER	ORIG. DATE	REFILL DATE	REFILL DATE	REFILL DATE	REFILL DATE
Ask client for medication history							

Dr. Thomas Fornier
78 Tea Rose Trail, Miami, FL 44718
463-555-8009

Name Lyndon Peterson Date 5/11

Address 325 Iris Blvd. Age 57

℞

Folic Acid 1.0 mg
ī PO BID #100

Refills 0

Dr. Thomas Fornier

5.9a

Dr. Theodore Russell
7999 NE 164 St., Miami, FL 44718
463-555-9596

Name Lyndon Peterson Date 5/11

Address 325 Iris Blvd. Age 57

℞

Efudex Cream 5%

Sig: Apply to Nose BID

#25 gm

Refills 0

Dr. Theodore Russell

5.9b

5.10

PT. NAME: **SUSAN WILLIAMS** GENDER: **F** ADDRESS: **452 HALL ST.** WEIGHT: **122** HEIGHT: **5′ 1″**

AGE: **48** DX: **COPD, TYPE 2 DM, THRUSH, ANEMIA** ALLERGY: **PCN, SULFA**

MEDICATION	SIG.	PRESCRIBER	ORIG. DATE	REFILL DATE	REFILL DATE	REFILL DATE	REFILL DATE
Allegra 60 mg #25	1 qd	Thomas	4/11	5/7	6/19		
Amaryl 4 mg #90	1 daily	Thomas	4/28				
Lotrisone Cr. 45 g	Apply bid	Thomas	2/16	6/7			
QVAR 40 mcg 7.3 g	Use ud	Thomas	2/1	3/9	4/13	5/16	

Dr. Erin Thomas
988 North Ridge, New York, NY 88364
813-555-7554

Name Susan Williams Date 8/18

Address 452 Hall St. Age 48

℞

Folic acid

1mg qd

#100

Generic

Refills 0

Dr. Erin Thomas

5.10a

Dr. Roy Verga, D.D.S.
12-South Ridge, New York, NY 88364
813-555-2957

Name Susan Williams Date 8/20

Address 452 Hall St. Age 48

℞

Nystatin Oral

Sig 6mL P.O. qid

S+S x10day

Disp # suff 10 days

LABEL

REFILL 1 TIMES

☐ NON-REPETATUR

Dr. Roy Verga, DDS

5.10b

5.11

PT. NAME: **LISA COOPER**	GENDER: **F**	ADDRESS: **688 GREEN ST.**	WEIGHT: **165**	HEIGHT: **5′ 10″**
AGE: **68**	DX: **RA, HTN, HRT, INSOMNIA, GERD**	ALLERGY: **PCN**		

MEDICATION	SIG.	PRESCRIBER	ORIG. DATE	REFILL DATE	REFILL DATE	REFILL DATE	REFILL DATE
Premarin 0.625 mg #90	I qd	Griffin	6/19	9/28			
Avapro 150 mg #30	I qd	Griffin	5/23	9/1	11/1		
Ambien 5 mg #30	I hs	Griffin	8/10	9/13	10/10		

Dr. Harvey Johns
5555 166th Terrace, Monterey, CA 38411
705-555-1232

Name Lisa Cooper Date 11/5

Address 688 Green St. Age 68

℞

Mobic 7.5

#14 [illegible]

Refills 0

Dr. Harvey Johns

5.11a

Dr. Doug Griffin
7611 147th Terrace, Monterey, CA 38411
705-555-6644

Name Lisa Cooper Date 11/5

Address 688 Green St. Age 68

℞

Zantac 300mg

#30

Sig: i qhs

Refills 0

Dr. Doug Griffin

5.11b

5.12

PT. NAME: **WILLIAM HOFFMAN** GENDER: **M** ADDRESS: **845 FANTASTIC ST.** WEIGHT: **173** HEIGHT: **5′ 10″**
AGE: **49** DX: **TYPE 2 DM, PSORIATIC ARTHRITIS, INSOMNIA** ALLERGY: **NKA**

MEDICATION	SIG.	PRESCRIBER	ORIG. DATE	REFILL DATE	REFILL DATE	REFILL DATE	REFILL DATE
Insulin Syr 1 cc #100	Use ud	Sauls	7/14				
Ambien 5 mg #30	1 hs	Sauls	8/10	9/13	10/9		
Motrin PM caplets #40	1 hs prn	OTC	6/1	7/8	8/5	9/2	10/4

Dr. Alfred Sauls
151212 S. High Rd., Chicago, IL 23875
954-555-1300

Name William Hoffman Date 10/18

Address 845 Fantastic St. Age 49

℞

Methotrexate 2.5 mg
#12

Sig: iii tabs po q week (Tues)

Refills 0

Dr. Alfred Sauls

5.12a

Dr. Alfred Sauls
151212 S. High Rd., Chicago, IL 23875
954-555-1300

Name William Hoffman Date 10/18

Address 845 Fantastic St. Age 49

℞

Folic Acid 1 mg
1 q day

#100

☒ Label

Refill [illegible] times

Dr. Alfred Sauls

5.12b

5.13 PT. NAME: **MARY SULLIVAN** AGE: **58** GENDER: **F** DX: **HTN, RA, ANXIETY** ADDRESS: **89 DEXTER AVE.** ALLERGY: **NKA** WEIGHT: **198** HEIGHT: **5′ 9″**

MEDICATION	SIG.	PRESCRIBER	ORIG. DATE	REFILL DATE	REFILL DATE	REFILL DATE	REFILL DATE
Maxzide 50/75 #30	I qd	Weiss	9/11				
Xanax 0.25 mg #5	I ud	Weiss	9/5				

Dr. Barry Weiss
901 Sheridan St., Austin, TX 90902
874-555-9000

Name Mary Sullivan Date 10/20

Address 89 Dexter Ave. Age 58

℞
Prednisone 10 mg
#50
iii daily x 3 days in AM
then ii daily in AM x 3 days
then i daily x 3 days

☐ Label

Refill ______ times

Dr. Barry Weiss

5.13a

Dr. Barry Weiss
901 Sheridan St., Austin, TX 90902
874-555-9000

Name Mary Sullivan Date 10/20

Address 89 Dexter Ave. Age 58

℞
PRILOSEC 20mg #25
Sig: i qd AM a bkfst

3X Refills

Dr. Barry Weiss

5.13b

5.14 PT. NAME: **GEORGE SMITH** AGE: **58** GENDER: **M** DX: **HTN, RA, DYSPEPSIA** ADDRESS: **145 NORTH AVE.** ALLERGY: **PCN** WEIGHT: **148** BMI: **24**

MEDICATION	SIG.	PRESCRIBER	ORIG. DATE	REFILL DATE	REFILL DATE	REFILL DATE	REFILL DATE
Altace 10 mg #60	1 bid	Robins	10/8				
Furosemide 20 mg #50	1 qd	Robins	10/8				
Prednisone 1 mg #CC	2 tabs bid with food	Samuels	9/30				

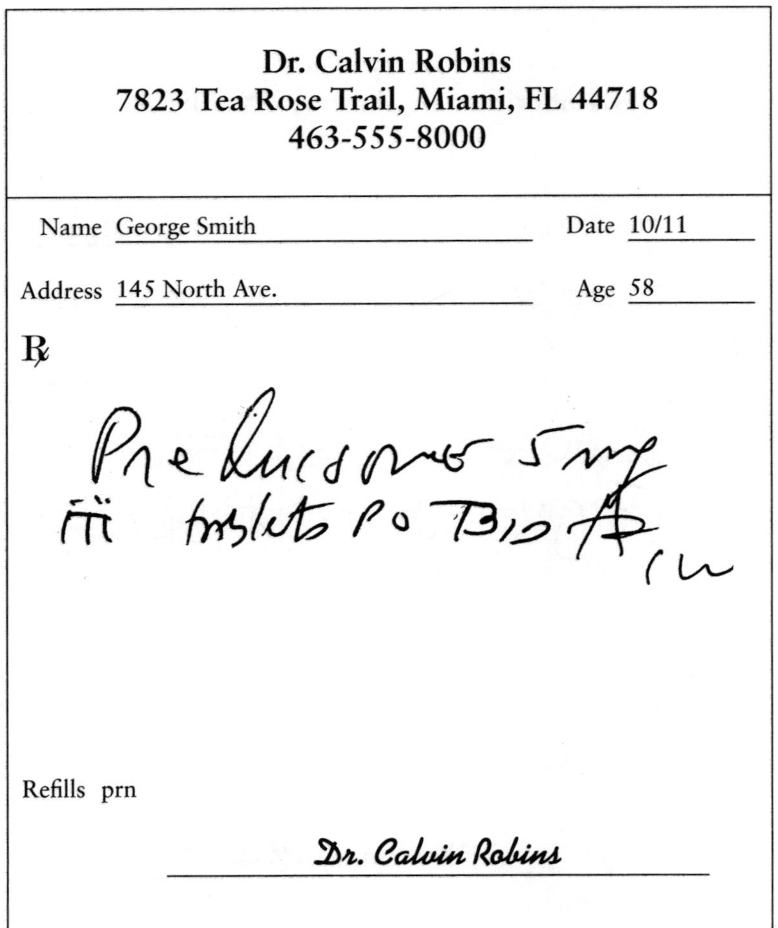
Dr. Calvin Robins
7823 Tea Rose Trail, Miami, FL 44718
463-555-8000

Name George Smith Date 10/11
Address 145 North Ave. Age 58
℞
Prednisone 5 mg
iii tablets PO BID ā c

Refills prn
Dr. Calvin Robins

5.14a

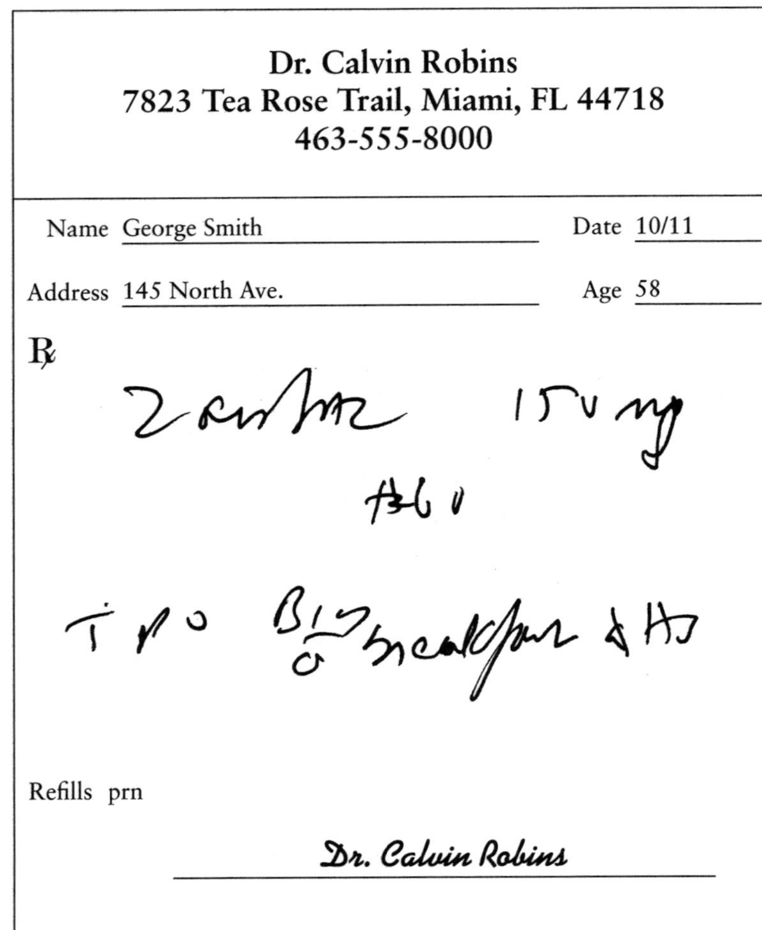
Dr. Calvin Robins
7823 Tea Rose Trail, Miami, FL 44718
463-555-8000

Name George Smith Date 10/11
Address 145 North Ave. Age 58
℞
Zantac 150 mg
#60
i PO BID ō breakfast & HS

Refills prn
Dr. Calvin Robins

5.14b

5.15 PT. NAME: **SEAN NELSON** AGE: **72** GENDER: **M** DX: **HTN, RA, RESPIRATORY INFECTION, BASAL CELL CARCINOMA** ADDRESS: **92 IBIS LANE** ALLERGY: **NKA** WEIGHT: **132** HX: **TENNIS INSTRUCTOR** BMI: **26**

MEDICATION	SIG.	PRESCRIBER	ORIG. DATE	REFILL DATE	REFILL DATE	REFILL DATE	REFILL DATE
Z-Pak	Take ud	Thomas	9/27				
Zestril 40 mg #90	1 daily	Thomas	10/12				
Biaxin XL 500 mg #20	1 bid	Thomas	10/24				

Dr. Erin Thomas
988 North Ridge, New York, NY 88364
813-555-7554

Name Sean Nelson Date 10/31

Address 92 Ibis Lane Age 72

℞

Prednisone 1 mg tabs
Sig 4 tabs po qd for 2 days
then 3 tabs po qd
#18

Refills 0

Dr. Erin Thomas

5.15a

Dr. Arthur Halpern
22 North Ridge, New York, NY 88364
813-555-0444

Name Sean Nelson Date 10/31

Address 92 Ibis Lane Age 72

℞

1% Efudex cr 25 gm
apply q week —
carefully to
(L) lower eyelid —
upper cheek — Avoid
eye

Refills 0

Dr Arthur Halpern

5.15b

5.16	PT. NAME: **FRED BROWN**	GENDER: **M**	ADDRESS: **9 EAGLE RUN**	WEIGHT: **149**	HEIGHT: **5′ 4″**
	AGE: **62**	DX: **PROSTATE CA, HTN, OA, UTI**	ALLERGY: **NKA**	HX: **SMOKER, SOCIAL DRINKER**	

MEDICATION	SIG.	PRESCRIBER	ORIG. DATE	REFILL DATE	REFILL DATE	REFILL DATE	REFILL DATE
Cipro 500 mg #30	I bid × 7 d, then I qd	Weiss	8/30	9/24			
Proscar 5 mg #90	I daily	Weiss	9/12				
Oxybutynin 5 mg #180	I tab tid	Weiss	7/7	9/5			
Sonata 10 mg #30	I cap hs	Weiss	9/12	10/14			
Zestril 10 mg #90	I tab qd	Weiss	2/2	5/10	8/16		

Dr. Barry Weiss
901 Sheridan St., Austin, TX 90902
874-555-9000

Name Fred Brown Date 10/15

Address 9 Eagle Run Age 62

℞

Casodex 50 mg #120

Sig ī po qd

Refills 2

Dr. Barry Weiss

5.16a

Dr. Barry Weiss
901 Sheridan St., Austin, TX 90902
874-555-9000

Name Fred Brown Date 10/15

Address 9 Eagle Run Age 62

℞

Celebrex 200mg

ī po qd

#30

REFILL (1) - 2 - 3 - NR - PRN

Dr. Barry Weiss

5.16b

5.17 PT. NAME: **DAVID WAGNER** AGE: **24** GENDER: **M** DX: **HIV, NEUROPATHY, OPPORTUNISTIC INFECTIONS (OI)** ADDRESS: **145 NORTH AVE.** ALLERGY: **PCN** WEIGHT: **113** HX: **"PROMISCUOUS" LIFESTYLE** BMI: **19**

MEDICATION	SIG.	PRESCRIBER	ORIG. DATE	REFILL DATE	REFILL DATE	REFILL DATE	REFILL DATE
Combivir #C	1 bid, bkfst and dinner	Robins	9/30				
Sustiva 600 mg #50	1 hs	Robins	9/30				
Lidocaine Viscous 2% 100 mL	1 tsp S-S prn	Robins	9/2	9/20			
Diflucan 100 mg #30	2 today, then 1 daily	Robins	8/24	9/20			
Bactrim DS #30	1 tab qd	Robins	9/2				

Dr. Calvin Robins
7823 Tea Rose Trail, Miami, FL 44718
463-555-8000

Name David Wagner Date 10/10

Address 145 North Ave. Age 24

℞

Megace
240u
10a HS

Refills 3

Dr. Calvin Robins

5.17a

Dr. Calvin Robins
7823 Tea Rose Trail, Miami, FL 44718
463-555-8000

Name David Wagner Date 10/10

Address 145 North Ave. Age 24

℞

Neurontin 200
#20 → Refill for #60 pr
1 po qhs

LABEL

REFILL PRN TIMES

☐ NON-REPETATUR

Dr. Calvin Robins

5.17b

5.18

PT. NAME: **HARRY MORRIS**	GENDER: **M**	ADDRESS: **80 ALTON RD.**	WEIGHT: **166**	HEIGHT: **5′ 8″**
AGE: **59**	DX: **GENERALIZED MYASTHENIA GRAVIS, HTN, SEVERE PAIN**	ALLERGY: **PCN, ASA**	HX: **YEARS OF FEELING TIRED**	

MEDICATION	SIG.	PRESCRIBER	ORIG. DATE	REFILL DATE	REFILL DATE	REFILL DATE	REFILL DATE
Prednisone 5 mg #60	I daily	Renosik	1/15	3/18	5/11	7/14	
Pyridostigmine Br 60 mg tabs #90	I tid	Renosik	2/20	3/19	4/19	5/20	6/20
Avapro 150 mg #30	I daily	Feldman	1/8	2/7	4/2	6/1	7/7
Nucynta 75 mg #30	I q 6 h prn pain	Feldman	4/8				

Dr. Michael Renosik
44 Orange Drive, New York, NY 88364
813-555-9993

Name Harry Morris Date 7/17

Address 80 Alton Rd Age 59

℞

Imuran 50 mg tab

ʒ: iii tab / day

#100

NR

Dr. Michael Renosik

5.18a

Dr. Michael Renosik
44 Orange Drive, New York, NY 88364
813-555-9993

Name Harry Morris Date 7/17

Address 80 Alton Rd Age 59

℞

Tylenol #3

ii po q4h prn

sixty

NR

Dr. Michael Renosik

DEA # BR1234563

5.18b

5.19 PT. NAME: **MELINDA GRANOX** AGE: **67** GENDER: **F** DX: **BREAST CA, HTN, GERD, OSTEOPOROSIS** ADDRESS: **77 BAYVIEW DR.** ALLERGY: **NKA** WEIGHT: **133** HX: **SMOKER FOR 20 YEARS** BMI: **24**

MEDICATION	SIG.	PRESCRIBER	ORIG. DATE	REFILL DATE	REFILL DATE	REFILL DATE	REFILL DATE
Propranolol 20 mg #120	1 bid	Davis	4/9	6/8	8/4	9/1	
Triamterene/HCTZ 37.5/25 mg tabs #30	1 daily in am	Davis	3/6	4/8			
Dicyclomine 10 mg #50	1 bid prn	Davis	4/8	8/9			
Cartia XT 120 mg #30	1 daily	Davis	5/8	6/9	7/3	8/1	9/1
Diazepam 5 mg #12	1 tid prn	Davis	4/9				
Diazepam 5 mg #50	1 tid prn	Davis	4/29	5/18	6/10	7/26	8/20

Dr. John Davis
61 NW 5 Ave., Monterey, CA 38411
705-555-0202

Name Melinda Granox Date 9/4

Address 77 Bayview Dr. Age 67

℞

Arimidex 1 mg

1 tab i QD

#30

☐ Do Not Refill

☒ Refill 6 Times

Dr. John Davis

5.19a

Dr. John Davis
61 NW 5 Ave., Monterey, CA 38411
705-555-0202

Name Melinda Granox Date 9/4

Address 77 Bayview Dr. Age 67

℞

Zantac 150 mg po qid

#50 (fifty)

Refill 2 times

Dr. John Davis

5.19b

5.20

PT. NAME: **MARIO ARIOLA** GENDER: **M** ADDRESS: **8809 CROPSEY AVE.** WEIGHT: **171** HEIGHT: **5′ 6″**

AGE: **68** DX: **RA, UTI, DRY EYES, MUSCLE PAIN, ED** ALLERGY: **NKA**

MEDICATION	SIG.	PRESCRIBER	ORIG. DATE	REFILL DATE	REFILL DATE	REFILL DATE	REFILL DATE
Cipro 500 mg #20	I bid	Spencer	10/7	7/20			
Viagra 100 mg #5	I before intercourse	Beale	5/9	8/20	10/30		
Systane eye drops 30 mL	As directed for dry eyes	Halcombe	3/6	6/9	8/1		
Zostrix HP 0.075% cream 60 g	Apply qid	OTC	2/6	4/8	5/9	7/8	9/19
Tylenol arthritis caplets #150	I tid prn	OTC	2/6	6/19	8/30		

Dr. Gwen Spencer
7000 Utopia Parkway, Jamaica, NY 11439
343-555-2221

Name Mario Ariola Date 12/6

Address 8809 Cropsey Ave. Age 68

℞

ENTER...NAME AFTER Rx ON LABEL	MG/CC	QUAN
Rx 1 Prednisone 60 mg SIG. po QD	20 mg tabs	150
Rx 2 Cytoxan 100 mg po SIG. QD	50 mg tab	60
Rx 3 Compazine 10 mg SIG. po QID prn		30
Rx 4 Folic Acid 1 mg po SIG. QD		30

No Refills

Dr. Gwen Spencer

5.20a

Dr. Harvey Greco
5000 Utopia Parkway, Jamaica, NY 11439
343-555-9295

Name Mario Ariola Date 12/6

Address 8809 Cropsey Ave. Age 68

℞

Macrobid #10

Sig: i bid pc.

Refill 0 times

Dr. Harvey Greco

5.20b

5.21

PT. NAME: **MARY REILAND** GENDER: **F** ADDRESS: **11 CENTER ST.** WEIGHT: **140** BMI: **30**

AGE: **74** DX: **HTN, "SUNSPOTS" (AK), HEART RHYHTM DISTURBANCE** ALLERGY: **NKA** HX: **SUNBATHER**

MEDICATION	SIG.	PRESCRIBER	ORIG. DATE	REFILL DATE	REFILL DATE	REFILL DATE	REFILL DATE
Norvasc 5 mg #30	1 daily	Rue	8/12	9/10	10/4		
Avalide 150/12.5 #60	1 daily	Rue	2/15	4/10	6/16	8/11	10/2
Metoprolol 25 mg #30	1 daily	Rue	5/8	6/9	7/1	8/30	10/15
Coumadin 5 mg #30	1 daily	Rue	9/20	10/19			
St. John's wort 300 mg #50	1 tid	OTC	11/1				

Dr. Paul Sinclair
2100 Broadway, Kansas City, MO 64110
463-555-0630

Name Mary Reiland Date 11/2

Address 11 Center St. Age 74

℞

EFFUDEX CREAM 5% SMALL TUBE.

SIG: APPLY TO LESION B.I.D.

NR

Dr. Paul Sinclair

5.21a

Dr. Cheryl Rue
1234 Parkview Place, St. Louis, MO 63112
947-555-4441

Name Mary Reiland Date 11/3

Address 11 Center St. Age 74

℞

Toprol XL 50 mg

#30

Sig i QD

☐ LABEL

REFILL two TIMES PRN NR

Dr. Cheryl Rue

5.21b

5.22

PT. NAME: **MARTHA HAUSER**	GENDER: **F**	ADDRESS: **33 GRAY ST.**	WEIGHT: **121**	HEIGHT: **5′**
AGE: **61**	DX: **PSORIATIC ARTHRITIS, HTN, ELEVATED CHOLESTEROL, OSTEOPOROSIS, SEVERE PAIN**	ALLERGY: **NKA**	HX: **RETIRED, ACTIVE IN CHARITABLE ORGANIZATION**	

MEDICATION	SIG.	PRESCRIBER	ORIG. DATE	REFILL DATE	REFILL DATE	REFILL DATE	REFILL DATE
Hydrocodone-APAP 5/325 #60	1–2 q 4 h prn pain	Johnson	3/9	4/2	5/3	6/8	7/14
Furosemide 40 mg #90	1 q am	Samet	2/6	5/16			
Lisinopril 10 mg #90	1 q am	Samet	2/6	5/16			
Vitamin D 1000 IU #90	1 q am	Samet	2/6	5/16			
Lipitor 10 mg #90	1 hs	Samet	2/6	5/16			
Methotrexate 2.5 mg #40	10 tabs per week	Johnson	6/3	7/1			
Fosamax Plus D 70 mg + 2800 U #4	1 tab per week	Samet	3/3	4/3	5/5	6/2	7/1

Dr. James Johnson
9103 Highland Ave., Madison, WI 85845
999-383-5748

Name Martha Hauser Date 8/1

Address 33 Gray St. Age 61

℞

Methotrexate 2.5 mg
#40

SIG: DAILY (10 WEEKLY) AS DIRECTED TIMES PER DAY

LABEL

RENEW 1 – 2 – 3 – (4) – NR

DO NOT USE SAFETY CAP

Dr. James Johnson

5.22a

Dr. James Johnson
9103 Highland Ave., Madison, WI 85845
999-383-5748

Name Martha Hauser Date 8/1

Address 33 Gray St. Age 61

℞

Oxycontin
20 mg po q TID
#21

DO NOT USE SAFETY CAP

No Refills

Dr. James Johnson

DEA # BJ1234563

5.22b

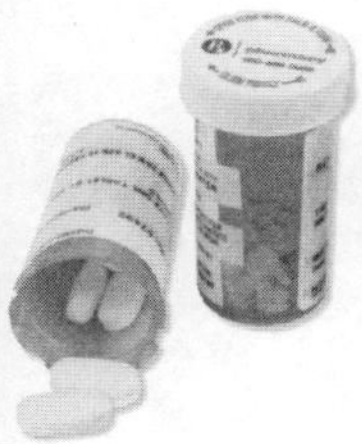

6 • GASTROENTEROLOGY

UPON COMPLETION OF THIS CHAPTER, THE STUDENT WILL BE ABLE TO:

- identify medication warnings associated with the use of certain drugs or drug classes in pregnant women.
- adjust the dose of certain renally excreted drugs (Zantac, Tagamet, etc.) by estimating the patient's renal function with the use of the formula for determining creatinine clearance.
- explain the mechanisms of action of the proton pump inhibitors and the histamine-2 receptor antagonists.
- explain the special counseling necessary for patients taking Tagamet and theophylline.
- counsel the patient on the different uses of histamine-2 receptor antagonists Rx, as well as OTC.
- explain pharmacologic differences between cimetidine and Cytotec.
- discuss the action of 5-aminosalicylic acid in the treatment of Crohn's disease and ulcerative colitis.
- describe the problems with substitution of various manufacturers' pancreatic enzyme products.

DRUG LIST

Amitiza
Azulfidine/Asacol/Asacol HD/Pentasa/Dipentum/Colazal/Lialda
Bentyl
Carafate
Compazine
Cytotec
Donnatal
Levsin
Librax
Lomotil
Pancreatic enzymes (Creon, Pancreaze, Ultrase MT, generic pancrelipase, etc.)
Pepcid
Prevacid/Prilosec/Aciphex/Nexium/Protonix/Zegerid/Dexilant
Reglan
Tagamet
Tigan
Zantac
Zofran/Kytril

• DRUG HOT POINTS

Amitiza
Increases intestinal fluid secretion
Stimulates bowel motility
Used for constipation predominant IBS
Used for chronic idiopathic constipation
Warning: diarrhea

Azulfidine (sulfasalazine)
Metabolites: 5-ASA and sulfapyridine
In lower Crohn's and ulcerative colitis, the 5-ASA (mesalamine) appears to be the active agent
5-ASA: 5-amino salicylic acid (not ASA)
Check for sulfa allergy, take with water
Compare with Asacol, Asacol HD, Dipentum, Pentasa, Colazal, and Lialda
Compare with Rowasa rectal suspension
Compare with Canasa suppositories

Bentyl
Take AC
Counsel male patients about urinary retention
Compare with Levsin for abdominal cramps

Carafate
Sucralfate: aluminum-sulfated sucrose
Protective layer at ulcer site (GI band-aid)
Take with water, AC
Separate from other drugs
Slurry: mix with water and swallow
Constipation warning
Also taken PC to coat the esophagus

Compazine
Phenothiazine indicated for nausea treatment
EPS potential
Suppositories, tablets, and injection
Compare with Zofran, Kytril
Tigan: moderately effective; DESI drug

Cytotec
Prostaglandin: increases GI mucus
Pregnancy warnings
Dispense with warning
No sharing of medications

Donnatal
Belladonna and phenobarbital
Anticholinergic cautions

Librax
Anticholinergic with benzodiazepine (chlordiazepoxide)
Cautions: driving, may be habit-forming
Caution: elderly men: BPH (↓ urine flow)

Lomotil (diphenoxylate with atropine sulfate)
C-V controlled drug
Narcotic: inhibits peristalsis
Atropine included to discourage abuse
Variable doses

Pancreatic enzymes (Creon, Pancreaze, Ultrase MT, generic pancrelipase, etc.)
Various formulations and contents
Variability in drug delivery
Substitution of products should be avoided

Pepcid
Blocks H_2 receptor on parietal cell
Advantages and disadvantages compared with antacids
Counseling on OTC form (Pepcid AC)
OTC combination with antacids (Pepcid Complete)

Prevacid/Prilosec
Shuts the proton pump in the parietal cell
Stops acid production
Dosing optimal: 30 minutes to 1 hour before breakfast or major meal of the day
Enteric-coated particles to protect the drug
Compare with Aciphex, Protonix, Nexium, and Dexilant
Compare with Zegerid (Rx and OTC)
Prilosec OTC: 20-mg tablets nonprescription
Prevacid 24-hr capsules nonprescription

Reglan
Useful in treating heartburn (GERD)
Stimulates peristalsis (GI prokinetic)
Indicated to treat diabetic gastroparesis
EPS side effects (dopamine blockade)
Double action: CTZ (antinausea) and GI tract
Take AC
Interaction with anticholinergic drugs when taken at the same time

• DRUG HOT POINTS (*continued*)

Tagamet
Frequent dosing
Antacid interaction (decreased absorption)
Inhibits metabolism of Coumadin and theophylline, increasing their effects
OTC: Tagamet HB 200 mg

Zantac
OTC is 75 mg and 150 mg, Rx is 150 mg and 300 mg
BID or HS (or 6 P.M.) dosing
Tablets, capsules, liquid, effervescent, etc.
Therapeutic vs. maintenance regimens
Adjust dose for elderly: estimate creatinine clearance with Cockroft & Gault formula
Compare with Pepcid (Rx and OTC)
Compare with Axid (Rx and OTC)

• QUESTIONS TO BE ANSWERED IN PREPARATION FOR CHAPTER 6 LAB

- Why is it important to dispense Cytotec in its original package?
- What is the role of misoprostol when it is prescribed with an NSAID?
- A person who is taking Donnatal as well as an OTC adrenergic receptor agonist, such as Sudafed (pseudoephedrine), may be at risk for experiencing a heart rhythm disturbance. Explain the mechanism of the disturbance, including the receptor(s) involved.
- If a patient takes 2 tsp QID of Donnatal Elixir, how many milligrams of phenobarbital did the patient receive in 1 day?
- Explain the reason why Bentyl is contraindicated in men who are using Hytrin, Cardura, Flomax, or Rapaflo for the treatment of BPH.
- What is the mechanism of action of Bentyl when treating spastic colon? The answer must mention the receptor that is involved.
- What is the name of the anticholinergic component and the benzodiazepine component in Librax?
- How many milligrams of narcotic are contained in each tablet of Lomotil?
- What is the purpose of the small amount of atropine sulfate contained in Lomotil?
- What are the side effects of atropine in an overdose?
- To which DEA schedule does Lomotil belong?
- Briefly explain the mechanism of action of Zantac and the other H_2 receptor blockers.
- Explain the mechanism and outcome of the interaction between Tagamet and Coumadin.
- How many milligrams of cimetidine are in each Tagamet HB tablet (OTC)?
- Explain what would happen if a Prilosec capsule was taken at the same time as an antacid product. Be specific regarding the capsule and contents.
- Concerning the proton pump, describe:
  - its function
  - its location
  - PPI mechanism of action
  - outcome of therapy
- What is the role of PPIs in risk reduction of NSAID-associated gastric ulcer?
- Briefly explain the mechanism of action of Reglan in the treatment of nausea and heartburn.
- Give the mechanism of action of Kytril and Zofran.
- Draw the structure of the active moiety of Azulfidine (as used in ulcerative colitis).
- Azulfidine may upset the stomach if taken in the same time frame as NSAIDs, including aspirin. Using the structure of Azulfidine as the basis for your answer, explain the nature of the interaction.
- What is the name of the sulfonamide component of the molecule of Azulfidine?
- Describe the difference or similarities in structural formulas between Azulfidine, Asacol, and Rowasa.
- Explain why Carafate should be taken before meals with water. Your answer must be based on the mechanism of action of Carafate.
- Focusing on the structural formula, explain the constipation that commonly occurs with the use of Carafate.
- A patient is experiencing tightness, or cramps, in the lower abdomen. The physician prescribes Levsin tablets 0.125 mg PO TID PRN. Which autonomic receptors are being affected? Is the drug acting as an agonist or as an antagonist at these receptors?
- Explain the mechanism of action of Amitiza.

• GASTROENTEROLOGY MEDICATION THERAPY MANAGEMENT QUESTIONS AND COMMENTS

- You are taking a medication for your intestinal condition. It is called Asacol HD. It is very important to keep taking it according to the doctor's instructions, even if you feel better.
- Your mother has been prescribed a new medication called Librax. She also takes another medication from another doctor called Donnatal. These two drugs are very similar. Taking both together might cause serious side effects. Would you mind waiting while I contact both offices to coordinate your mom's medications?
- Your doctor has prescribed a drug for nausea. It is Compazine. When you take it, please watch for any unusual movement disorders with your tongue, lips, or any other part of the body and report it to the doctor.
- The physician ordered your medication, a product that is called a proton pump inhibitor. It was written for one tablet daily. If the physician did not specify the time, this medication works best if it is taken a half to 1 hour before breakfast, or before the largest meal of the day if you do not have a regular breakfast.
- Your physician ordered famotidine and omeprazole. It is very important to remember that omeprazole must be taken early in the day, and famotidine to be taken later in the day. That way, both medications will work better.
- Your doctor ordered a medication for your stomach called Cytotec. It is extremely important that you do not share this medication with anyone else, especially with a woman who is pregnant or of childbearing age.
- I notice that you say that Tigan has not been as effective as you would like. There are other drugs for nausea that might be more appropriate for you. Would you mind if I contact the physician to discuss alternate medications?
- You have been taking Donnatal, as well as other medications, from your doctor for many years. This medication might interact with other drugs. Please contact your doctor to ask if we could discuss alternate medications that do not have these interactions.
- You have stated that since you have been taking Reglan, you have had serious diarrhea. Would it be okay with you if I contact the physician to discuss the problem and make recommendations for alternate medications?
- Your mother has been taking Reglan or metoclopramide for a few months, and now, I notice that when she is in the pharmacy, she appears to be chewing gum, even though there is no chewing gum in her mouth. I feel that it is urgent that we contact the prescriber to alert him or her to this potentially serious problem and discuss alternative therapy.
- I understand that you have been experiencing serious tiredness since you have started taking Reglan. Please allow me to contact your doctor to discuss this.
- You have been prescribed both Bentyl and Reglan by your doctor. Were you informed that these two medications should not be taken at the same time? They may not work if taken that way.
- You mention that your tablet medication called sucralfate is hard to swallow. I can call your doctor to recommend the liquid form or the tablets can be placed in a glass of water, mixed well with a spoon, and swallowed as a drink.
- You have said that your medication called Zegerid is not working to control heartburn. Are you taking it on an empty stomach, with lots of water? That will make it work best.

6.1

PT. NAME: **JENNIFER COOK**	GENDER: **F**	ADDRESS: **500 SE 2ND ST.**	WEIGHT: **138**	BMI: **27**
AGE: **38**	DX: **ULCERATIVE COLITIS**	ALLERGY: **NKA**	HX: **GI PROBLEMS SINCE YOUTH**	

MEDICATION	SIG.	PRESCRIBER	ORIG. DATE	REFILL DATE	REFILL DATE	REFILL DATE	REFILL DATE
Cipro 500 mg #28	I bid × 14 d	Gramling	6/10				
Flagyl 250 mg #90	I tid ud	Gramling	3/12	5/30	6/18		

Dr. Leo Gramling
300 Orange Ave., Fresno, CA 38411
705-555-6000

Name Jennifer Cook Date 6/20

Address 500 SE 2nd St. Age 38

℞

CANASA SUPP

Sig: i PR q HS

X 1 mos

Refills 4

Dr. L. Gramling

6.1a

Dr. Leo Gramling
300 Orange Ave., Fresno, CA 38411
705-555-6000

Name Jennifer Cook Date 6/20

Address 500 SE 2nd St. Age 38

℞

ASA COL 400 mg tab

Sig: iii po TID

X 1 mos

Refills 4

Dr. L. Gramling

6.1b

6.2

PT. NAME: **DON GREEN** AGE: **52**
GENDER: **M**
DX: **ULCERATIVE COLITIS, CHOLESTEROL, BPH, ALLERGIC RHINITIS**
ADDRESS: **654 IBIS CT.** ALLERGY: **NKA**
WEIGHT: **152** BMI: **28**

MEDICATION	SIG.	PRESCRIBER	ORIG. DATE	REFILL DATE	REFILL DATE	REFILL DATE	REFILL DATE
Flomax 0.4 mg #60	1 hs	Isaacs	1/27	3/6	4/19	5/6	
Asacol 400 mg #180	2 tid	Eisenberg	3/7	4/10	5/6		
Claritin 10 mg #20	1 qd	OTC	2/5	3/8			
Lipitor 10 mg #60	1 qd	Isaacs	3/3	4/2	5/3		

Dr. Howard Isaacs
1115 Turnaround Lane, Detroit, MI 64789
343-555-7000

Name Don Green Date 5/20

Address 654 Ibis Ct. Age 52

℞

Lomotil
Disp # 200
Sig: As directed

Refills 2

Dr. Howard Isaacs

DEA# AI1234563

6.2a

Dr. Marilyn Zoeller
45 Alabama Place, Detroit, MI 64789
343-555-7771

Name Don Green Date 5/18

Address 654 Ibis Ct. Age 52

℞

diphenoxylate 2mg tab
#100
Sig: as dir

N.R.

Dr. Marilyn Zoeller

DEA# AZ1234563

6.2b

6.3

PT. NAME: **JOHN JONES** AGE: **45**
GENDER: **M**
DX: **OA, GERD, NERVES, CONSTIPATION, DIARRHEA**
ADDRESS: **854 GREEN ST.**
ALLERGY: **SULFA, THIAZIDES, CODEINE, LASIX**
WEIGHT: **162**
HEIGHT: **5′ 8″**

MEDICATION	SIG.	PRESCRIBER	ORIG. DATE	REFILL DATE	REFILL DATE	REFILL DATE	REFILL DATE
Percocet 5/325 #C	1 tid prn	Keller	4/26				
Dulcolax Laxative tabs #C	1 hs	OTC	4/10	5/20	6/18		
Ativan 1 mg #50	1 bid prn	Keller	4/6	6/5			
Percocet 5/325 #C	1 tid prn	Keller	6/2				

Dr. Barry Weiss
901 Sheridan St., Austin, TX 90902
874-555-9000

Name John Jones Date 6/20

Address 854 Green St. Age 45

℞

Zantac 300 mg
#60
Sig: i tab h.s. daily

Refills 1

Dr. Barry Weiss

6.3a

Dr. Barry Weiss
901 Sheridan St., Austin, TX 90902
874-555-9000

Name John Jones Date 6/20

Address 854 Green St. Age 45

℞

Lomotil
Disp # 100
Take 1 qid PRN

Refills 1

Dr. Barry Weiss

DEA# AW1234563

6.3b

6.4

PT. NAME: **ELIZABETH MEYER**
AGE: **70**
GENDER: **F**
DX: **CA, HIGH TRIGLYCERIDES, DYSPEPSIA, CONSTIPATION, NAUSEA, VOMITING**
ADDRESS: **53 IRIS BLVD.**
ALLERGY: **NKA**
WEIGHT: **122**
HEIGHT: **5′ 3″**

MEDICATION	SIG.	PRESCRIBER	ORIG. DATE	REFILL DATE	REFILL DATE	REFILL DATE	REFILL DATE
Oxycontin 80 mg #60	I bid	Halloway	8/17				
Oxycodone 5 mg #60	I q 8 h prn pain	Halloway	7/25				
Lopid 600 mg #60	I bid	Isaacs	4/12	6/I	7/9	9/2	
Bisacodyl 5 mg #C	I hs	Halloway	8/30				
Oxycodone 5 mg #C	I q 8 h prn pain	Halloway	8/14				

Dr. Janet Halloway
4414 W Bridge Rd., San Francisco, CA 40001
154-555-8558

Name Elizabeth Meyer Date 9/4

Address 53 Iris Blvd. Age 70

℞ Compazine Supp 25mg
#15
Sig 1 Supp PR
q8h PRN

Refills 0

Dr. Janet Halloway

6.4a

Dr. Janet Halloway
4414 W Bridge Rd., San Francisco, CA 40001
154-555-8558

Name Elizabeth Meyer Date 9/4

Address 53 Iris Blvd. Age 70

℞ Pepcid 40mg
#30
Sig i p.o. q h.s.

☐ Label

Refill 3 times PRN NR

Dr. Janet Halloway

6.4b

6.5 PT. NAME: **MICHAEL BRYANT** AGE: **50** GENDER: **M** DX: **OA, HTN, GERD, ANXIETY, HIGH TRIGLYCERIDES** ADDRESS: **684 HURRICANE ALLEY** ALLERGY: **NKA** WEIGHT: **152** BMI: **28**

MEDICATION	SIG.	PRESCRIBER	ORIG. DATE	REFILL DATE	REFILL DATE	REFILL DATE	REFILL DATE
Monopril 10 mg #30	1 qd	Griffin	8/14	9/16	10/30		
Lopid 600 mg #60	1 bid	Griffin	6/20	7/26	8/17		
OTC Maalox Liquid 12 oz	5 mL prn	Griffin	5/12	5/20	6/30	8/12	
Mobic 7.5 mg #30	1 q am	Griffin	10/30				
Valium 5 mg #L	1 hs prn	Griffin	5/9	8/19	10/5		

Dr. Donna Johns
7000 SW 1st Ave., Santa Fe, NM 54545
766-555-9097

Name Michael Bryant Date 11/4

Address 684 Hurricane Alley Age 50

℞

Tagamet 200 mg #30
Sig: ī bid for and burning
or heartburn

Refills ad lib

Dr. Donna Johns

6.5a

Dr. Donna Johns
7000 SW 1st Ave., Santa Fe, NM 54545
766-555-9097

Name Michael Bryant Date 11/4

Address 684 Hurricane Alley Age 50

℞

Doxepin 25 mg
ī po q hs
#30

Refills 1

Dr. Donna Johns

6.5b

6.6

PT. NAME: **LINDA RIVERA**	GENDER: **F**	ADDRESS: **1984 GREEN ST.**	WEIGHT: **230**	BMI: **31**
AGE: **52**	DX: **PUD, GERD, SKIN FUNGUS, NAUSEA**	ALLERGY: **SULFA**	HX: **SMOKER, SOCIAL DRINKER**	

MEDICATION	SIG.	PRESCRIBER	ORIG. DATE	REFILL DATE	REFILL DATE	REFILL DATE	REFILL DATE
Zantac 150 mg #90	1 bid	Connell	4/12	6/20			
Librax #90	1 hs	Connell	4/12	6/20			
Pepto Bismol 8 oz	30 mL (2 tbs) prn	OTC	3/12	5/20	6/14		
Nizoral Cream 30 g	Apply prn itch	Capland	5/1				

Dr. Tim Connel
122 S. Joyce St., Arlington, VA 98887
247-555-9911

Name Linda Rivera Date 7/20

Address 1984 Green St. Age 52

℞

Donnatal

#C

Sig: 1/2 ac & hs prn

Refills 3

Dr. Tim Connell

6.6a

Dr. Tim Connel
122 S. Joyce St., Arlington, VA 98887
247-555-9911

Name Linda Rivera Date 7/20

Address 1984 Green St. Age 52

℞

Compazine Supps 25mg

i supp pr q 8h prn

#10

Refills 3

Dr. Tim Connell

6.6b

6.7	PT. NAME: **MARK OLSON**	GENDER: **M**	ADDRESS: **774 FANTASTIC ST.**	WEIGHT: **188**	BMI: **29**
	AGE: **28**	DX: **IBS, NERVES, GERD, ABDOMINAL CRAMPS**	ALLERGY: **NKA**	HX: **HYPERACTIVE, SALESMAN**	

MEDICATION	SIG.	PRESCRIBER	ORIG. DATE	REFILL DATE	REFILL DATE	REFILL DATE	REFILL DATE
Claritin 10 mg #20	1 qd	Keller	4/12	6/19			
Diazepam 5 mg #60	1 bid prn	Yountz	3/15	6/24			
Reglan 5 mg #90	1 tid ac	Yountz	5/12	6/1	6/16	7/1	
Kaopectate 12 oz	30 mL tid	OTC	5/15	5/30	6/13	6/28	

Dr. Daniel Keller
5007 Turtle Drive, Miami, FL 98887
247-555-9876

Name Mark Olson Date 7/12

Address 774 Fantastic St. Age 28

℞

Bentyl 20mg
#100
Sig: i tab QID (a.c. & h.s.)

Refills prn

Dr. Daniel Keller

6.7a

Dr. Doris White
38 Turtle Drive, Miami, FL 98887
247-555-1000

Name Mark Olson Date 7/11

Address 774 Fantastic St. Age 28

℞

VALium 5mg
#30 (Thirty)
Sig: i p.o. q h.s. prn

REFILL ...Ø... TIMES

Dr. Doris White

6.7b

6.8 PT. NAME: **LISA MILLER** AGE: **62** GENDER: **F** DX: **HTN, HEARTBURN, DANDRUFF, BACK PAIN** ADDRESS: **522 ELEPHANT DR.** ALLERGY: **NKA** WEIGHT: **144** HEIGHT: **5′ 2″**

MEDICATION	SIG.	PRESCRIBER	ORIG. DATE	REFILL DATE	REFILL DATE	REFILL DATE	REFILL DATE
Nizoral Shampoo 2% 120 mL	Use prn	Daniels	5/18	7/26			
Atenolol 50 mg #30	1 qd	Griffin	10/11				
Anacin tabs #C	1 prn	OTC	6/4	6/20	7/18	8/22	9/30

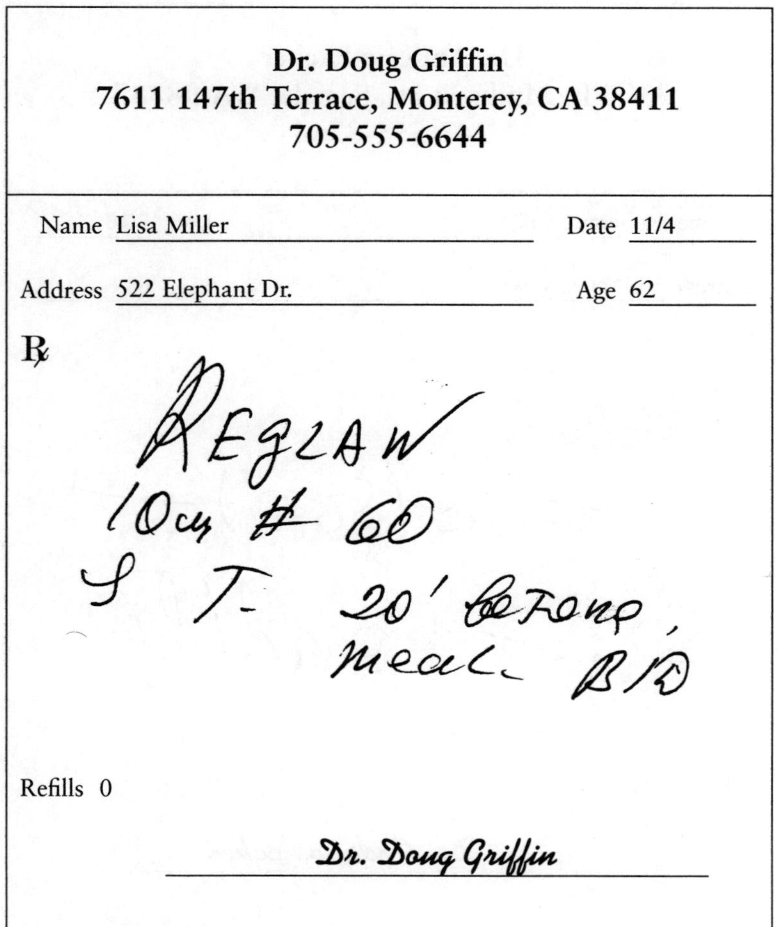

Dr. Doug Griffin
7611 147th Terrace, Monterey, CA 38411
705-555-6644

Name Lisa Miller Date 11/4

Address 522 Elephant Dr. Age 62

℞

Reglan
10mg #60
Sig T 20′ before
meal BID

Refills 0

Dr. Doug Griffin

6.8a

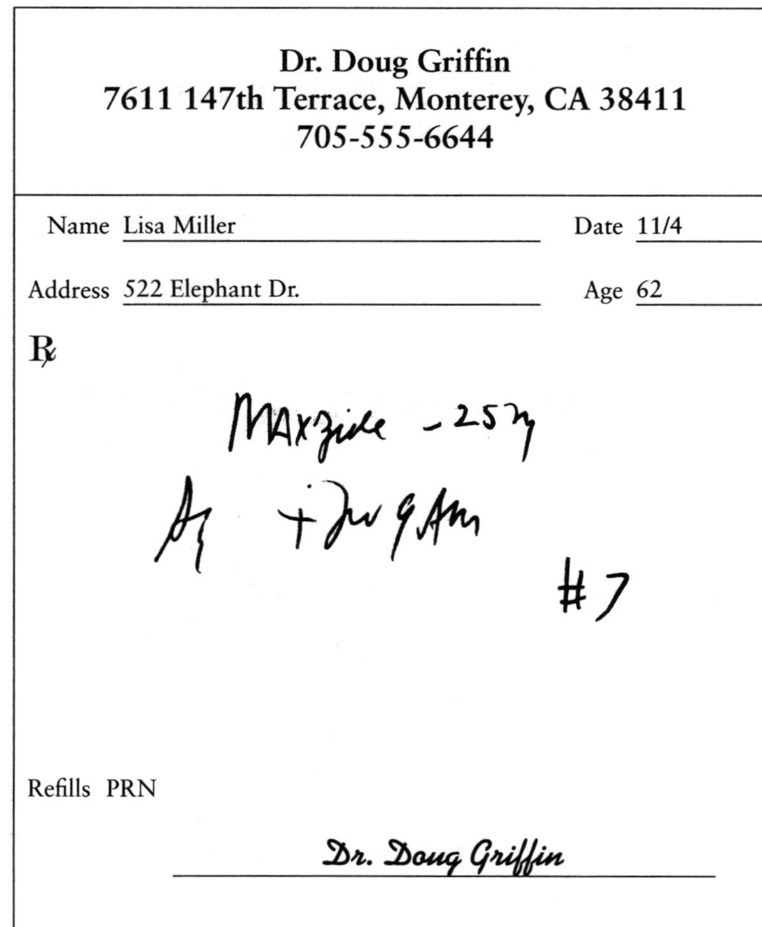

Dr. Doug Griffin
7611 147th Terrace, Monterey, CA 38411
705-555-6644

Name Lisa Miller Date 11/4

Address 522 Elephant Dr. Age 62

℞

Maxzide -25mg
Sig i po q AM
#7

Refills PRN

Dr. Doug Griffin

6.8b

6.9

PT. NAME: **ROBERTA COOK**	GENDER: **F**	ADDRESS: **333 OLIVE WAY**	WEIGHT: **225**	BMI: **34**
AGE: **63**	DX: **GERD, COPD, NAUSEA, INSOMNIA, ABDOMINAL CRAMPS**	ALLERGY: **NKA**	HX: **HEAVY SMOKER (75 PACK-YEARS: 1.5 PACKS/DAY FOR 50 YEARS)**	

MEDICATION	SIG.	PRESCRIBER	ORIG. DATE	REFILL DATE	REFILL DATE	REFILL DATE	REFILL DATE
Advair Diskus 250/50 mcg #60	Use bid	Eisen	2/10	4/5	6/12		
Restoril 15 mg #10	1 hs	Eisen	4/6	6/4	8/14		
Pepcid AC 10 mg #60	1 bid prn acid	OTC	4/6	5/3	6/6	7/9	8/8

Dr. John Wallington
2100 E. Madison St., Seattle, WA 98887
247-555-9000

Name Roberta Cook Date 8/20

Address 333 Olive Way Age 63

℞

Tigan Caps, 300 mg
#15
Label: 1 cap po tid a.c
prn nausea or
vomiting

Refills x 1

Dr. John Wallington

6.9a

Dr. Andrew Packer
3300 E. Madison St., Seattle, WA 98887
247-555-8764

Name Roberta Cook Date 8/10

Address 333 Olive Way Age 63

℞

Librax
#60 (Sixty) —
Sig: i po qd/PRN

Refills ad lib

Dr. Andrew Packer

6.9b

6.10

PT. NAME: **MARY MCCOY** AGE: **38**
GENDER: **F**
DX: **DYSPEPSIA, VERY ANXIOUS, SPASTIC COLON, PANCREATIC INSUFFICIENCY**
ADDRESS: **71 CAPITOL AVE.**
ALLERGY: **ASA**
WEIGHT: **105**
HX: **NERVOUS FOR YEARS**
HEIGHT: **5′ 3″**

MEDICATION	SIG.	PRESCRIBER	ORIG. DATE	REFILL DATE	REFILL DATE	REFILL DATE	REFILL DATE
Creon 12,000 U capsules #C	1 cap tid during meals	Johns	1/6	2/4			

Dr. Donna Johns
7000 SW 1st Ave., Santa Fe, NM 54545
766-555-9097

Name Mary McCoy Date 2/20

Address 71 Capitol Ave. Age 38

℞

Carafate 1gm
#100
T po QID (½° AC + HS)

Refill 6 times

Dr. Donna Johns

6.10a

Dr. Donna Johns
7000 SW 1st Ave., Santa Fe, NM 54545
766-555-9097

Name Mary McCoy Date 2/20

Address 71 Capitol Ave. Age 38

℞

1) Vistaril 25mg #100 ī q TID
2) Bentyl 10mg #100 ī q TID

Refill 3 times

Dr. Donna Johns

6.10b

6.11

PT. NAME: **TIMOTHY BLACK**	GENDER: **M**	ADDRESS: **555 TULANE AVE.**	WEIGHT: **189**	HEIGHT: **5′ 10″**
AGE: **48**	DX: **OA, TYPE 2 DM, HEARTBURN, STOMACH CRAMPS, DIARRHEA**	ALLERGY: **NKA**	HX: **SMOKER, ETOH**	

MEDICATION	SIG.	PRESCRIBER	ORIG. DATE	REFILL DATE	REFILL DATE	REFILL DATE	REFILL DATE
Ecotrin 325 mg #C	I prn pain	OTC	1/20	2/1	4/15		
Surfak 240 mg #C	I hs	Brown	1/12				
Zantac 150 mg #60	I bid	Brown	2/12	3/10	4/15		
Metformin 850 mg #C	I tid	Brown	1/15	2/18	3/20	4/19	5/17
Imodium A–D caplets #24	I bid	OTC	1/20	2/10	2/25	3/15	4/31

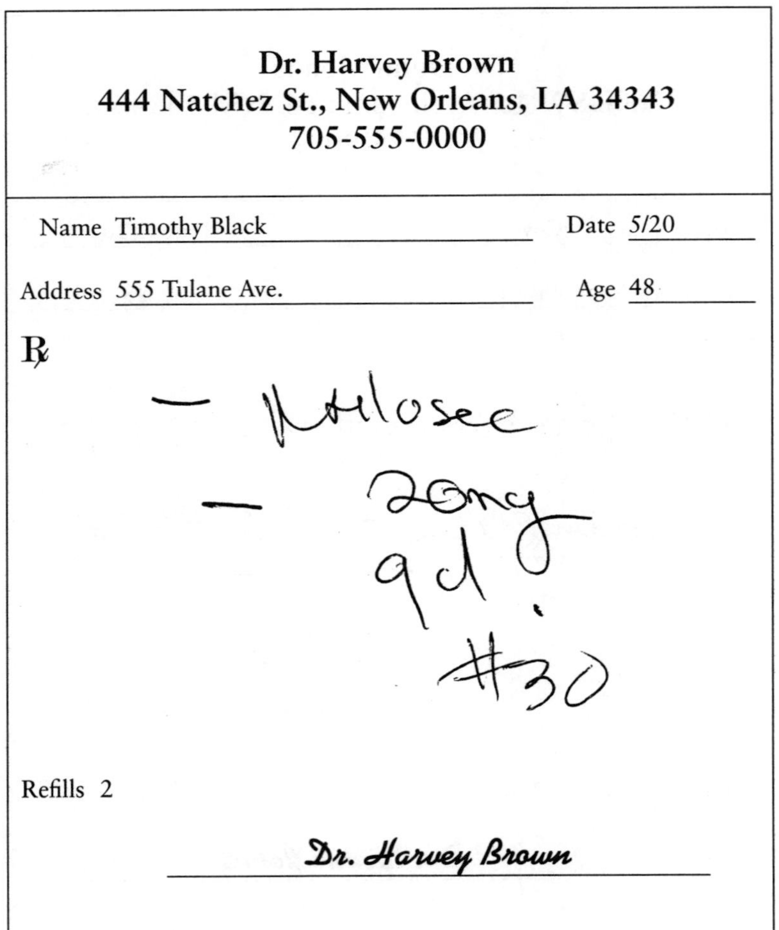

Dr. Harvey Brown
444 Natchez St., New Orleans, LA 34343
705-555-0000

Name Timothy Black Date 5/20

Address 555 Tulane Ave. Age 48

℞

Prilosec
20mg
qd
#30

Refills 2

Dr. Harvey Brown

6.11a

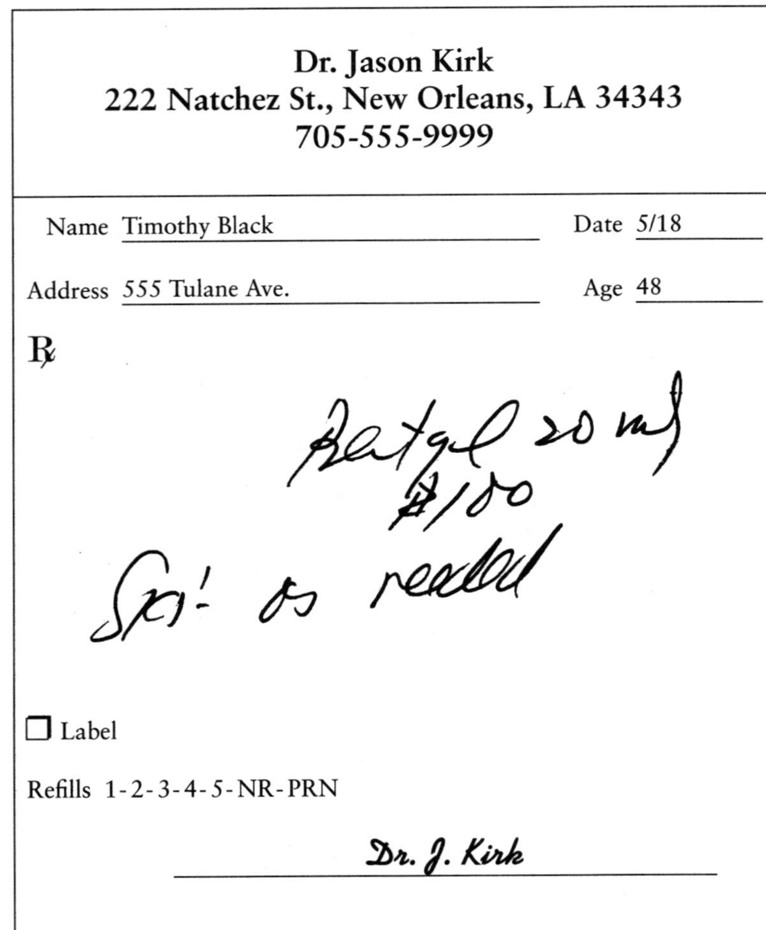

Dr. Jason Kirk
222 Natchez St., New Orleans, LA 34343
705-555-9999

Name Timothy Black Date 5/18

Address 555 Tulane Ave. Age 48

℞

Ratgel 20 ml
#100
Sig: as needed

❐ Label

Refills 1-2-3-4-5-NR-PRN

Dr. J. Kirk

6.11b

6.12

PT. NAME: **SUSAN HANSEN**	GENDER: **F**	ADDRESS: **224 ALBERTY CIR.**	WEIGHT: **126**	HEIGHT: **5′ 2″**
AGE: **64**	DX: **UC, HYPOTHYROID, HTN**	ALLERGY: **SULFA**	NOTE: ASK ABOUT THYROID MEDICATIONS	

MEDICATION	SIG.	PRESCRIBER	ORIG. DATE	REFILL DATE	REFILL DATE	REFILL DATE	REFILL DATE
Prednisone 10 mg #50	4 qd ud	Zoeller	8/23	11/18			
Colyte with Flavor Packs 4000 mL	Use ud	Zoeller	7/26				

Dr. Howard Isaacs
1115 Turnaround Lane, Detroit, MI 64789
343-555-7000

Name Susan Hansen Date 11/23

Address 224 Alberty Cir. Age 64

℞

Donnatal tab #50
Sig: i tid ac

Refills 2

Dr. Howard Isaacs

6.12a

Dr. Marilyn Zoeller
45 Alabama Place, Detroit, MI 64789
343-555-7771

Name Susan Hansen Date 11/23

Address 224 Alberty Cir. Age 64

℞

① ~~Rowasa enema #14 i qhs~~
② Canasa suppos #24 i qd AM

Refills 2

Dr. Marilyn Zoeller

6.12b

6.13

PT. NAME: **SHARON DAVIS** | GENDER: **F** | ADDRESS: **14 HALL ST.** | WEIGHT: **190** | BMI: **24**

AGE: **64** | DX: **HTN, GERD, TYPE 2 DM, FUNGAL SKIN INFECTION, ACUTE SINUS INFECTION** | ALLERGY: **NKA**

MEDICATION	SIG.	PRESCRIBER	ORIG. DATE	REFILL DATE	REFILL DATE	REFILL DATE	REFILL DATE
Nizoral Cream 15 g	Apply bid	Isaacs	9/26	10/20			
Cipro 500 mg #20	1 bid	Green	11/16				
Amaryl 4 mg #30	1 qd	Green	8/11	9/10	10/10	11/11	
Sudafed 30 mg #24	1 tid for sinus and drip	OTC	4/6	5/7	7/5	10/9	
Capoten 25 mg #60	1 bid	Green	8/11	10/6			

Dr. Donna Johns
7000 SW 1st Ave., Santa Fe, NM 54545
766-555-9097

Name Sharon Davis Date 11/20

Address 14 Hall St. Age 64

℞

Aciphex 20mg
#30
Sig: i daily

Refills 3

Dr. Donna Johns

6.13a

Dr. Ira Greene
2000 W. 8 Ave., Santa Fe, NM 54545
766-555-1230

Name Sharon Davis Date 11/19

Address 14 Hall St. Age 64

℞

GLUCOPHAGE
500mg # 90
1 TID c̄ Food

Refills 2

Dr. Ira Greene

6.13b

6.14

PT. NAME: **CHARLES SMITH** AGE: **42** GENDER: **M** DX: **IBS, OA** ADDRESS: **33 W BOOTH ST.** ALLERGY: **PCN** WEIGHT: **245** HX: **CONSTRUCTION WORKER, BAD DIET** HEIGHT: **6′** BMI: **33**

MEDICATION	SIG.	PRESCRIBER	ORIG. DATE	REFILL DATE	REFILL DATE	REFILL DATE	REFILL DATE
Percocet 5/325 #30	1 q 4 h prn	Keller	8/16				
Percocet 5/325 #30	1 q 4–6 h prn	Keller	10/20				
Ultram 50 mg #C	1 q 6 h prn	Keller	5/20	7/22	8/29		
Bufferin tabs #130	2 prn pain	OTC	2/22	4/16	7/30		
APAP 500 mg #250	1–2 prn pain	OTC	2/20	5/5			

Dr. Frank Crosby
555 Pino Rd., Santa Fe, NM 33999
247-555-9777

Name Charles Smith Date 11/16

Address 33 W Booth St. Age 42

℞

Levsin/SL
Disp #30
Sig: i–ii tabs sublingually q 4°, max 12 daily for IBS

Refills 3

Dr. Frank Crosby

6.14a

Dr. Harris Akra
858 Pino Rd., Santa Fe, NM 33999
247-888-6666

Name Charles Smith Date 11/14

Address 33 W Booth St. Age 42

℞

Donnatal Liquid
5–10cc c̄ 30cc Mylanta
prn Disp: 8oz

☐ Label

Refills 1 Times PRN NR

Dr. Harris Akra

6.14b

6.15

PT. NAME: **ANDREA KELLY** GENDER: **F** ADDRESS: **474 HURRICANE ALLEY** WEIGHT: **158** HEIGHT: **5′ 9″**

AGE: **41** DX: **DYSPEPSIA, OA, MIGRAINES, ABDOMINAL CRAMPS** ALLERGY: **NKA** HX: **ETOH, LIKES CHINESE FOOD**

MEDICATION	SIG.	PRESCRIBER	ORIG. DATE	REFILL DATE	REFILL DATE	REFILL DATE	REFILL DATE
Fioricet #30	1 q 4–6 h prn	Griffin	11/7	11/14	11/22		
Xanax 0.5 mg	1/2 tab tid prn	Griffin	8/4	9/20	11/18		
Prevacid 30 mg #30	1 qd	Griffin	11/7				
ASA 5 grains (325 mg) #250	1–2 prn HA	OTC	5/12	8/30	12/1		

Dr. Doug Griffin
7611 147th Terrace, Monterey, CA 38411
705-555-6644

Name Andrea Kelly Date 12/2

Address 474 Hurricane Alley Age 41

℞

Prilosec
#XXX
Sig: one daily

Refills 5

Dr. Doug Griffin

6.15a

Dr. Doug Griffin
7611 147th Terrace, Monterey, CA 38411
705-555-6644

Name Andrea Kelly Date 12/2

Address 474 Hurricane Alley Age 41

℞

Levsin 0.125 mg
twenty
Sig ii q 4 prn for colicky pain

☑ Label

Refill N/C times PRN NR

Dr. Doug Griffin

6.15b

6.16

PT. NAME: **KEITH JOHNSON** | GENDER: **M** | ADDRESS: **92 IBIS LANE** | WEIGHT: **150** | BMI: **23**
AGE: **42** | DX: **CROHN'S DISEASE, ALLERGIES, NERVES** | ALLERGY: **NKA**

MEDICATION	SIG.	PRESCRIBER	ORIG. DATE	REFILL DATE	REFILL DATE	REFILL DATE	REFILL DATE
Zyrtec 10 mg #30	1 prn qd	Isaacs	2/29	7/11	8/11		
Lorazepam 1 mg #90	1 q 8 h prn	Isaacs	7/11	8/11	11/9		
Azulfidine 500 mg #90	1 tid	Isaacs	8/12	9/13	10/9	11/11	

Dr. Howard Isaacs
1115 Turnaround Lane, Detroit, MI 64789
343-555-7000

Name Keith Johnson Date 11/12

Address 92 Ibis Lane Age 42

℞

Purinethol (6-MP) 50mg
Disp #50
Sig: i qd

Call for Refills

Dr. Howard Isaacs

6.16a

Dr. Howard Isaacs
1115 Turnaround Lane, Detroit, MI 64789
343-555-7000

Name Keith Johnson Date 11/12

Address 92 Ibis Lane Age 42

℞

PEPSID 20mg #60
i DAILY

Call for Refills

Dr. Howard Isaacs

6.16b

6.17

PT. NAME: **BRIAN CARLSON**	GENDER: **M**	ADDRESS: **9 EAGLE RUN**	WEIGHT: **144**	HEIGHT: **5′ 4″**
AGE: **68**	DX: **OA, GERD, IBS, CHOLESTEROL**	ALLERGY: **NKA**	HX: **STOCKBROKER, HIGH-STRUNG**	

MEDICATION	SIG.	PRESCRIBER	ORIG. DATE	REFILL DATE	REFILL DATE	REFILL DATE	REFILL DATE
Pravachol 20 mg #30	I qd	Robins	1/3	2/1	3/6	4/4	
Percocet 2.5/325 #C	I qid prn	Green	8/29				
Librax #60	I cap bid	Robins	7/22	9/12			

Dr. Calvin Robins
7823 Tea Rose Trail, Miami, FL 44718
463-555-8000

Name Brian Carlson Date 9/15

Address 9 Eagle Run Age 68

℞

Lomotil 2.5mg
#30
Sig tabs II qid for diarrhea

Refills 0

Dr. Calvin Robins

6.17a

Dr. Calvin Robins
7823 Tea Rose Trail, Miami, FL 44718
463-555-8000

Name Brian Carlson Date 9/15

Address 9 Eagle Run Age 68

℞

Prilosec 20 T qd #30

REPEAT / TIMES

N.R.______________

Dr. Calvin Robins

6.17b

6.18

PT. NAME: **BRIAN MARTIN** AGE: **42** | GENDER: **M** DX: **PUD, IBS, HYPOTHYROID** | ADDRESS: **3975 BLACK DR.** ALLERGY: **NKA** | WEIGHT: **179** HX: **DYSPEPTIC SINCE CHILDHOOD** | BMI: **31**

MEDICATION	SIG.	PRESCRIBER	ORIG. DATE	REFILL DATE	REFILL DATE	REFILL DATE	REFILL DATE
Xanax 0.25 mg #50	1 bid prn	Thomas	9/22	11/15			
Maalox susp. 12 oz	2 tbs prn	OTC	8/12	9/23	10/15	11/15	
Synthroid 0.1 mg #90	1 q am	Thomas	4/1	7/5	10/8		

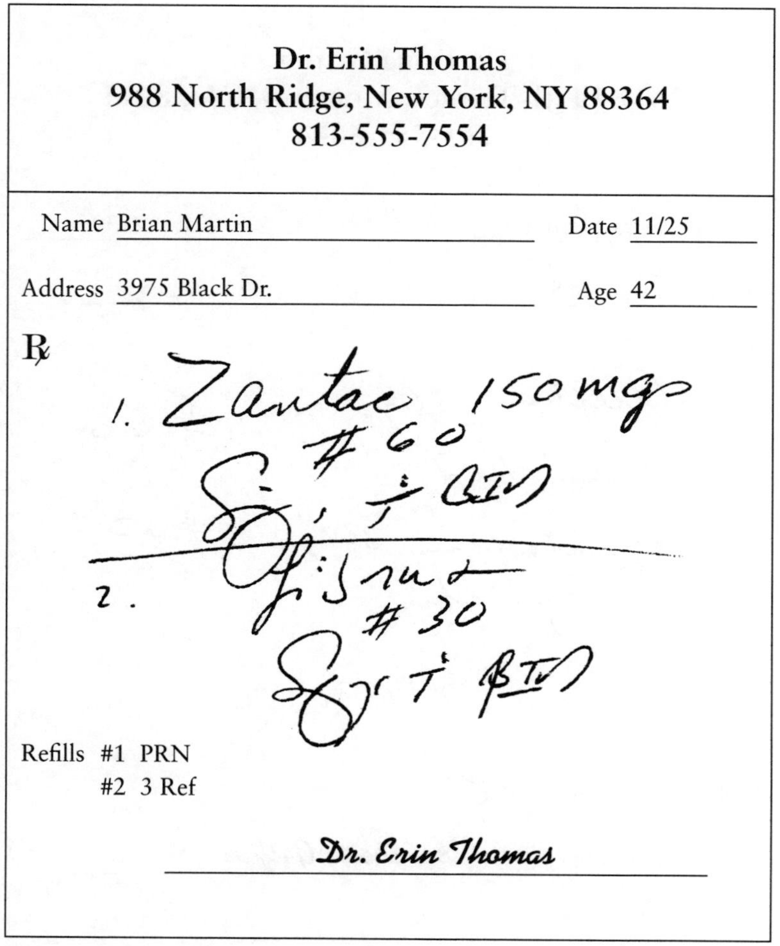
Dr. Erin Thomas
988 North Ridge, New York, NY 88364
813-555-7554

Name Brian Martin Date 11/25
Address 3975 Black Dr. Age 42

℞
1. Zantac 150 mgs #60 Sig: i QID
2. [illegible] #30 Sig: i BID

Refills #1 PRN
#2 3 Ref

Dr. Erin Thomas

6.18a

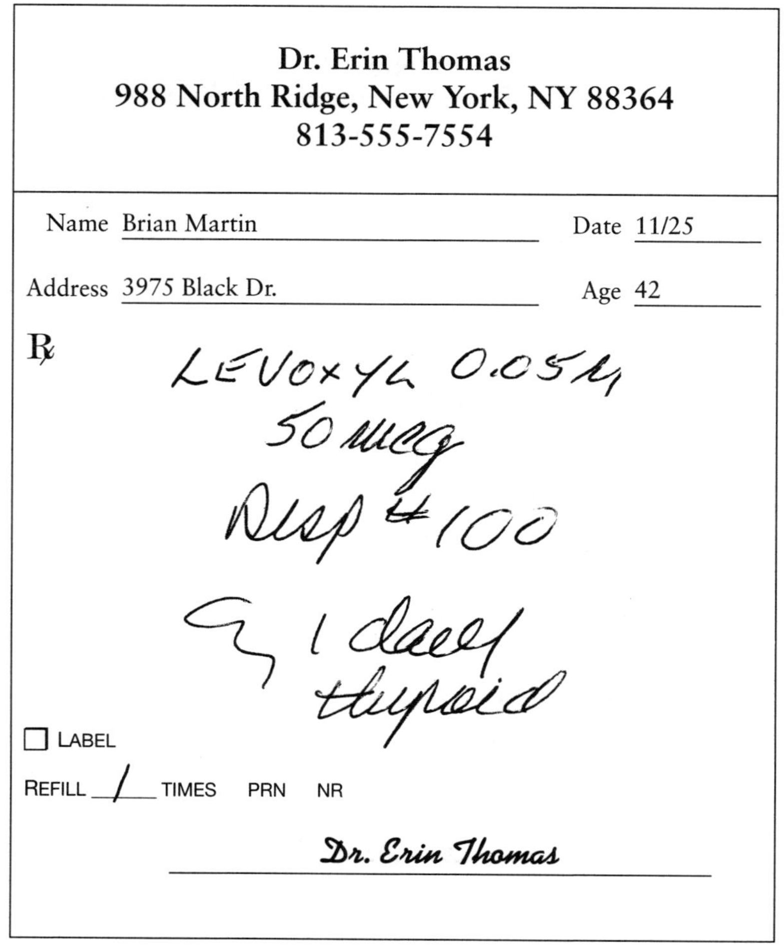
Dr. Erin Thomas
988 North Ridge, New York, NY 88364
813-555-7554

Name Brian Martin Date 11/25
Address 3975 Black Dr. Age 42

℞
LEVOXYL 0.05 mg 50 mcg
Disp #100
Sig: 1 daily thyroid

☐ LABEL
REFILL 1 TIMES PRN NR

Dr. Erin Thomas

6.18b

6.19

PT. NAME: **ERICA MARTINEZ** GENDER: **F** ADDRESS: **61 GREEN ST.** WEIGHT: **122** BMI: **21**

AGE: **53** DX: **LOWER CROHN'S, IBS, ACNE VULGARIS, HEARTBURN** ALLERGY: **PCN** HX: **SURGICAL RESECTION OF INTESTINES**

MEDICATION	SIG.	PRESCRIBER	ORIG. DATE	REFILL DATE	REFILL DATE	REFILL DATE	REFILL DATE
Prednisone 5 mg #30	Take ud	Griffin	8/30	10/18			
Retin-A Microgel 0.04% 45 g	Apply ud	Eisenberg	6/21	10/20			

Dr. Doug Griffin
7611 147th Terrace, Monterey, CA 38411
705-555-6644

Name Erica Martinez Date 10/30

Address 61 Green St. Age 53

℞

Asacol 400 mg
#
Sig: iiii po tid

Bentyl 10 mg
#60
Sig: i po q6° prn

Refills 2

Dr. Doug Griffin

6.19a

Dr. Doug Griffin
7611 147th Terrace, Monterey, CA 38411
705-555-6644

Name Erica Martinez Date 10/30

Address 61 Green St. Age 53

℞

Aciphex 20 mg #60
i po bid
Ranitidine 300 mg #30
i po qhs

LABEL

REFILL 1 - 2 - 3 - 4 - 5 - NR - PRN (circled)

Dr. Doug Griffin

6.19b

6.20

PT. NAME: **MICHAEL MARTINS** GENDER: **M** ADDRESS: **500 SE 2ND ST.** WEIGHT: **159** BMI: **26**
AGE: **62** DX: **THYROID, OA, GERD, CONSTIPATION, BACTERIAL INFECTION** ALLERGY: **NKA**

MEDICATION	SIG.	PRESCRIBER	ORIG. DATE	REFILL DATE	REFILL DATE	REFILL DATE	REFILL DATE
Synthroid 0.1 mg #90	1 qd	Sauls	8/7				
Ibuprofen 800 mg #30	1 q 6–8 h prn pain	Sauls	10/20				
Amoxicillin 500 mg #21	1 q 8 h	Green	11/2				
Prilosec 20 mg #30	1 bid	Sauls	9/15	10/1			
Zantac 300 mg #50	1 hs	Sauls	9/15				

Dr. Alfred Sauls
151212 S. High Rd., Chicago, IL 23875
954-555-1300

Name Michael Martins Date 11/30

Address 500 SE 2nd St. Age 62

℞

Reglan 10 mg tab
one P.O. Q 6 hrs P.R.N.

30

Refills 1

Dr. Alfred Sauls

6.20a

Dr. Alfred Sauls
151212 S. High Rd., Chicago, IL 23875
954-555-1300

Name Michael Martins Date 11/30

Address 500 SE 2nd St. Age 62

℞

Protonix 40 mg
#30
Sig: i po QD

Refills 1

Dr. Alfred Sauls

6.20b

6.21

PT. NAME: **CHERYL ABBEY** AGE: **68**
GENDER: **F** DX: **DYSPEPSIA, HTN, TYPE 2 DM, VERTIGO, HIGH CHOLESTEROL, DEPRESSION**
ADDRESS: **99 GOLD ST.** ALLERGY: **NKA**
WEIGHT: **146** HX: **FORMER SMOKER**
HEIGHT: **5′ 7″**

MEDICATION	SIG.	PRESCRIBER	ORIG. DATE	REFILL DATE	REFILL DATE	REFILL DATE	REFILL DATE
Lipitor 10 mg #30	1 qd	Maxson	3/5	4/3	5/4	6/5	7/5
Metformin 500 mg #60	1 bid	Maxson	6/1	7/5			
Januvia 100 mg #30	1 qd	Maxson	7/1				
Bupropion HCl SR 150 mg #30	1 bid	Drachman	5/2	6/1	7/1		

Dr. Mark Green
200 Peach Ave., Fresno, CA 38411
705-555-9944

Name Cheryl Abbey Date 7/15

Address 99 Gold St. Age 68

℞

Nexium 40 mg
T po daily
#30

☐ LABEL

REFILL 8 TIMES PRN NR

Dr. Mark Green

6.21a

Dr. Agnes Maxson
100 Peach Ave., Fresno, CA 38411
705-555-0971

Name Cheryl Abbey Date 7/15

Address 99 Gold St. Age 68

℞

Norvasc 2.5 mg
#60
1 tab daily

Refills 4

Dr. Agnes Maxson

6.21b

6.22

PT. NAME: **IRENE PRINCE** | GENDER: **F** | ADDRESS: **22 NE 4TH AVE.** | WEIGHT: **139** | HEIGHT: **5′ 4″**

AGE: **52** | DX: **NERVOUS, IBS, DIARRHEA, INSOMNIA** | ALLERGY: **PCN, ASA** | HX: **HIGH-STRUNG**

MEDICATION	SIG.	PRESCRIBER	ORIG. DATE	REFILL DATE	REFILL DATE	REFILL DATE	REFILL DATE
Restoril 7.5 mg #30	1 hs	Kovack	6/21				
Protonix 40 mg #30	1 tab 30 min ac bkfst	Kovack	6/21				
Hyoscyamine 0.375 mg ER tabs #30	1 prn spasm	Kovack	4/5	5/3	6/1		

Dr. Drew Kovack
90 Brighton Lane, Detroit, MI 64789
343-555-8810

Name Irene Prince Date 7/7

Address 22 NE 4 Ave. Age 52

℞

lomotil
#50
1 tablet po q4-6h
prn

Refills 5

Dr. Drew Kovack

6.22a

Dr. Drew Kovack
90 Brighton Lane, Detroit, MI 64789
343-555-8810

Name Irene Prince Date 7/7

Address 22 NE 4 Ave. Age 52

℞

LibRAX
#25
i BID

NR

Dr. Drew Kovack

DEA# AK 1234563

6.22b

6.23

PT. NAME: **SUSAN TOONKEL** GENDER: **F** ADDRESS: **10 GREEN ST.** WEIGHT: **122** HEIGHT: **5′ 1″**

AGE: **55** DX: **NERVES, PUD, DIARRHEA, URI, FACE SURGERY** ALLERGY: **LASIX, CODEINE**

MEDICATION	SIG.	PRESCRIBER	ORIG. DATE	REFILL DATE	REFILL DATE	REFILL DATE	REFILL DATE
Ambien 10 mg #30	1 hs	Lien	7/9	8/9	9/8		
Z-Pak	Take ud	Lien	8/1				
Lomotil #18	1–2 tid prn diarrhea	Lien	8/9				
Tobradex eye drops 5 mL	1 drop in od tid	Tenzer	6/9				
Atarax 25 mg #60	1 bid	Lien	8/17				

Dr. Horace Baumberg
4 Sheridan St., Austin, TX 90902
874-555-0022

Name Susan Toonkel Date 9/9

Address 10 Green St. Age 55

℞

Zofran ODT 8mg
#2 (two)
Sig: Take 2 tabs
1 hour prior
surgery let
dissolve on tongue

Medrol dose
pack Take
as directed

Dr. Horace Baumberg

6.23a

Dr. Horace Baumberg
4 Sheridan St., Austin, TX 90902
874-555-0022

Name Susan Toonkel Date 9/9

Address 10 Green St. Age 55

℞

Prilosec 20 mg
60
1 tab daily

Refills 1

Dr. Horace Baumberg

6.23b

6.24 PT. NAME: **STEVE WELCH** AGE: **30** GENDER: **M** DX: **SURGERY, ADHD, INSOMNIA** ADDRESS: **5 NORTH BEACH DR.** ALLERGY: **PCN** WEIGHT: **166** BMI: **28**

MEDICATION	SIG.	PRESCRIBER	ORIG. DATE	REFILL DATE	REFILL DATE	REFILL DATE	REFILL DATE
Strattera 25 mg #30	I qd	Glasser	4/8	5/7	6/6	7/4	
Restoril 15 mg #30	I hs	Glasser	2/9	3/8	4/6	5/6	6/8

Dr. Jane Flanigan
44 Mason St., San Francisco, CA 40001
154-555-3331

Name Steve Welch Date 7/10

Address 5 North Beach Drive Age 30

℞ Zofran 8mg
Sig – rapidly dissolving tablet the morning of surgery
Disp #2

REFILL 0 TIMES

Dr. Jane Flanigan

6.24a

Dr. Jane Flanigan
44 Mason St., San Francisco, CA 40001
154-555-3331

Name Steve Welch Date 7/10

Address 5 North Beach Drive Age 30

℞ Vicodin tabs
#30
i q 4-6 h prn severe pain

Refills 0

Dr. Jane Flanigan

6.24b

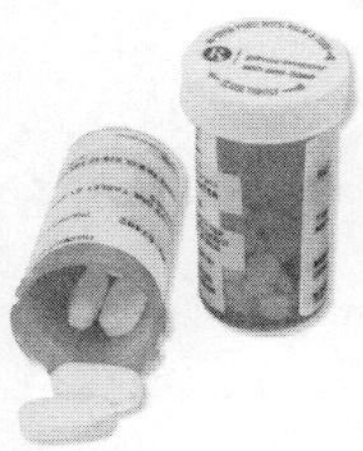

7 • GENITOURINARY

UPON COMPLETION OF THIS CHAPTER, THE STUDENT WILL BE ABLE TO:

- counsel male patients on the proper use of Viagra and other products for the treatment of erectile dysfunction.
- ensure that the patient understands the importance of taking certain potent drugs with food to minimize gastrointestinal side effects.
- ensure that the patient understands that large volumes of water must be ingested when taking certain medications.
- give advice to patients who have urinary obstruction regarding the anticholinergic side effects of OTC cold pills and other OTCs.
- explain the significance of maintaining low urine pH in patients receiving methenamine antimicrobial products.
- counsel patients regarding certain medications that discolor urine and feces.

DRUG LIST

Adcirca
Avodart
Caverject
Cialis
Detrol
Enablex
Flomax
Jalyn
Levitra
Levsin
Methenamine
MUSE
Nitrofurantoin
Noroxin
Oxybutynin (Oral: Ditropan; Topical: Oxytrol, Gelnique)
Proscar
Pyridium
Rapaflo
Revatio
Sanctura
Toviaz
Uroxatral
Viagra
VESIcare

• DRUG HOT POINTS

Detrol
Antispasmodic for bladder instability
Similar strategies as for Ditropan
Regular and long-acting formulations

Ditropan
Antispasmodic for bladder instability
Oral: regular and XL formulations
Topical: Oxytrol patch, Gelnique gel (less dry mouth)
Compare with Detrol formulations
Strategies to treat urinary incontinence
- Limit caffeine, drink less in P.M.
- Create time for urination

Caution: narrow-angle glaucoma
Compare with Enablex, Sanctura, VESIcare, and Toviaz

Flomax
Inhibits alpha$_{1A}$ receptor (urinary tract): less activity on vascular receptors
Indicated for treatment of BPH
Compare with Uroxatral and Rapaflo
Combination product: Jalyn (dutasteride plus tamsulosin)
Caution: "floppy iris syndrome"

Levsin
L-Hyoscyamine: anticholinergic
Urinary tract and GI antispasmodic
Drying agent for terminally ill
Oral tablets, SL, long acting, drops, elixir

Methenamine combinations
Urinary tract anticholinergic, antibacterial, and analgesic
May discolor urine, take with water, ensure low urine pH

Methenamine products: Hiprex (methenamine hippurate, methenamine mandelate)
Converted to formaldehyde (urine pH ↓5.5)
Acid urine: use cranberry juice or vitamin C
Sulfa interaction
Tablets are hygroscopic

MUSE
*M*edicated *U*rethral *S*ystem for *E*rection
PGE$_1$ treatment for erectile dysfunction
Urethral insertion of medicated pellet
Vasodilates vascular beds, causes erection
Administration techniques (urinate first)
Store unopened product at 36° to 46° F
Caution: priapism (erection lasting >6 hours)
Compare with Caverject

Nitrofurantoin
Antimicrobial for urinary tract infections only
Large flakes (macroparticles): less GI upset
Acute or chronic use
Caution: pulmonary adverse effects
Caution: G6PD-deficient patients
Take with food or milk
Renal function should be monitored
Contraindicated if creatinine clearance is less than 60 mL/minute

Noroxin
Quinolone antimicrobial
No polyvalent cations
For UTIs and intestinal infections
Compare with Cipro

Proscar
Inhibits 5-α reductase, reduces formation of active form of testosterone (DHT)
Pregnant women: advise not to handle the active ingredient (broken tablets)
OTC counseling (Avoid first-generation antihistamines and alpha-agonists.)
May have to wait 6 months or more for results
Best results in men with larger prostates
Propecia (1 mg) for male pattern baldness
Compare with Avodart

• DRUG HOT POINTS (*continued*)

Pyridium
Topical analgesic on urinary tract mucosa
Take with food and water
Urine color change

Viagra (Sildenafil)
Oral therapy for ED (erectile dysfunction)
Inhibits PDE-5, enhances effect of NO
In renally impaired and elderly: 25-mg tabs
Available in 25-, 50-, and 100-mg tabs
Nitrate interaction: potentially fatal fall in BP
Nitrates: Isordil, Nitro SL, ISMO, Imdur, amyl nitrite, Nitrolingual Pumpspray, Nitro-Dur, etc.
Caution: pilots—blue-green colors, altered
Cardiovascular status should be considered
Counsel: report symptoms such as angina, dizziness
Cimetidine and erythromycin inhibit hepatic metabolism of Viagra (↑ levels)
Caution: black market, mail order, unsupervised use
Caution: alpha-1 blockers
Compare with Cialis and Levitra
Compare with Revatio
Compare with Adcirca

• QUESTIONS TO BE ANSWERED IN PREPARATION FOR CHAPTER 7 LAB

- What is the mechanism of action of Viagra?
- Which class of medication is contraindicated with Viagra?
- How is MUSE administered?
- How is Caverject administered?
- Describe the pharmacologic differences between Ditropan and Levsin.
- What are some exercises that can be done by the person with urinary incontinence?
- Describe the different forms of urinary incontinence.
- What is the mechanism of action of the methenamine products?
- What is the outcome of the drug interaction between sulfonamides and methenamine?
- What urinary pH is optimal for Hiprex to work?
- What is the active agent that is formed as a metabolite of Hiprex?
- What is the mechanism of action of nitrofurantoin?
- What are some cautions concerning the use of nitrofurantoin?
- Which PDE-5 (phosphodiesterase type 5) inhibitor is the longest acting?
- What two forms of nitrofurantoin are contained in Macrobid capsules?
- What is the benefit of doing Kegel exercises for a patient at risk for urinary incontinence?
- How does Proscar work?
- Describe the "floppy iris syndrome" associated with tamsulosin.
- Compare the dose of Flomax and Rapaflo.
- Describe the caution with the use of alpha-blockers and PDE-5 inhibitors.
- If a prescription is written for Viagra 25 mg PO q 8 h, what is the probable therapeutic purpose?
- Generally, how long would it take for a patient to experience results with the use of Proscar?
- Which group of men will likely not have good results with the use of Proscar?
- Can Proscar be combined with an alpha-1 blocker such as terazosin?
- Which dietary cautions should be exercised with the use of Noroxin?
- Which auxiliary labels should be attached to the prescription bottle of Noroxin?
- What is the mechanism of action of Pyridium?
- Which auxiliary labels should be used with Pyridium?
- Pharmacologically, how does Flomax differ from Cardura, Minipress, and Hytrin?
- What is the difference between Avodart and Proscar?
  - —milligram strength
  - —selectivity in enzyme (5-alpha reductase) inhibition
- Which vitamin is commonly prescribed with methenamine products with the intention of lowering urinary pH?
- Compare the action of Toviaz to that of Detrol.
- How does MUSE differ from Caverject?
- Compare the recommended po doses of Revatio and Adcirca.
- What is the name of an OTC product that contains phenazopyridine?

• GENITOURINARY MEDICATION THERAPY MANAGEMENT QUESTIONS AND COMMENTS

- Did your doctor mention that this medication called oxybutynin might cause dry mouth?
- I notice that you have stopped taking the pills for urinary incontinence. You have reported that the dry mouth is too distressing. Would you like me to call your doctor and recommend a similar product in the form of a patch or a gel to be applied to the skin? That would be easier than taking pills and would reduce dry mouth and constipation.
- Your doctor has given you a medication to reduce urinary incontinence. Please remember not to take any OTC or nonprescription products without consulting with us first. The most problematic ones would be some antihistamines, sleeping pills, allergy pills, and others.
- Your physician has prescribed Viagra. Are you aware of the problem with nitrates and alpha-blockers? Would you like a list of these products to avoid?
- Your prescription medicine for Macrobid should be taken with food. Please remember to drink plenty of water each day. Did the doctor tell you to return for a chest checkup? Please call the doctor if you experience any difficulty in breathing.
- I notice that you are taking a pill called an "alpha-blocker." Please remember to report this to your eye doctor for your records for eye care, especially if you ever have cataract surgery.
- Your doctor prescribed Flomax. The prescription states to take one a day. Please remember to take the medication at 8 P.M. promptly. This will give you time to empty your bladder before bedtime and get a good night's sleep.
- Also, when taking this medication, remember to stand up very slowly. Your body needs time to adjust to it.
- Your doctor prescribed a medicine called methenamine. Please remember to avoid any antacids while using this. Did the doctor recommend that you take vitamin C each day?
- You have recently been taking Bactrim DS, and now, your new prescription is for methenamine. Did your doctor inform you that these two medications cannot be taken at the same time?
- I notice that you have been taking Proscar (or Avodart) for a few weeks. Please stay on your medication. Sometimes it takes weeks or months to see the results.
- Your doctor has prescribed a pill for urinary irritation. It is called Pyridium. Did the doctor tell you that your urine would probably turn red or orange? The color has no bad effects.
- I notice that you are purchasing an OTC or nonprescription product that contains phenazopyridine. Is your doctor aware that you are experiencing a urinary tract problem? It would be best to see a urologist before using that product. It might hide or mask a more serious infection.
- Your doctor has prescribed Noroxin for infection. It is related to Cipro. Please remember not to take it with any milk products, calcium, milk of magnesia, antacids, vitamins, or minerals without consulting us.
- Are you aware of the exercises called Kegel exercises? They are designed to strengthen the muscles at the floor of the pelvis and help decrease your problem with urine leaking.
- Would you like information about these exercises? I can print them for you.
- Many patients with urinary incontinence or obstruction have found that a technique called "double voiding" works well for their problem. Would you like some literature on this helpful technique?
- There are many lifestyle issues that we should talk about concerning your urinary problems. Would you like to have a discussion about these? It would help to make your medications work better.

7.1

PT. NAME: **MARTHA PEREZ** GENDER: **F** ADDRESS: **7584 GREEN AVE.** WEIGHT: **160** HEIGHT: **5′ 5″**

AGE: **64** DX: **CHOLESTEROL, OA, URINARY INCONTINENCE, INSOMNIA** ALLERGY: **PCN** HX: **SMOKER, 50 PACK-YEARS**

MEDICATION	SIG.	PRESCRIBER	ORIG. DATE	REFILL DATE	REFILL DATE	REFILL DATE	REFILL DATE
Celebrex 200 mg #30	1 bid	Sauls	6/14	6/30			
Lipitor 10 mg #30	1 qd	Sauls	4/4	5/4	6/5	7/5	
Alprazolam 0.25 mg #30	1 prn sleep	Sauls	1/4	6/4			

Dr. Alfred Sauls
151212 S High Rd., Chicago, IL 23875
954-555-1300

Name Martha Perez Date 8/4

Address 7584 Green Ave. Age 64

℞

Ditropan 5mg
#30
Sig 1/2 tab AM &
1/2 tab hs

Refills 5

Dr. Alfred Sauls

7.1a

Dr. Alfred Sauls
151212 S High Rd., Chicago, IL 23875
954-555-1300

Name Martha Perez Date 8/4

Address 7584 Green Ave. Age 64

℞

Halcion 0.25
#30
T po prn sleep

N.R.

Dr. Alfred Sauls

7.1b

7.2

PT. NAME: **ALEXANDRA LARSON**	GENDER: **F**	ADDRESS: **2940 LEXTER DR.**	WEIGHT: **130**	HEIGHT: **5′ 2″**
AGE: **61**	DX: **HTN, DEPRESSION, URINARY INCONTINENCE, OA, INSOMNIA**	ALLERGY: **EGGS**	HX: **"ACTS STRANGE" (REPORTED BY FAMILY MEMBER)**	

MEDICATION	SIG.	PRESCRIBER	ORIG. DATE	REFILL DATE	REFILL DATE	REFILL DATE	REFILL DATE
Sonata 10 mg #30	1 hs	Thomas	8/26	9/15			
Celexa 20 mg #20	1/2 tab qd	Jones	6/29	8/3	9/22		
Risperdal 0.25 mg #15	1/2 tab hs	Jones	6/29	7/28	8/28	9/28	
Zestoretic 10/12.5 mg #30	1 qd	Thomas	6/2	7/1	8/1	9/1	

Dr. Erin Thomas
988 North Ridge, New York, NY 88364
813-555-7554

Name Alexandra Larson Date 9/30

Address 2940 Lexter Dr. Age 61

℞

Ditropan 2.5 mg
T po Bid
[illegible]

Refills 5

Dr. Erin Thomas

7.2a

Dr. Ben Jones
32 South Ridge, New York, NY 88364
813-555-7330

Name Alexandra Larson Date 9/28

Address 2940 Lexter Dr. Age 61

℞

Bayer Aspirin 5 gr
[illegible] tab T-TT Bid
prn pain

REFILL 1 - 2 - 3 - NR - PRN
LABEL WITH NAME OF MEDICATION DISPENSED

#100

Dr. Ben Jones

7.2b

7.3

PT. NAME: **KAREN ANDERSON** GENDER: **F** ADDRESS: **1906 ANDERSON PARKWAY** WEIGHT: **121** HEIGHT: **5′ 6″**
AGE: **68** DX: **HTN, UTI, PERIPHERAL ARTERY DISEASE, NASAL ALLERGY** ALLERGY: **NKA** HX: **SOCIAL DRINKER**

MEDICATION	SIG.	PRESCRIBER	ORIG. DATE	REFILL DATE	REFILL DATE	REFILL DATE	REFILL DATE
Ambien 5 mg #30	1 hs	Griffin	2/15	3/20			
Bumex 2 mg #60	1 bid	Griffin	2/15	3/10	4/15		
Plavix 75 mg #60	1 qd	Griffin	1/30	3/28			
Allegra 60 mg #60	1 bid prn	Griffin	3/4	4/15			

Dr. Doug Griffin
7611 147th Terrace, Monterey, CA 38411
705-555-6644

Name Karen Anderson Date 4/16

Address 1906 Anderson Parkway Age 68

℞

Bactrim DS
ii BID
QS 7 Days

☐ LABEL

REFILL Ø TIMES PRN NR

Dr. Doug Griffin

7.3a

Dr. Doug Griffin
7611 147th Terrace, Monterey, CA 38411
705-555-6644

Name Karen Anderson Date 4/16

Address 1906 Anderson Parkway Age 68

℞

Pyridium
200mg PO TID
c̄ meals QS 3 Days

☐ LABEL

REFILL Ø TIMES PRN ~~NR~~

Dr. Doug Griffin

7.3b

7.4

PT. NAME: **AMANDA SMITH** GENDER: **F** ADDRESS: **31 PHILLIP LANE** WEIGHT: **192** HEIGHT: **5′ 7″** BMI: **30**
AGE: **59** DX: **CONSTIPATION, UTI, DYSPEPSIA** ALLERGY: **PCN** HX: **SEDENTARY LIFESTYLE**

MEDICATION	SIG.	PRESCRIBER	ORIG. DATE	REFILL DATE	REFILL DATE	REFILL DATE	REFILL DATE
Dulcolax Laxative 5 mg #C	1 qd	Weiss	5/20	7/29	8/29		
Milk of Magnesia 12 oz	1 tbs hs, 1 tsp prn	OTC	5/12	6/10	7/30	8/29	

Dr. Barry Weiss
901 Sheridan St., Austin, TX 90902
874-555-9000

Name Amanda Smith Date 10/30

Address 31 Phillip Lane Age 59

℞

Pyridium 200
T po tid
#20

Refills 0

Dr. Barry Weiss

7.4a

Dr. Barry Weiss
901 Sheridan St., Austin, TX 90902
874-555-9000

Name Amanda Smith Date 10/30

Address 31 Phillip Lane Age 59

℞

Levaquin 250
T po qd
#5

Refills 0

Dr. Barry Weiss

7.4b

7.5	PT. NAME: **CHRISTOPHER KELLER** AGE: **72**	GENDER: **M** DX: **GLAUCOMA, DEMENTIA, HTN, MUSCLE PAIN, BPH**	ADDRESS: **3906 LEE PARKWAY** ALLERGY: **NKA**	WEIGHT: **140**	BMI: **28**

MEDICATION	SIG.	PRESCRIBER	ORIG. DATE	REFILL DATE	REFILL DATE	REFILL DATE	REFILL DATE
Norflex 100 mg #60	I bid	Robins	7/17	8/23	9/16		
Betimol 0.5% 10 mL	I gtt ou bid	Smith	4/10	6/8	8/12		
HCTZ 25 mg #90	I qd	Robins	6/2	8/22			
KCL 10 mEq #90	I qd	Robins	6/2	8/22			
Mobic 7.5 mg #30	I qd	Green	5/20	6/30			

Dr. Calvin Robins
7823 Tea Rose Trail, Miami, FL 44718
463-555-8000

Name Christopher Keller Date 9/21

Address 3906 Lee Parkway Age 72

℞

Viagra 50 mg

#30

Sig T as directed

Refills 1

Dr. Calvin Robins

7.5a

Dr. Calvin Robins
7823 Tea Rose Trail, Miami, FL 44718
463-555-8000

Name Christopher Keller Date 9/21

Address 3906 Lee Parkway Age 72

℞

Hytrin 1.0 mg #60

Sig T PO hs

Refills 1

Dr. Calvin Robins

7.5b

7.6 PT. NAME: **DANIEL REILEY** AGE: **60** GENDER: **M** DX: **CHRONIC UTI, HTN, DANDRUFF, SKIN RASH (HIVES)** ADDRESS: **492102 GREEN BLVD.** ALLERGY: **NKA** WEIGHT: **155** BMI: **27**

MEDICATION	SIG.	PRESCRIBER	ORIG. DATE	REFILL DATE	REFILL DATE	REFILL DATE	REFILL DATE
Cardizem CD 180 mg #30	1 qd	Thomas	3/28	4/26	5/30		
Claritin 10 mg #30	1 qd prn	Thomas	3/25	4/26	6/28		
Nizoral Shampoo 2% 120 mL	Use ud	Thomas	5/30	6/20			
Bactrim DS #28	1 bid	Thomas	6/20				

Dr. Erin Thomas
988 North Ridge, New York, NY 88364
813-555-7554

Name Daniel Reiley Date 6/29

Address 492102 Green Blvd. Age 60

℞

Hyprex
1g i po BID
#100

Refills 1

Dr. Erin Thomas

7.6a

Dr. Erin Thomas
988 North Ridge, New York, NY 88364
813-555-7554

Name Daniel Reiley Date 6/29

Address 492102 Green Blvd. Age 60

℞

HCTZ 12.5mg – #30
Sig: i po qd

☐ LABEL

REFILL 1 TIMES

Dr. Erin Thomas

7.6b

7.7	PT. NAME: **DANIEL GREEN**	GENDER: **M**	ADDRESS: **7201 MINORS LANE**	WEIGHT: **149**	HEIGHT: **5′ 10″**
	AGE: **62**	DX: **HTN, UTI, OA, ANGINA, ED, INSOMNIA**	ALLERGY: **NKA**		

MEDICATION	SIG.	PRESCRIBER	ORIG. DATE	REFILL DATE	REFILL DATE	REFILL DATE	REFILL DATE
Tylenol No. 3 #20	I q 4–6 h prn	Griffin	4/12	5/20			
Z-Pak	Take ud	Griffin	3/12				
Restoril 30 mg #30	I hs	Griffin	2/28	4/20			
Imdur 60 mg #30	I qd	Griffin	2/25	3/25	4/25		

Dr. Doug Griffin
7611 147th Terrace, Monterey, CA 38411
705-555-6644

Name Daniel Green Date 5/28

Address 7201 Minors Lane Age 62

℞ [illegible] 20 bid
#20
Sig: 1 p bid
~~dz~~

Rp Capoten 12.5
#30
Sig: 1 p daily

Refills 0

Dr. Doug Griffin

7.7a

Dr. Jack Karns
720 150th Terrace, Monterey, CA 38411
705-555-3000

Name Daniel Green Date 5/26

Address 7201 Minors Lane Age 62

℞ VIAGRA 100 mg
#10
ut dicta

Refills 0

Dr. Jack Karns

7.7b

7.8

PT. NAME: **BOB ERIKSON**
AGE: **55**
GENDER: **M**
DX: **HTN, BPH, INSOMNIA, DEEP VEIN THROMBOSIS**
ADDRESS: **894 MALL ST.**
ALLERGY: **NKA**
WEIGHT: **249**
HX: **ETOH**
HEIGHT: **6′**
BMI: **34**

MEDICATION	SIG.	PRESCRIBER	ORIG. DATE	REFILL DATE	REFILL DATE	REFILL DATE	REFILL DATE
Coumadin 5 mg #30	I q am	Sauls	3/5	4/4	5/4		
Amoxicillin 500 mg #28	I qid	Green, DDS	4/20				
Sonata 5 mg #30	I hs	Sauls	3/15	4/8			
Norvasc 5 mg #30	I qd	Sauls	4/29	5/20			
Ginkgo biloba 60 mg #90	I bid	OTC	1/5	2/1	3/1		

Dr. Alfred Sauls
151212 S High Rd., Chicago, IL 23875
954-555-1300

Name Bob Erikson Date 5/27

Address 894 Mall St. Age 55

℞

Flomax 0.4 mg

#90

i p.o. qs

Refills 3

Dr. Alfred Sauls

7.8a

Dr. Alfred Sauls
151212 S High Rd., Chicago, IL 23875
954-555-1300

Name Bob Erikson Date 5/27

Address 894 Mall St. Age 55

℞

Proscar (10 D)

Sig - i qd

Refills 3

Dr. Alfred Sauls

7.8b

7.9

PT. NAME: **DAVID WILSON**
AGE: **71**
GENDER: **M**
DX: **BPH, HTN, PERENNIAL RHINITIS, HEMORRHOIDS, ANXIETY, DRY EYES**
ADDRESS: **771 NO. 9TH AVE.**
ALLERGY: **PCN**
WEIGHT: **178**
HX: **SMOKER FOR 57 YEARS**

MEDICATION	SIG.	PRESCRIBER	ORIG. DATE	REFILL DATE	REFILL DATE	REFILL DATE	REFILL DATE
HCTZ 25 mg #90	I q am	Das	4/10				
Xanax 0.25 mg #90	I prn	Das	6/22	8/22			
Centrum Silver #C	I qd	OTC	2/2	5/10	8/22		
HypoTears 15 mL	I drop ou prn	OTC	4/20	5/29	8/16		
Coricidin HBP Cold & Flu # 24	I bid for allergy	OTC	3/6	5/8	7/9		

Dr. Raj Das
901 E Freemont, Pocatello, ID 80902
874-222-3333

Name David Wilson Date 10/5

Address 771 No. 9 Ave. Age 71

℞

Flomax 0.4mg
#120
Sig ii tab po qhs

Refills 2

Dr. Raj Das

7.9a

Dr. Raj Das
901 E Freemont, Pocatello, ID 80902
874-222-3333

Name David Wilson Date 10/5

Address 771 No. 9 Ave. Age 71

℞

Anusol HC Suppositories
Sig: i (R) BID

#28

☐ SUBSTITUTION ALLOWED
☐ PRIOR APPROVAL REQUIRED
☑ REFILL 1 TIMES
☐ LABEL

Dr. Raj Das

7.9b

7.10 PT. NAME: **JENNIFER KLEIN** AGE: **59** GENDER: **F** DX: **A-FIB, ANGINA, HTN, BACK PAIN, URINARY INCONTINENCE** ADDRESS: **1920 W. RENO AVE.** ALLERGY: **NKA** WEIGHT: **140** HEIGHT: **5′ 8″**

MEDICATION	SIG.	PRESCRIBER	ORIG. DATE	REFILL DATE	REFILL DATE	REFILL DATE	REFILL DATE
Anusol HC suppository #10	use bid	Pray	10/7				
Norvasc 10 mg #30	1 qd	Pray	8/21	9/18	10/13		
Coumadin 5 mg #30	1 q am	Pray	7/20	8/11	8/31		
Coumadin 1 mg #30	1 q am	Pray	7/20	8/11	8/31		
Tylenol Extra Strength caplets #C	2 tid for headaches	OTC	8/2	8/29	9/15		

Dr. H. Norman Pray
555 N Walker Ave., Oklahoma City, OK 39333
463-555-1111

Name Jennifer Klein Date 10/15

Address 1920 W Reno Ave. Age 59

℞

Ditropan
5 mg po
TID
#60

Refills 0

Dr. H. N. Pray

7.10a

Dr. H. Norman Pray
555 N Walker Ave., Oklahoma City, OK 39333
463-555-1111

Name Jennifer Klein Date 10/15

Address 1920 W Reno Ave. Age 59

℞

Ultram 5mg

50

Sig: i po q 4-6h prn pain

☒ Label

Refill NR times

Dr. H. N. Pray

7.10b

7.11

PT. NAME: **KAREN GREEN**	GENDER: **F**	ADDRESS: **445 LINCOLN AVE.**	WEIGHT: **130**	BMI: **28**
AGE: **62**	DX: **URINARY INCONTINENCE, ANGINA, HTN, OA, SKIN FUNGUS**	ALLERGY: **PCN**	HX: **SMOKER, 1 PACK PER WEEK**	

MEDICATION	SIG.	PRESCRIBER	ORIG. DATE	REFILL DATE	REFILL DATE	REFILL DATE	REFILL DATE
Norvasc 10 mg #30	1 qd	Thomas	10/3				
Nitro Patch 0.3 mg/hr # 30	Apply am, remove hs	Thomas	6/3	8/21			
Lotrisone Cream 45 g	Apply bid × 2 weeks	Thomas	6/3	7/13	8/31	10/13	

Dr. Erin Thomas
988 North Ridge, New York, NY 88364
813-555-7554

Name Karen Green Date 10/20

Address 445 Lincoln Ave. Age 62

℞

Levsin-SL Tablet

Sig: i or ii every 4 hours as needed for bladder control

Disp. #30

Refills 1

Dr. Erin Thomas

7.11a

Dr. Jay Ash
22 W. Broadway, New York, NY 88364
813-555-3341

Name Karen Green Date 10/21

Address 445 Lincoln Ave. Age 62

℞

Clinoril 200 mg

#20

i BID c̄ meals

[illegible]

☐ Label

Refill ______ times PRN NR

Do Not Substitute ☐

Dr. Jay Ash

7.11b

7.12 PT. NAME: **JONATHAN BROWN** AGE: **64** GENDER: **M** DX: **CHF, ED, HTN, ANGINA** ADDRESS: **1 MAIN ST.** ALLERGY: **NKA** WEIGHT: **188** HX: **SOCIAL DRINKER** HEIGHT: **5′ 11″**

MEDICATION	SIG.	PRESCRIBER	ORIG. DATE	REFILL DATE	REFILL DATE	REFILL DATE	REFILL DATE
Coreg 3.125 mg #30	1 bid 8 am and 8 pm	Griffin	4/3	5/22	7/5	9/21	
Lanoxin 0.25 mg #30	1 qd	Griffin	4/3	5/22	7/5		
K-Dur 20 mEq #30	1 qd	Griffin	4/3	5/22	7/5	8/7	
Lasix 40 mg #30	1 qd	Griffin	4/3	5/22	7/5	8/7	
Vitamin E 1000 IU #C	1 bid	OTC	6/1	7/2	8/5	9/1	

Dr. Alfred Eisenstadt
1123 Mercer St., Princeton, NJ 38383
705-555-4444

Name Jonathan Brown Date 9/25

Address 1 Main St. Age 64

℞

Viagra 100mg
#8 ī PO 1h pre-Sex

Refills 2

Dr. Alfred Eisenstadt

7.12a

Dr. Alice Griffin
33 Tiger Rd. Princeton, NJ 38383
705-555-1934

Name Jonathan Brown Date 9/27

Address 1 Main St. Age 64

℞

Nitrostat 0.4mg
4x25
Sig: 1 tab sublingually at onset
max 3 tab w/15 min

Dr. Alice Griffin

7.12b

7.13

PT. NAME: **JONATHAN SWANSON** GENDER: **M** ADDRESS: **42 SPRING ST.** WEIGHT: **229** BMI: **30**
AGE: **56** DX: **TYPE 2 DM, INSOMNIA, HTN, BPH** ALLERGY: **SHELLFISH, EGGS** HX: **ADDICTED TO NICOTINE GUM**

MEDICATION	SIG.	PRESCRIBER	ORIG. DATE	REFILL DATE	REFILL DATE	REFILL DATE	REFILL DATE
Glucophage 500 mg #60	I bid	Knorr	5/24	7/8	8/2		
Warfarin 5 mg #30	I M, W, F, Sat, Sun	Knorr	6/29	8/11	10/1		
Ambien 10 mg #30	I hs	Knorr	8/5	9/10			
Norvasc 5 mg #30	I qd	Knorr	6/29	7/22	8/15	9/18	

Dr. Alfred Sauls
151212 S High Rd., Chicago, IL 23875
954-555-1300

Name Jonathan Swanson Date 11/12

Address 42 Spring St. Age 56

℞

FLOMAX 0.4 mg
Sig: cap ii hs –
#60

Refills 6

Dr. Alfred Sauls

7.13a

Dr. Alfred Sauls
151212 S High Rd., Chicago, IL 23875
954-555-1300

Name Jonathan Swanson Date 11/12

Address 42 Spring St. Age 56

℞

COUMADIN 5.0 mg
Sig: 1 TABLET M–F
1/2 TABLET SAT–SUN
Disp: #45

Refills 6

Dr. Alfred Sauls

7.13b

7.14

PT. NAME: **KATHERINE SMITH** AGE: **78** GENDER: **F** DX: **HTN, CHOLESTEROL, OA, UTI** ADDRESS: **498 E 11TH ST.** ALLERGY: **NKA** WEIGHT: **120** HX: **RECURRENT UTI** HEIGHT: **5′ 3″**

MEDICATION	SIG.	PRESCRIBER	ORIG. DATE	REFILL DATE	REFILL DATE	REFILL DATE	REFILL DATE
Pravachol 40 mg #30	I qd	Weiss	5/5	6/1	7/17	8/20	
Vicoprofen #100	I qid prn, severe pain only	Weiss	4/19	6/16	8/1		
Adalat CC 60 mg #30I	I qd	Weiss	3/14	4/12	5/30		
Afrin Nasal Spray	prn runny nose	OTC	7/14	7/28	8/3	8/10	8/24

Dr. Barry Weiss
901 Sheridan St., Austin, TX 90902
874-555-9000

Name Katherine Smith Date 8/25

Address 498 E 11th St. Age 78

℞

Macrobid

#20

T BID

Refill 6 times

Dr. Barry Weiss

7.14a

Dr. Barry Weiss
901 Sheridan St., Austin, TX 90902
874-555-9000

Name Katherine Smith Date 8/25

Address 498 E 11th St. Age 78

℞

Lasix 40 mg

#30

Sig i q am

Refill prn times

Dr. Barry Weiss

7.14b

7.15 PT. NAME: **JUSTINE ANDERSON** AGE: **67** GENDER: **F** DX: **THYROID, OA, GERD, URINARY INCONTINENCE** ADDRESS: **4620 FRAME WAY** ALLERGY: **NKA** WEIGHT: **149** HX: **SMOKER FOR 50 YEARS** BMI: **29**

MEDICATION	SIG.	PRESCRIBER	ORIG. DATE	REFILL DATE	REFILL DATE	REFILL DATE	REFILL DATE
Synthroid 0.05 mg #30	1 qd	Robins	4/8	6/9	7/28	10/7	
Zantac 150 mg #C	1 bid	Robins	1/12	2/14	5/12	8/4	10/6
Motrin IB tablets #C	1 tid prn	OTC	4/6	6/9	8/20	10/6	
Excedrin Extra Strength caplets #100	1–2 prn headache	OTC			Buys in food store		
Oxybutynin 5 mg #C	1 tid prn	Robins	1/20	4/12	6/30	8/26	9/30
Diazepam 2 mg #30	1 hs prn sleep	Robins	4/20	5/21	7/5	9/20	

Dr. Calvin Robins
7823 Tea Rose Trail, Miami, FL 44718
463-555-8000

Name Justine Anderson Date 10/17

Address 4620 Frame Way Age 67

℞

Detrol Tab 2mg PO
QD

#30

Refills 6

Dr. Calvin Robins

7.15a

Dr. Calvin Robins
7823 Tea Rose Trail, Miami, FL 44718
463-555-8000

Name Justine Anderson Date 10/17

Address 4620 Frame Way Age 67

℞

Motrin 800 mg tab
Sig ī tab po. BID prn
Disp #30 tab

☑ Label

Refill X1 (one) times

Dr. Calvin Robins

7.15b

7.16

PT. NAME: **KRISTEN CLARK**	GENDER: **F**	ADDRESS: **909 KEATS AVE.**	WEIGHT: **140**	BMI: **24**
AGE: **58**	DX: **UTI, HTN, GI**	ALLERGY: **NKA**	HX: **BINGE ALCOHOL DRINKER**	

MEDICATION	SIG.	PRESCRIBER	ORIG. DATE	REFILL DATE	REFILL DATE	REFILL DATE	REFILL DATE
Lomotil #30	2 q 6 h prn	Thomas	9/25	10/15			
Lopressor 50 mg #30	1/2 tab bid	Thomas	3/8	10/20			
Amoxicillin 500 mg #15	1 tid	Eisenberg	7/18				

Dr. Erin Thomas
988 North Ridge, New York, NY 88364
813-555-7554

Name Kristen Clark Date 10/25

Address 909 Keats Ave. Age 58

℞

Macrodantin 50 g
#45
ī po QD c/ dinner

Refills 0

Dr. Erin Thomas

7.16a

Dr. Erin Thomas
988 North Ridge, New York, NY 88364
813-555-7554

Name Kristen Clark Date 10/25

Address 909 Keats Ave. Age 58

℞

Cytotec 200 μg

Sig: ½ tabs po TID c̄ meals
#100

Refill 1 - 2 - 3 - NR - PRN

☐ NO SUBSTITUTION

LABEL CONTENTS

Dr. Erin Thomas

7.16b

7.17 PT. NAME: **MICHELLE MITCHELL** AGE: **43** GENDER: **F** DX: **COPD, INSOMNIA, UTI, TENSION HA** ADDRESS: **8625 STIRLING RD.** ALLERGY: **NKA** WEIGHT: **168** HEIGHT: **5′ 9″**

MEDICATION	SIG.	PRESCRIBER	ORIG. DATE	REFILL DATE	REFILL DATE	REFILL DATE	REFILL DATE
Restoril 30 mg #90	1 hs prn	Griffin	2/15	5/20			
Advair Diskus 250/50 mcg #60	1 puff q 12 h	Griffin	7/30				

Dr. Doug Griffin
7611 147th Terrace, Monterey, CA 38411
705-555-6644

Name Michelle Mitchell Date 8/2

Address 8625 Stirling Rd. Age 43

℞

NoRoxin 400
i bid
#14

Refills 0

Dr. Doug Griffin

7.17a

Dr. Doug Griffin
7611 147th Terrace, Monterey, CA 38411
705-555-6644

Name Michelle Mitchell Date 8/2

Address 8625 Stirling Rd. Age 43

℞

Fioricet #30
as needed

Refills 3

Dr. Doug Griffin

7.17b

7.18 PT. NAME: **MARIA JOHNSON** AGE: **62** GENDER: **F** DX: **HRT, OSTEOPOROSIS, URINARY INCONTINENCE, CONSTIPATION** ADDRESS: **900 PENNSYLVANIA AVE.** ALLERGY: **NKA** WEIGHT: **120** HEIGHT: **5′ 4″** BMI: **20**

MEDICATION	SIG.	PRESCRIBER	ORIG. DATE	REFILL DATE	REFILL DATE	REFILL DATE	REFILL DATE
Imipramine 10 mg #30	1 qd	Griffin	9/20	10/18			
Climara Patch 0.05 mg/24 hr #4	Apply weekly ud	Smith	7/5	8/3	9/1		
Fosamax 70 mg #4	1 weekly	Griffin	8/28	10/2			
MiraLAX powder 17.9 oz	1 capful in 8 oz water q 3 d	Griffin	9/5	10/19			

Dr. Doug Griffin
7611 147th Terrace, Monterey, CA 38411
705-555-6644

Name Maria Johnson Date 10/20

Address 900 Pennsylvania Ave. Age 62

℞

Ditropan #30

Sig: up to i QID

☐ Label

Refill PRN times

Dr. Doug Griffin

7.18a

Dr. J. Smith
21 38th Terrace, Monterey, CA 38411
705-555-3300

Name Maria Johnson Date 10/20

Address 900 Pennsylvania Ave. Age 62

℞

Premarin Vag Cream

[illegible]

P.R.N.

Dr. J. Smith

7.18b

7.19 PT. NAME: **MELISSA THOMAS** AGE: **54** GENDER: **F** DX: **HTN, GERD, URINARY URGE INCONTINENCE** ADDRESS: **7021 MARKSMAN DR.** ALLERGY: **PCN** WEIGHT: **225** HX: **ALCOHOL ABUSE** BMI: **32**

MEDICATION	SIG.	PRESCRIBER	ORIG. DATE	REFILL DATE	REFILL DATE	REFILL DATE	REFILL DATE
Elavil 10 mg #50	I alternating with 2 qd	Sauls	8/7	8/30	9/26	10/23	
Prilosec 20 mg #30	I cap 30 min ac bkfst	Sauls	4/18	5/30	7/10		
Prevacid 15 mg #20I	I q am	Sauls	7/19				
Hygroton 25 mg #30	I am on M, W, F	Sauls	4/5	6/20	8/10		

Dr. Alfred Sauls
151212 S High Rd., Chicago, IL 23875
954-555-1300

Name Melissa Thomas Date 10/25

Address 7021 Marksman Dr. Age 54

℞

Ditropan XL 5 mg

#30

i p.o. daily

Refills 6

Dr. Alfred Sauls

7.19a

Dr. Alfred Sauls
151212 S High Rd., Chicago, IL 23875
954-555-1300

Name Melissa Thomas Date 10/25

Address 7021 Marksman Dr. Age 54

℞

[illegible]-20

#100

Sig: i B.I.D.

P.R.N.

Dr. Alfred Sauls

7.19b

7.20 PT. NAME: **MARSHA RUIZ** AGE: **63** GENDER: **F** DX: **ANXIETY, OA, URINARY INCONTINENCE, NEURALGIA, MUSCLE SPASM, HIGH LDL CHOLESTEROL** ADDRESS: **23 SKEDOO ST.** ALLERGY: **ASA** WEIGHT: **130** HX: **ETOH** HEIGHT: **5′ 2″**

MEDICATION	SIG.	PRESCRIBER	ORIG. DATE	REFILL DATE	REFILL DATE	REFILL DATE	REFILL DATE
Amitriptyline 25 mg #50	1 tab hs	Remington	5/4	6/30	7/28	9/15	10/20
Gabapentin 300 mg #30	1 cap tid	Remington	11/5				
Gabapentin 300 mg #C	1 cap tid	Remington	11/15	12/15	1/12		
Ibuprofen 600 mg #60	1 tab tid	Panaveli	8/3	9/4			
Methadone 10 mg #60	1 tab bid	Panaveli	9/9				

Dr. Jarvis Remington
33 S. Brotherly Blvd., Chicago, IL 23875
954-555-7777

Name Marsha Ruiz Date 2/2

Address 23 Skedoo St Age 63

℞

Detrol LA 4 mg

#30

i qday

☑ LABEL

REFILL 4x TIMES PRN NR

Dr. Jarvis Remington

7.20a

Dr. Jarvis Remington
33 S. Brotherly Blvd., Chicago, IL 23875
954-555-7777

Name Marsha Ruiz Date 2/2

Address 23 Skedoo St Age 63

℞

Lipitor

10 mg

#90

i qpm

☑ LABEL

REFILL 4x TIMES PRN NR

Dr. Jarvis Remington

7.20b

7.21 PT. NAME: **JANICE GRAY** AGE: **74** GENDER: **F** DX: **GERD, HTN, UI, BACK PAIN, INSOMNIA** ADDRESS: **888 NE 22 LANE** ALLERGY: **NKA** WEIGHT: **131** HX: **SMOKER FOR MANY YEARS** HEIGHT: **5′ 6″**

MEDICATION	SIG.	PRESCRIBER	ORIG. DATE	REFILL DATE	REFILL DATE	REFILL DATE	REFILL DATE
Nexium 40 mg #60	1 bid, half hour ac bkfst & dinner	White	6/7	7/3	8/5	9/4	
HCTZ 25 mg #15	1/2 tab q am	White	6/7	7/6	8/7	9/6	
Flexeril 5 mg #30	1 tid	White	7/29	8/15	9/30		
Lunesta 1 mg #30	1 hs prn sleep	White	8/5	9/30			

Dr. Harry White
6 NE 4 Terr., Manchester, NH 90944
766-555-3332

Name Janice Gray Date 10/2

Address 888 NE 22 Lane Age 74

℞

Vesicare 5 mg

[illegible] #90

T daily

Dr. Harry White

7.21a

Dr. Harry White
6 NE 4 Terr., Manchester, NH 90944
766-555-3332

Name Janice Gray Date 10/2

Address 888 NE 22 Lane Age 74

℞

Norvasc 2.5

#60

Take i BID

Dr. Harry White

7.21b

7.22

PT. NAME: **ROY MARTIN**	GENDER: **M**	ADDRESS: **320 WHITCOLM BLVD.**	WEIGHT: **179**	HEIGHT: **5′ 10″**
AGE: **66**	DX: **GOUT, TYPE 2 DM, BPH, HTN, INSOMNIA, ED**	ALLERGY: **NKA**	HX: **FORMER NAVY MAN, WORKS AS A CARPENTER**	

MEDICATION	SIG.	PRESCRIBER	ORIG. DATE	REFILL DATE	REFILL DATE	REFILL DATE	REFILL DATE
Allopurinol 100 mg #30	I qd	Terry	12/13	1/11			
Metformin 500 mg #60	I bid, am and pm	Terry	10/5	11/3	12/1	1/3	2/1
Flomax 0.4 mg #30	I at 8 pm for urine flow	Terry	1/9				
Lisinopril 5 mg #30	I q am for blood pressure	Terry	10/5	11/3	1/28		

Dr. Ivan Terry
30 NW Steeler Drive, Pittsburgh, PA 33322
994-555-4477

Name Roy Martin Date 2/2

Address 320 Whitcolm Blvd Age 66

℞

Cialis 20 ʒ
#10

ʒ ½ – 1 tab
po q 48° prn

Refills 5x

Dr. Ivan Terry

7.22a

Dr. Jane Melfo
8 NW Bus Drive, Pittsburgh, PA 33322
994-555-6541

Name Roy Martin Date 2/2

Address 320 Whitcolm Blvd Age 66

℞

AMBIOW 10 ʒ
#30

ʒ 1 tablet Daily – QHS

Refills NR

Dr. Jane Melfo

7.22b

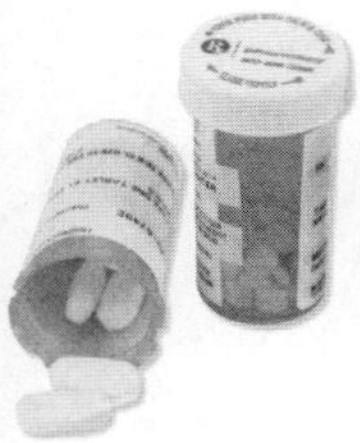

• ANTIMICROBIALS 8

UPON COMPLETION OF THIS CHAPTER, THE STUDENT WILL BE ABLE TO:

- counsel patients on the proper administration of medicines to children (droppers, measured teaspoonfuls, etc.).
- discuss the reasons for developing a system whereby the expiration dates of medications (especially antibiotics) are checked on a regular schedule.
- identify dietary requirements associated with antibiotic usage.
- explain to the patient or caregiver why certain antibiotics must be used exactly as prescribed, and for the *full course of treatment*, even though the symptoms subside.
- list drug interactions involving Sporanox (itraconazole), antacids, H_2-receptor antagonists, other agents, and strategies for avoiding the interactions.
- be knowledgeable about the dental prophylaxis dose for the prevention of bacterial endocarditis and the correct dosage regimens of antibiotics.
- discuss the mechanisms of action of various anti-infective agents.
- identify certain antibiotics (tetracycline, Cipro) that may cause adverse effects in young patients.

DRUG LIST

- Amoxicillin/Ampicillin/Augmentin
- Bactrim
- Ceclor/Keflex/Ceftin
- Cipro/Levaquin/Avelox
- Clindamycin
- Dapsone
- Dicloxacillin
- Erythromycin/Biaxin/Zithromax/Ketek
- Flagyl
- Fuzeon
- Griseofulvin
- Isentress
- Isoniazid (INH)
- Lamisil
- Nizoral/Sporanox/Diflucan/Vfend
- Nucleoside and nonnucleoside reverse transcriptase inhibitors
- Pen VK
- Protease inhibitors
- Rifampin
- Selzentry
- Tetracycline/Doxycycline/Minocycline/Demeclocycline
- Unasyn/Timentin/Zosyn
- Zovirax/Valtrex/Famvir/Denavir

DRUG HOT POINTS

Amoxicillin/Augmentin
Amoxicillin: extended-spectrum penicillin, preferred for prophylaxis of bacterial endocarditis after dental procedure
Augmentin: clavulanic acid inhibits β-lactamase enzymes, extending antibiotic spectrum
Take for full course of treatment
Take Augmentin pc, check for PCN allergy
Tablets: do not break Augmentin
Compare with Unasyn, Timentin, Zosyn

Ampicillin
Complete full course of therapy
Take a full glass of water with each dose
Take at even intervals (q 6 h) four times a day vs. amoxicillin (q 8 h) three times a day
Watch for rash, itching, hives, severe diarrhea

Bactrim
Single strength and DS
Dose based on trimethoprim component
Take with lots of water; stay out of sun
Compare with dapsone (sometimes used in sulfa-intolerant patients)

Cipro/Levaquin/Avelox
Inhibit microbial DNA gyrase
Used for UTI and other infections
Interaction with antacids (Mg, Ca, Al)

Dicloxacillin
Penicillinase-resistant penicillin
Take on an empty stomach
Take for the full course of treatment
Usual adult dose:
250 mg PO qid (q 6 h) × 10 days
Check for penicillin allergy

Diflucan
Broad-spectrum antifungal
CYP-450 inhibitor—crosses BBB—qd dosing
Compare with Vfend, amphotericin B

Entry Inhibitors
1. **Fusion inhibitor** Fuzeon: SUB-Q. Pain at injection site. Rotate sites.
2. **CCR5 coreceptor inhibitor** Selzentry: PO for patients with CCR5 coreceptor strains (Trofile assay needed. Very costly.)

Erythromycin
Take with food or water
Delayed GI effects: diarrhea and cramps
QID = q 6 h (doses equally spaced)
Interaction with oral contraceptives
Compare with Clindamycin

Flagyl
Three indications: trichomonas, intestinal parasites, anaerobic infections
No alcohol—disulfiram reaction

Griseofulvin
Take with largest meal of day (fatty foods)
Photosensitivity
Hepatic enzyme inducer

Integrase inhibitor: Isentress
Prevents integration of HIV DNA into host cell genome

Isoniazid (INH)
Anti-TB agent compliance hepatotoxicity
Take pyridoxine (B_6)

Keflex
Complete full course of therapy
Take with food or milk (GI upset)
Compare with Ceclor, Ceftin, and other cephalosporins

Lamisil
Mechanism of action, patient counseling

Nizoral
Gastric pH <3; take with Coca-Cola Classic (pH 2.5) to acidify gastric contents (increase absorption)
Topical preparations: cream, shampoo
CYP-450 inhibitor (also Diflucan and Sporanox)

Nucleoside/nucleotide reverse transcriptase inhibitors, nonnucleoside reverse transcriptase inhibitors, protease inhibitors
Compliance with multiple therapy
Atripla: low pill burden
Compassion and appropriate patient interaction

• DRUG HOT POINTS (*continued*)

Pen VK
Take for full course of treatment, even if better
Best taken on empty stomach (↑ absorption)
Check for PCN allergy
Do not take for every "runny nose" or "cold"

Rifampin
Indications: TB, meningococcal carriers
Take qd, 1 hour AC or 2 hours PC
Red urine, CYP-450 inducer

Tetracycline/Doxycycline/Minocycline/Demeclocycline
Take tetracycline on empty stomach
Doxycycline/minocycline can be taken without regard to food
Warning: phototoxicity (stay out of the sun)
Demeclocycline used to treat SIADH

Zithromax
Compare with Biaxin
Tablets: 250 mg, 500 mg, and 600 mg, suspension, powder, Z-Pak
MAC prophylaxis: two 600-mg tabs once a week
Dental prophylaxis, other uses
Compare with Ketek

Zovirax/Valtrex/Famvir/Denavir
Nucleoside analogs, antiviral: oral, IV, topical
Herpes simplex, zoster
Counsel: compliance
Herpes is contagious

• QUESTIONS TO BE ANSWERED IN PREPARATION FOR CHAPTER 8 LAB

- What is the mechanism of action of Zithromax?
- What is the PO dose of Zithromax in the prophylaxis of MAC in an AIDS patient?
- What is the PO adult dose of Biaxin for prophylaxis of bacterial endocarditis for dental procedures?
- What is the usual adult dosing regimen (milligram per dose, times per day, duration of treatment) of Dicloxacillin for the treatment of a skin infection caused by penicillinase-producing *Staphylococcus aureus*?
- What is the dosing regimen for Lamisil tablets in the treatment of fungal infections of the toenail?
- What would be the outcome if a person started taking a new prescription for griseofulvin after being stabilized on Coumadin?
- Give some reasons why Diflucan could be considered a better choice than Nizoral in the treatment of topical fungal infections and systemic fungal infections.
- Why is it recommended that a person take a cola drink, specifically Coca-Cola Classic, with each PO dose of Nizoral or Sporanox?
- Name some dietary cautions to be given to the patient taking tetracyclines and fluoroquinolones.
- Describe important counseling tips to be given to the person taking PO erythromycin products.
- Explain the interaction between Coumadin and the following products: Sporanox, Nizoral, or Diflucan.
- If a patient's chart shows an allergy to PCN (penicillin), which agent(s) and dosing regimen(s) would be appropriate for the prophylaxis of bacterial endocarditis after dental procedures?
- Give the complete PO dosing regimen for the dental prophylaxis of bacterial endocarditis for a patient who is allergic to PCN and who has experienced severe diarrhea when taking clindamycin.
- Viread is a nucleotide reverse transcriptase inhibitor. How does this differ from a nucleoside reverse transcriptase inhibitor?
- What is the PO dose and regimen for Diflucan for the treatment of vaginal candidiasis?
- How does the mechanism of action of Fuzeon differ from that of Selzentry?
- Explain why a patient with HIV requires a Trofile assay when Selzentry is being considered as a therapeutic agent?
- What is the name of the primary antibiotic in Augmentin?
- What is the reason for combining clavulanic acid (the potassium salt) with amoxicillin in the formulation of Augmentin?
- What is the reason why a 500-mg Augmentin tablet cannot be broken in half to make a 250-mg dose?
- Why is amoxicillin preferred over ampicillin as PO prophylaxis therapy for dental procedures?
- What is an advantage of Levaquin over Cipro?
- Your client is taking birth control pills (oral contraceptives) and presents you with a new prescription for rifampin. How would you counsel her?
- Your customer calls you reporting that his urine is bright red. He just started using rifampin. How would you advise him?
- What are the indicated uses for rifampin?
- Name a vitamin that must be taken with isoniazid, and explain the reason for this requirement.
- Compare and contrast the mechanism of action, formulations, dosing regimens, and advantages of Zovirax, Famvir, Valtrex, and Denavir.
- What are the calculations used in the dosing of Bactrim?
- Biaxin is used in the treatment of active duodenal ulcer associated with *Helicobacter pylori*. Describe the following:
    - *H. pylori* double therapy
    - *H. pylori* triple therapy
- What is the role of dapsone in the HIV patient who is intolerant to sulfonamides?

• QUESTIONS TO BE ANSWERED IN PREPARATION FOR CHAPTER 8 LAB *(continued)*

- Compare and contrast the structural formulas of dapsone and the sulfonamide component in Bactrim.
- What is an important dietary warning for the patient who takes Flagyl?
- Sporanox is sometimes used as "pulse therapy" in the treatment of fingernail fungus. Explain the dosing strategy for this treatment.
- Why must Sporanox capsules never be substituted for the solution?
- What advantage does voriconazole have over fluconazole?
- What are the differences between Ceftin and Keflex?
- What are the ingredients in Atripla?

• ANTIMICROBIALS MEDICATION THERAPY MANAGEMENT QUESTIONS AND COMMENTS

- Did your doctor tell you to take all the medication for the full period?
- What type of reaction did you have when you experienced an allergy to medication in the past?
- Please notice that your prescription for a sulfa drug has a caution about staying out of the sun and taking the medication with a full glass of water each time. It also means that twice a day should be every 12 hours.
- This antimicrobial tablet should not be taken with milk, calcium, milk of magnesia, minerals, vitamins with minerals, and antacids. Please contact us to discuss dietary cautions.
- Would you like to have a discussion about proper skin and nail hygiene? Your medication is designed to treat a yeast or fungus. The proper hygiene would help the medication give better results and prevent future infections.
- Your doctor prescribed Flagyl, or metronidazole. Did the doctor mention that you should drink no alcohol while you are taking this medication?
- You are taking a potent medication for your condition. You have mentioned that you are HIV positive. Did the doctor mention that nonprescription herbals and alternative medications should be avoided? They have a potential to inactivate your HIV medications.
- Your doctor has prescribed some powerful medications for your condition. Taking them correctly and not missing any will give good results. Would you like to consult with us and discuss a weekly pill reminder? Then, we can discuss lifestyle issues.
- You are receiving a medication called rifampin. You will notice that your urine and other body fluids will be colored red. This is not to be alarmed about. Did you tell your doctor about any other medications that you take from other prescribers? Rifampin has the potential to inactivate many other medications.
- It is very important that you take your medication for the skin viral infection correctly. Would you like to discuss methods for remembering the schedule, as well as lifestyle issues?
- Your doctor prescribed isoniazid (INH) for your condition. Please remember to take vitamin B_6 or pyridoxine (25-, 50-, or 100-mg tablets) once a day. This will prevent nerve problems from the INH medication. It would be good for us to discuss all your other medications privately to make sure that you know what they do and how important each one is.
- Your doctor prescribed Reyataz. Did he or she mention that this medication should be taken only when there is normal acid in the stomach? If you have heartburn, let's discuss how you can treat this problem with a class of drugs called histamine-2 blockers. They must be taken many hours apart from Reyataz.
- I notice that you have been experiencing recurrent yeast infections. Let's discuss what has been happening and if you should see a specialist in treating infections.
- Your child is receiving a strong medication to stop infection. It is critical that you make sure that each dose is given to him on time and for the full duration of therapy. If for any reason the medication is stopped early, even though he feels good, the infection has a high risk of returning—only the next time it might be unstoppable.

8.1

PT. NAME: **STEPHEN WILLIAMS**	GENDER: **M**	ADDRESS: **987 WATER WAY**	WEIGHT: **173**	BMI: **30**
AGE: **63**	DX: **HTN, OA, TENSION HEADACHE**	ALLERGY: **ASA**	HX: **SOCIAL DRINKER**	

MEDICATION	SIG.	PRESCRIBER	ORIG. DATE	REFILL DATE	REFILL DATE	REFILL DATE	REFILL DATE
Calan SR 240 mg #90	I qd	Weiss	2/4	5/18	10/12		
Zestril 40 mg #90	I qd	Weiss	2/4	5/18	10/12		
Prednisone 5 mg #50	I bid × 5 d then I qd	Weiss	10/14				

Dr. Barry Weiss
901 Sheridan St., Austin, TX 90902
874-555-9000

Name Stephen Williams Date 11/13

Address 987 Water Way Age 63

℞

Biaxin XL 500 mg
i po BID
#20

Refills 0

Dr. Barry Weiss

8.1a

Dr. David Finch
444 Sheridan St., Austin, TX 90902
874-555-6565

Name Stephen Williams Date 11/1

Address 987 Water Way Age 63

℞

Fiorinal
Dis Tabs #20
Sig i Tab prn pain

Refills 5x

Dr. David Finch

DEA# AD 1234563

8.1b

8.2 PT. NAME: **KEVIN JACKSON** AGE: **2** GENDER: **M** DX: **THRUSH, SKIN INFECTION, RESPIRATORY INFECTION, BRONCHOSPASM** ADDRESS: **477 CLUB RD.** ALLERGY: **NKA** WEIGHT: **30**

MEDICATION	SIG.	PRESCRIBER	ORIG. DATE	REFILL DATE	REFILL DATE	REFILL DATE	REFILL DATE
Albuterol 2 mg/5 mL 120 mL	1/2 tsp q 8 h	Robins	10/27				
Amoxil 125 mg/5 mL susp. 150 mL	1 tsp q 8 h × 10 d	Robins	6/15				
Poly-Vi-Flor 0.25 mg/mL	1 dropperful daily	Robins	5/20				
Nizoral Cream 15 g	Apply qd × 2 wks	Robins	4/6				

Dr. Calvin Robins
7823 Tea Rose Trail, Miami, FL 44718
463-555-8000

Name Kevin Jackson Date 10/31

Address 477 Club Rd. Age 2

℞

Nystatin Solution
1cc in ea side of
mouth
qid
1wk

Refills 0

Dr. Calvin Robins

8.2a

Dr. Calvin Robins
7823 Tea Rose Trail, Miami, FL 44718
463-555-8000

Name Kevin Jackson Date 10/31

Address 477 Club Rd. Age 2

℞

Bactroban
ointment
15 gm tube
apply to affected
area QD

☐ LABEL

REFILL 2 TIMES PRN NR

Dr. Calvin Robins

8.2b

8.3

PT. NAME: **SARA LEWIS**	GENDER: **F**	ADDRESS: **437 ALONZO SMITH RD.**	WEIGHT: **140**	BMI: **26**
AGE: **73**	DX: **ANGINA, GERD, HTN, OA, INFECTION**	ALLERGY: **NKA**	HX: **SMOKER: 60 PACK-YEARS**	

MEDICATION	SIG.	PRESCRIBER	ORIG. DATE	REFILL DATE	REFILL DATE	REFILL DATE	REFILL DATE
Lopressor 50 mg #60	1/2 bid	Thomas	2/5	4/2	7/12		
Nitro-Dur 0.2 mg/h #30	Apply to chest wall am, remove hs	Thomas	3/1	5/1	7/12		
Lotrisone cream 45 g	Apply to AA tid	Thomas	1/24	6/29			
Atarax 10 mg #30	1 q 8 h prn	Thomas	2/20	6/15			
Sucralfate 1 g #90	1 tab in water tid ac	Thomas	6/20				

Dr. Erin Thomas
988 North Ridge, New York, NY 88364
813-555-7554

Name Sara Lewis Date 7/14

Address 437 Alonzo Smith Rd. Age 73

℞

Levaquin 500
1 po QD
#14

Refills 1

Dr. Erin Thomas

8.3a

Dr. Jose Munoz
4-South Ridge, New York, NY 88364
813-555-3199

Name Sara Lewis Date 7/12

Address 437 Alonzo Smith Rd. Age 73

℞

celebrex 200 mg
i po QD prn
#50

REFILL 1 ☐ 2 ☐ 3 ☐ 4 ☐ NR ☐
LABEL ☐

Dr. Jose Munoz

8.3b

8.4

PT. NAME: **GAIL HILL** | AGE: **28** | GENDER: **F** | DX: **INSOMNIA, UPPER RESPIRATORY INFECTIONS, MIGRAINE HEADACHE** | ADDRESS: **3975 BLACK DR.** | ALLERGY: **SULFA** | WEIGHT: **149** | HX: **ETOH, 3 CHILDREN** | BMI: **31**

MEDICATION	SIG.	PRESCRIBER	ORIG. DATE	REFILL DATE	REFILL DATE	REFILL DATE	REFILL DATE
Valium 2 mg #30	1 hs	Griffin	2/23	3/24	4/26	5/24	7/20
Sudafed 30 mg #24	1 tid prn sinus	Griffin	2/10	7/27			
Erythromycin 250 mg #28	1 tab qid pc	Griffin	2/10				
Ortho-Novum 7/7/7 #28	ud	Evans	6/1	7/1	8/1		

Dr. Doug Griffin
7611 147th Terrace, Monterey, CA 38411
705-555-6644

Name Gail Hill Date 8/2

Address 3975 Black Dr. Age 28

℞

Erythromycin 250. qid x 5 days
dispense 20

Ref: Non-Rep

Dr. Doug Griffin

8.4a

Dr. Doug Griffin
7611 147th Terrace, Monterey, CA 38411
705-555-6644

Name Gail Hill Date 8/2

Address 3975 Black Dr. Age 28

℞

Frova 2.5mg #1 packet.

Sig: take as directed

LABEL

REFILL prn TIMES

Dr. Doug Griffin

8.4b

8.5

PT. NAME: **ELIZABETH MEYER** GENDER: **F** ADDRESS: **53 IRIS BLVD.** WEIGHT: **123** BMI: **27**
AGE: **64** DX: **GLAUCOMA, HTN, ACNE** ALLERGY: **NKA**

MEDICATION	SIG.	PRESCRIBER	ORIG. DATE	REFILL DATE	REFILL DATE	REFILL DATE	REFILL DATE
Furosemide 20 mg #90	1 q am	Sauls	2/4	5/16			
Vasotec 5 mg #90	1 q am	Sauls	2/4	5/12			
Locoid cream 0.1% 45 g	Apply bid	Sauls	4/4	7/24			
Betoptic S 0.25% 15 mL	1 gtt ou bid	Benjamin	3/21	7/24	10/9		
Brimonidine 0.2% 10 mL	1 gtt bid	Benjamin	3/21	7/24	10/9		

Dr. Alfred Sauls
151212 S High Rd., Chicago, IL 23875
954-555-1300

Name Elizabeth Meyer Date 11/20

Address 53 Iris Blvd. Age 64

℞

Nizoral Cream

apply daily

Refill ______ times

Dr. Alfred Sauls

8.5a

H. Rudolph Porter
885 NE High Rd., Chicago, IL 23875
954-555-2222

Name Elizabeth Meyer Date 11/15

Address 53 Iris Blvd. Age 64

℞

Tetracycline 500 mg

Sig i po qd

Disp #30

Refill 1 times

Dr. H. Porter

8.5b

8.6	PT. NAME: **MICHAEL BRYANT**	GENDER: **M**	ADDRESS: **684 HURRICANE ALLEY**	WEIGHT: **162**	BMI: **31**
	AGE: **52**	DX: **HTN, ACNE VULGARIS, ACNE ROSACEA, HEADACHE**	ALLERGY: **PCN**		

MEDICATION	SIG.	PRESCRIBER	ORIG. DATE	REFILL DATE	REFILL DATE	REFILL DATE	REFILL DATE
Atenolol 25 mg #30	1 qd	Weiss	7/6	8/7	9/5		
Metrogel 1% 60 g	Apply qd	Black	8/21				

Dr. Barry Weiss
901 Sheridan St., Austin, TX 90902
874-555-9000

Name Michael Bryant Date 10/20

Address 684 Hurricane Alley Age 52

℞

Solodyn 115MG

Sig i PO Daily

#30

Refills 0

Dr. Barry Weiss

8.6a

Dr. Marvis Black
102 Tower St., Austin, TX 90902
874-555-3321

Name Michael Bryant Date 10/21

Address 684 Hurricane Alley Age 52

℞

Celebrex 100 mg #30

i bid PRN Headache

☐ LABEL

~~REFILL~~ 11 TIMES PRN NR

Dr. Marvis Black

8.6b

8.7

PT. NAME: **GLENN SMITH** GENDER: **M** ADDRESS: **1984 GREEN ST.** WEIGHT: **215** BMI: **26**
AGE: **52** DX: **INFECTIONS, JOCK ITCH** ALLERGY: **IODINE, SHELLFISH** HX: **AIRLINE PILOT**

MEDICATION	SIG.	PRESCRIBER	ORIG. DATE	REFILL DATE	REFILL DATE	REFILL DATE	REFILL DATE
Amoxicillin 500 mg #21	1 tid until gone	Robins	11/13				
Ciloxan 0.3% sol. 5 mL	1 gtt od qid	Jackson	6/16				

Dr. Calvin Robins
7823 Tea Rose Trail, Miami, FL 44718
463-555-8000

Name Glenn Smith Date 12/4
Address 1984 Green St. Age 52

℞
FLAGYL 250 MG
#40
Sig ii BID X10D
NO ETOH

Refills 0

Dr. Calvin Robins

8.7a

Dr. Calvin Robins
7823 Tea Rose Trail, Miami, FL 44718
463-555-8000

Name Glenn Smith Date 12/4
Address 1984 Green St. Age 52

℞
Lotrisone Cream
Apply as indicated

N.R.

Dr. Calvin Robins

8.7b

8.8

PT. NAME: **MARK OLSON** GENDER: **M** ADDRESS: **774 FANTASTIC ST.** WEIGHT: **189** BMI: **31**

AGE: **42** DX: **GERD, FUNGAL SKIN INFECTIONS, HEADACHE, NASAL ALLERGIES** ALLERGY: **NKA** HX: **TENNIS INSTRUCTOR**

MEDICATION	SIG.	PRESCRIBER	ORIG. DATE	REFILL DATE	REFILL DATE	REFILL DATE	REFILL DATE
Zantac 150 mg #30	1 q pm	Thomas	4/20	5/23			
Claritin 10 mg #20	1 qd prn	Thomas	2/12	3/14	5/20		
Maalox Susp. 12 oz	1 tsp prn heartburn	OTC	1/5	3/6	5/1	5/28	
Lotrimin AF cream 12 g	tid to rash	OTC	5/9				
Aleve #60	1 tab bid	OTC	4/4	5/21			

Dr. Erin Thomas
988 North Ridge, New York, NY 88364
813-555-7554

Name Mark Olson Date 5/30

Address 774 Fantastic St. Age 42

℞

Ketoconazole

#30 200mg

Sig. tab. i q.d.

Refills: Ne Repatur

Dr. Erin Thomas

8.8a

Dr. Jerry Price
4400 East Ridge, New York, NY 88364
813-555-1936

Name Mark Olson Date 5/29

Address 774 Fantastic St. Age 42

℞

Esgic #28

Sig. i tab po q4h prn

3×

Dr. Jerry Price

8.8b

8.9	PT. NAME: **JAMES SMITH**	GENDER: **M**	ADDRESS: **500 SE 2ND ST.**	WEIGHT: **180**	BMI: **27**
	AGE: **28**	DX: **BACTERIAL INFECTION OF FINGER, COUGH**	ALLERGY: **SULFA**	HX: **CARPENTER**	

MEDICATION	SIG.	PRESCRIBER	ORIG. DATE	REFILL DATE	REFILL DATE	REFILL DATE	REFILL DATE
Robitussin DM 4 oz	5 mL (1 tsp) tid	Isaacs	4/19				

Dr. Howard Isaacs
1115 Turnaround Lane, Detroit, MI 64789
343-555-7000

Name James Smith Date 4/30

Address 500 SE 2nd St. Age 28

℞

Dicloxacillin 500 mg
#20
Sig: ī qid

LABEL (circled)
NO REFILL
REFILL 1 TIMES

Dr. Howard Isaacs

8.9a

Dr. Howard Isaacs
1115 Turnaround Lane, Detroit, MI 64789
343-555-7000

Name James Smith Date 4/30

Address 500 SE 2nd St. Age 28

℞

Bactroban cream #1
Apply as indicated

Dr. Howard Isaacs

8.9b

8.10

PT. NAME: **DON MICHAELS**	GENDER: **M**	ADDRESS: **654 IBIS CT.**	WEIGHT: **198**	BMI: **34**
AGE: **65**	DX: **HTN, INFECTION, COUGH, CONSTIPATION, ANXIETY**	ALLERGY: **CODEINE**	HX: **GROCERY STORE CLERK**	

MEDICATION	SIG.	PRESCRIBER	ORIG. DATE	REFILL DATE	REFILL DATE	REFILL DATE	REFILL DATE
Capoten 25 mg #60	I bid	Weiss	4/12				
Lasix 20 mg #30	I q am	Weiss	4/12				
Lorazepam 0.5 mg #30	I/2 tab q am and pm	Weiss	3/I				
Metamucil, Original Coarse Milled 72 doses	I tsp qd in water	OTC	2/2	4/5			

Dr. Barry Weiss
901 Sheridan St., Austin, TX 90902
874-555-9000

Name Don Michaels Date 4/15

Address 654 Ibis Ct. Age 65

℞

Bactrim Susp. 16 oz

Sig: ʒ iv BID

Refills 0

Dr. Barry Weiss

8.10a

Dr. Barry Weiss
901 Sheridan St., Austin, TX 90902
874-555-9000

Name Don Michaels Date 4/15

Address 654 Ibis Ct. Age 65

℞

Tessalon Perle

#20

Sig i tab p.o. q8h

☐ LABEL

REFILL 3 TIMES

Dr. Barry Weiss

8.10b

8.11

PT. NAME: **JOHN MARTIN** GENDER: **M** ADDRESS: **854 S BLACKBURN ST.** WEIGHT: **152** BMI: **24**
AGE: **68** DX: **COPD** ALLERGY: **PCN** HX: **SMOKER FOR 50 YEARS**

MEDICATION	SIG.	PRESCRIBER	ORIG. DATE	REFILL DATE	REFILL DATE	REFILL DATE	REFILL DATE
Prednisone 5 mg #C	1 q am	Isaacs	4/12	7/20			
Theophylline SR 300 mg #60	1 q 12 h	Isaacs	4/6	5/2	6/6		
Serevent Diskus #60	ud q 12 h	Isaacs	4/6	5/2	6/3	7/8	

Dr. Janet Halloway
4414 W Bridge Rd., San Francisco, CA 40001
154-555-8558

Name John Martin Date 7/30

Address 854 S Blackburn St. Age 68

℞

Biaxin 500mg
Sig i po bid
Disp #10

Refills 0

Dr. Janet Halloway

8.11a

Dr. Janet Halloway
4414 W Bridge Rd., San Francisco, CA 40001
154-555-8558

Name John Martin Date 7/30

Address 854 S Blackburn St. Age 68

℞

Promethazine VC c̄ Codeine
Elixir
8 fl oz
Sig: 2 teaspoonful T.I.D.

Refill N/C times

Dr. Janet Halloway
DEA# AH1234563

8.11b

8.12 PT. NAME: **GLENN MEYER** AGE: **70** GENDER: **M** DX: **CHF, POST MI, HTN, URI** ADDRESS: **53 IRIS BLVD.** ALLERGY: **SULFA** WEIGHT: **161** HX: **RETIRED TEACHER** BMI: **29**

MEDICATION	SIG.	PRESCRIBER	ORIG. DATE	REFILL DATE	REFILL DATE	REFILL DATE	REFILL DATE
Furosemide 40 mg #60	I q am	Griffin	3/20	5/10	7/12		
Prilosec 20 mg #60	I cap 1/2 hr ac bkfst	Griffin	5/1	6/12	7/12		
Nitro-Dur 0.2 mg/hr #30	Apply to cw in am, d/c hs	Griffin	5/13	6/24	7/28		
Coumadin 5 mg #60	I q am	Griffin	5/13				
Benadryl 25 mg #24	I hs	OTC	4/12	5/20			

Dr. Donna Johns
7000 SW 1st Ave., Santa Fe, NM 54545
766-555-9097

Name Glenn Meyer Date 7/30

Address 53 Iris Blvd. Age 70

℞

Erythromycin 250mg
#28
Sig: 2 tabs. b.i.d. to help control infection

Refills 3

Dr. Donna Johns

8.12a

Ely Veterinary Clinic
6000 SW 2nd Ave., Santa Fe, NM 54545
766-555-7373

Name Precious Meyer—Cat (Feline) Date 7/28

Address 53 Iris Blvd. Age 5

℞

Phenobarb 1/4 gr. #100
SIG: Give
1 tablet in am
or
2 tablets in pm.

Dx: Seizures

Richard Ely, DVM
DEA# AE1234563

8.12b

8.13

PT. NAME: **JOHN BRYANT** | AGE: **40** | GENDER: **M** | DX: **ASTHMA, FREQUENT INFECTIONS, POSITIVE PPD** | ADDRESS: **684 HURRICANE ALLEY** | ALLERGY: **CODEINE** | WEIGHT: **178** | HX: **MULTIPLE SEX PARTNERS** | HEIGHT: **5′ 9″**

MEDICATION	SIG.	PRESCRIBER	ORIG. DATE	REFILL DATE	REFILL DATE	REFILL DATE	REFILL DATE
Metronidazole 500 mg #7	1 bid	Keller	10/18				
Proventil HFA 6.7 g	2 puffs tid PRN	Keller	9/16	10/28	11/17		
Serevent Diskus #60	Use ud	Keller	11/7				

Dr. Daniel Keller
5007 Turtle Drive, Miami, FL 98887
247-555-9876

Name John Bryant Date 11/20

Address 684 Hurricane Alley Age 40

℞ (1) Zovirax (400mg)
Sig: i BID
#40

(2) Zovirax ointment (5%)
Sig: For local use
AED
#15 Gm

Refills 1

Dr. Daniel Keller

8.13a

Dr. Daniel Keller
5007 Turtle Drive, Miami, FL 98887
247-555-9876

Name John Bryant Date 11/20

Address 684 Hurricane Alley Age 40

℞ INH 300 mg
#100
Sig: T tab QD as directed

Refills 1

Dr. Daniel Keller

8.13b

8.14

PT. NAME: **CAROL RIVERA** GENDER: **F** ADDRESS: **184 GREEN ST.** WEIGHT: **126** BMI: **24**

AGE: **45** DX: **ALLERGIES, "INFECTIONS," COPD, THRUSH** ALLERGY: **ASA, SULFA, YELLOW DYE #5 (TARTRAZINE)** HX: **SMOKER; THINKING ABOUT QUITTING**

MEDICATION	SIG.	PRESCRIBER	ORIG. DATE	REFILL DATE	REFILL DATE	REFILL DATE	REFILL DATE
Claritin 10 mg #30I	I qd prn	Keller	4/22	5/15	6/I	7/24	
Flonase Nasal Spray 16 g	ud once qd	Keller	5/15	8/15			
Flovent HFA 220 mcg 12 g	ud twice qd	Keller	5/15	8/15			

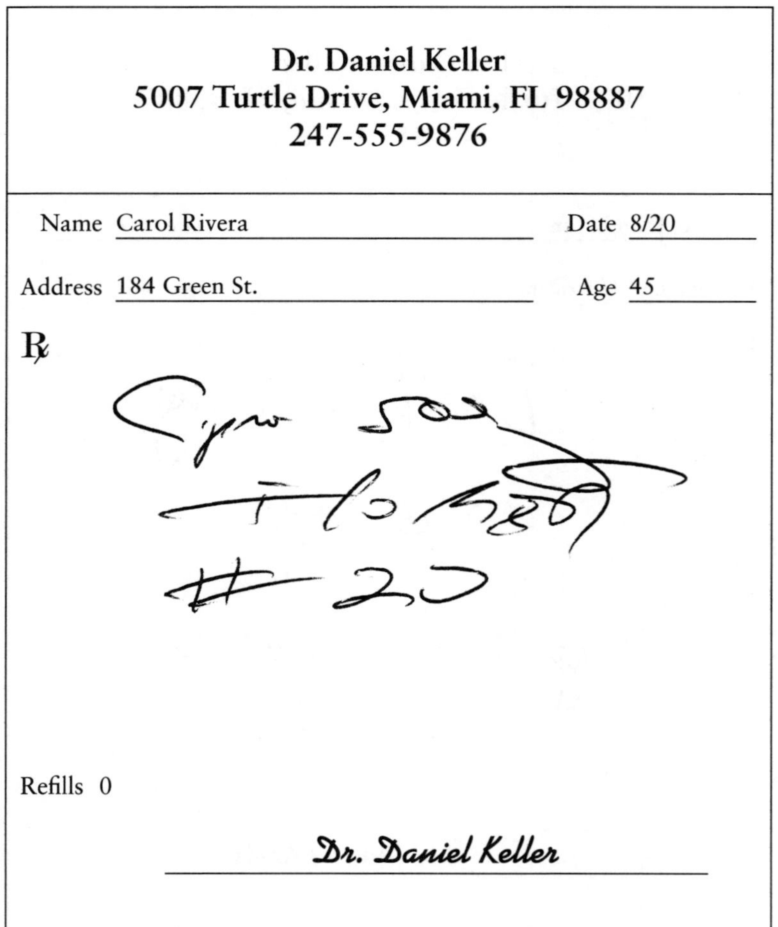

Dr. Daniel Keller
5007 Turtle Drive, Miami, FL 98887
247-555-9876

Name Carol Rivera Date 8/20

Address 184 Green St. Age 45

℞

Refills 0

Dr. Daniel Keller

8.14a

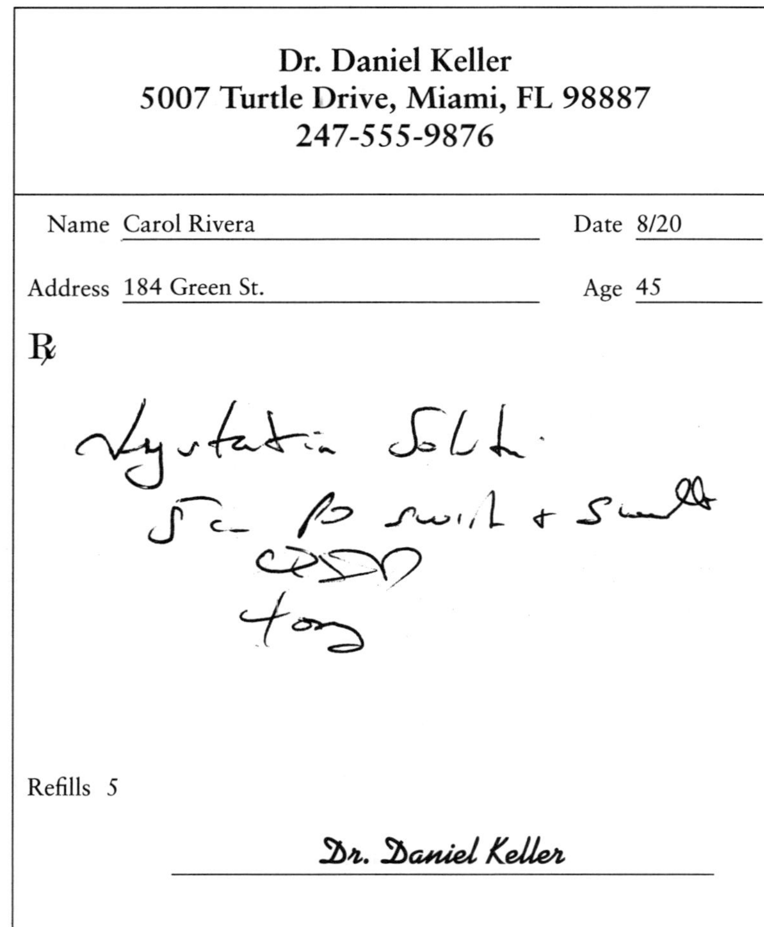

Dr. Daniel Keller
5007 Turtle Drive, Miami, FL 98887
247-555-9876

Name Carol Rivera Date 8/20

Address 184 Green St. Age 45

℞

Refills 5

Dr. Daniel Keller

8.14b

8.15

PT. NAME: **JEANNE OLSON**	GENDER: **F**	ADDRESS: **774 FANTASTIC ST.**	WEIGHT: **156**	HEIGHT: **5′ 2″**
AGE: **40**	DX: **PAIN, INSOMNIA, FUNGAL INFECTION**	ALLERGY: **SULFA**	HX: **SMOKER, TRYING TO QUIT**	

MEDICATION	SIG.	PRESCRIBER	ORIG. DATE	REFILL DATE	REFILL DATE	REFILL DATE	REFILL DATE
Ultram 50 mg # LX	I q 8 h	Griffin	9/29	11/1	12/1		
Naprosyn 500 mg # XXV	I bid pc	Griffin	6/29	7/3	8/9	9/12	9/14
Elavil 10 mg #30	I hs	Griffin	6/2	9/23			

Dr. Doug Griffin
7611 147th Terrace, Monterey, CA 38411
705-555-6644

Name Jeanne Olson Date 12/8

Address 774 Fantastic St. Age 40

℞

Diflucan 100mg
Disp: (10) ten - tabs
Sig: ii tabs STAT & i tab daily until gone

Refills 1

Dr. Doug Griffin

8.15a

Dr. Doug Griffin
7611 147th Terrace, Monterey, CA 38411
705-555-6644

Name Jeanne Olson Date 12/8

Address 774 Fantastic St. Age 40

℞

Mycolog cream
#15 gm tube
apply BID

Dr. Doug Griffin

8.15b

8.16

PT. NAME: **LISA ANN JONES** GENDER: **F** ADDRESS: **5132 GIRAFFE DR.** WEIGHT: **132** HEIGHT: **5′ 4″**

AGE: **62** DX: **IBS, ALLERGIES, HEARTBURN, BACK PAIN, TENSION HEADACHE, RESPIRATORY INFECTION** ALLERGY: **PCN** HX: **BRAND NAME ONLY**

MEDICATION	SIG.	PRESCRIBER	ORIG. DATE	REFILL DATE	REFILL DATE	REFILL DATE	REFILL DATE
Zyrtec 10 mg #30	1 qd	Isaacs	7/29	10/4	11/29		
Bentyl 10 mg #90	1 prn	Isaacs	9/8	9/29	11/6		
Fioricet #100	1 ud	Isaacs	8/29	10/30			
Aciphex 20 mg #30	1 qd	Isaacs	8/9	9/29	11/6		

Dr. Daniel Kohl
5007 Turtle Drive, Miami, FL 98887
247-555-9876

Name Lisa Ann Jones Date 11/30

Address 5132 Giraffe Dr. Age 62

℞

Azithromax #6
2 to start then
one daily

N. Rep

Dr. Daniel Kohl

8.16a

Dr. Daniel Kohl
5007 Turtle Drive, Miami, FL 98887
247-555-9876

Name Lisa Ann Jones Date 11/30

Address 5132 Giraffe Dr. Age 62

℞

Celebrex 200 mg
qd #30

N. Rep

Dr. Daniel Kohl
DEA# AK1234563

8.16b

8.17

PT. NAME: **CAROLINE COOK**
AGE: **60**
GENDER: **F**
DX: **HIGH CHOLESTEROL, NERVES, OA, OTITIS EXTERNA, ORAL SURGERY FOR GUM INFECTION**
ADDRESS: **1558 DEXTER AVE.**
ALLERGY: **PCN**
WEIGHT: **138**
HX: **SOCIAL DRINKER**
BMI: **23**

MEDICATION	SIG.	PRESCRIBER	ORIG. DATE	REFILL DATE	REFILL DATE	REFILL DATE	REFILL DATE
Ibuprofen 400 mg #30	I tid	Sauls	9/18				
Alprazolam 0.5 mg #30	I tid	Sauls	8/3	9/1			
Zocor 40 mg #30	I qd	Sauls	7/5	8/4	9/12	10/12	

Dr. Jack Berman, DDS
7000 SW 1st Ave., Santa Fe, NM 54545
766-555-9097

Name Caroline Cook Date 10/15
Address 1558 Dexter Ave. Age 60

℞

Cipro 500 mg
Metronidazole 500 mg
#16 for each
Sig 1 bid of each until gone

Refills 0

Dr. Jack Berman, DDS

8.17a

Dr. Ron Dix
28-NW 39 Ave., Santa Fe, NM 54545
766-555-1130

Name Caroline Cook Date 10/15
Address 1558 Dexter Ave. Age 60

℞

CORTISPORIN
Otic Solution
10 ml
Sig: 4 gtts in the Rt. ear TID.

Refill 4 times

Dr. Ron Dix

8.17b

8.18

PT. NAME: **MATHEW JOHNSON** GENDER: **M** ADDRESS: **71 CAPITOL AVE.** WEIGHT: **CHECK WITH PARENTS**
AGE: **5** DX: **INFECTION AND YEAST INFECTION IN CORNERS OF MOUTH** ALLERGY: **NKA**

MEDICATION	SIG.	PRESCRIBER	ORIG. DATE	REFILL DATE	REFILL DATE	REFILL DATE	REFILL DATE
Poly Vitamin with Fluoride 0.25 mg/mL 50 mL	1 mL po daily	Griffin	4/18	12/6			

Dr. Doug Griffin
7611 147th Terrace, Monterey, CA 38411
705-555-6644

Name Mathew Johnson Date 12/12

Address 71 Capitol Ave. Age 5

℞

Amoxil
250mg/TE
100E
3/4 tsp po tid
x 10 days

Refills 0

Dr. Doug Griffin

8.18a

Dr. Doug Griffin
7611 147th Terrace, Monterey, CA 38411
705-555-6644

Name Mathew Johnson Date 12/12

Address 71 Capitol Ave. Age 5

℞

LOTRISONE CREAM
15 gm
Sig BID to corners of mouth

☐ LABEL

REFILL 3 TIMES PRN NR

Dr. Doug Griffin

8.18b

8.19

PT. NAME: **ANTHONY THOMAS**	GENDER: **M**	ADDRESS: **575 REDWOOD WAY**	WEIGHT: **152**	BMI: **28**
AGE: **48**	DX: **INFECTIONS, NERVES, DYSPEPSIA, INSOMNIA**	ALLERGY: **SULFA**	HX: **LOW INCOME, GENERICS ON EVERYTHING**	

MEDICATION	SIG.	PRESCRIBER	ORIG. DATE	REFILL DATE	REFILL DATE	REFILL DATE	REFILL DATE
Amitriptyline 10 mg #30	1 qd	Jones	11/27				
Alprazolam 1 mg #90	1 tid	Jones	11/27				
Ranitidine 150 mg #60	2 qd	Jones	11/27				

Dr. Howard Isaacs
1115 Turnaround Lane, Detroit, MI 64789
343-555-7000

Name Anthony Thomas Date 11/29

Address 575 Redwood Way Age 48

℞

Augmentin 875 g
#28

Sig: i tab po bid

Refills 0

Dr. Howard Isaacs

8.19a

Dr. Howard Isaacs
1115 Turnaround Lane, Detroit, MI 64789
343-555-7000

Name Anthony Thomas Date 11/29

Address 575 Redwood Way Age 48

℞

Klonopin
0.5 mg po iii HS
#45

Refills 0

Dr. Howard Isaacs

8.19b

8.20	PT. NAME: **KATHERINE SMITH**	GENDER: **F**	ADDRESS: **2524 CANADIAN CIR.**	WEIGHT: **120**	BMI: **24**
	AGE: **73**	DX: **HTN, ANGINA, URI, LEG CRAMPS AT NIGHT**	ALLERGY: **NKA**	HX: **SMOKER, ETOH**	

MEDICATION	SIG.	PRESCRIBER	ORIG. DATE	REFILL DATE	REFILL DATE	REFILL DATE	REFILL DATE
Clonidine 0.2 mg #60	I bid	Johns	5/25	6/22	7/21	8/20	9/25
Imdur 30 mg #60	I bid	Johns	7/7	8/9	9/11	10/4	
Quinine Sulfate 324 mg #30	I hs	Johns	6/19	10/10			
NTG 0.4 mg #25	ud	Johns	7/7	10/11			

Dr. Donna Johns
7000 SW 1st Ave., Santa Fe, NM 54545
766-555-9097

Name Katherine Smith Date 10/20

Address 2524 Canadian Cir. Age 73

℞

Ceftin 250
Sig T BID
#14

☐ Fill Prescription Generically

Refills 0

Dr. Donna Johns

8.20a

Dr. Donna Johns
7000 SW 1st Ave., Santa Fe, NM 54545
766-555-9097

Name Katherine Smith Date 10/20

Address 2524 Canadian Cir. Age 73

℞

Tussi Organidin
Elixir
4oz
i-ii tsp Q4-6°
PRN
cough

Refills x 1

Dr. Donna Johns

DEA# AJ1234563

8.20b

8.21

PT. NAME: **TAMARA DAVIDSON** GENDER: **F** ADDRESS: **4154 HALL ST.** WEIGHT: **123** BMI: **22**
AGE: **30** DX: **AIDS, TOXOPLASMOSIS, THRUSH** ALLERGY: **PCN** HX: **IV DRUG USER, PROSTITUTE**

MEDICATION	SIG.	PRESCRIBER	ORIG. DATE	REFILL DATE	REFILL DATE	REFILL DATE	REFILL DATE
Zithromax 600 mg #4	2 tabs (1200 mg) po every Tuesday	Forrest	8/10				
Bactrim DS (800/160 mg) #60	1 tab qd	Forrest	8/10				
Daraprim 25 mg #90	3 tabs qd	Forrest	8/10				
Sulfadiazine 500 mg #C	2 tid	Forrest	8/10				
Folinic Acid 5 mg #C	1 tab bid	Forrest	8/10				
Truvada #30	1 tab once a day	Forrest	8/10				
Sustiva 600 mg #30	1 tab hs	Forrest	8/10				

Dr. John Forrest
5007 Turtle Drive, Miami, FL 98887
247-555-9876

Name Tamara Davidson Date 8/30

Address 4154 Hall Street Age 30

℞ Diflucan #15
100 mg
Sig: ii 1st day
Then i q AM

Refill 0 Times

☒ Label

Substitution Allowed Dr. John Forrest, M.D.

Prior Approval Required ______, M.D.

8.21a

Orville Midkiff, MD
5009 Turtle Drive, Miami, FL 98887
247-555-9800

Name Tamara Davidson Date 8/30

Address 4154 Hall Street Age 30

℞ MMX susp.
100 cc Mycostatin Susp
100 cc Mylanta
100 cc Xylocaine (viscous)
swish + swallow
ii tsp
po QID
#300cc

☐ DO NOT REFILL
☒ REFILL 1 TIMES

Dr. O. Midkiff

8.21b

8.22

PT. NAME: **CHARLENE JACKSON** GENDER: **F** ADDRESS: **218 CALIFORNIA ST.** WEIGHT: **AVERAGE (NOT AVAILABLE)**
AGE: **42** DX: **STD, URI, MULTIPLE INFECTIONS** ALLERGY: **NKA** HX: **MULTIPLE PARTNERS, SULFA INTOLERANT**

MEDICATION	SIG.	PRESCRIBER	ORIG. DATE	REFILL DATE	REFILL DATE	REFILL DATE	REFILL DATE
Claritin 10 mg #30	Use ud	Ng	5/3				
Dapsone 100 mg #30	1 bid	Ng	5/3				

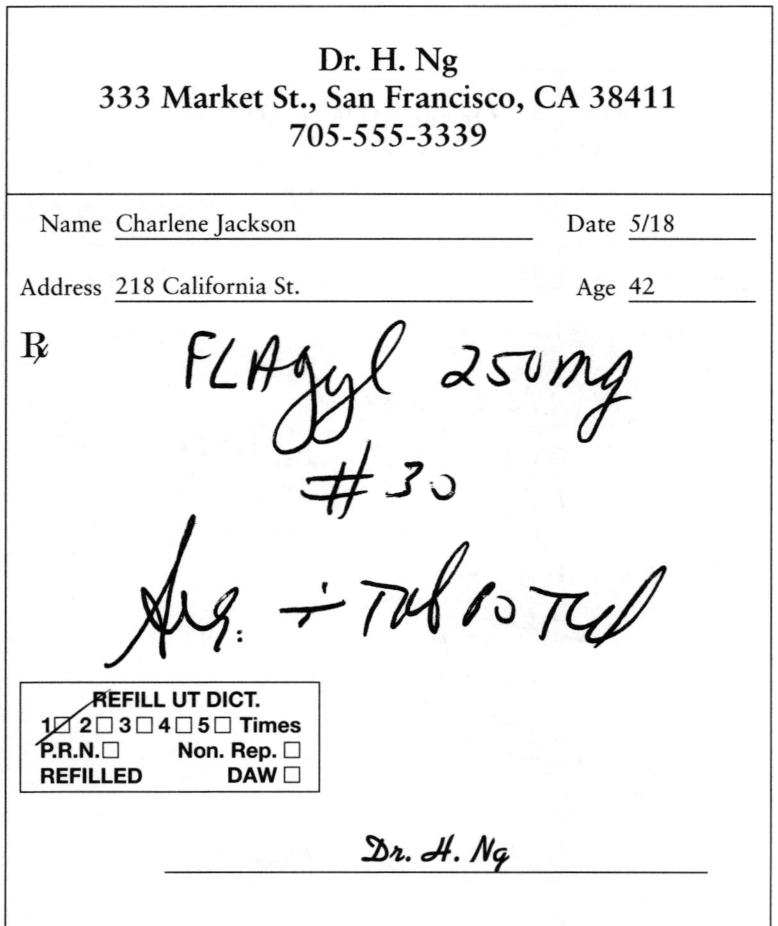
Dr. H. Ng
333 Market St., San Francisco, CA 38411
705-555-3339
Name Charlene Jackson Date 5/18
Address 218 California St. Age 42
℞ FLAgyl 250mg
#30
Sig: i Tab po TID
REFILL UT DICT.
1☒ 2☐ 3☐ 4☐ 5☐ Times
P.R.N.☐ Non. Rep. ☐
REFILLED DAW ☐
Dr. H. Ng

8.22a

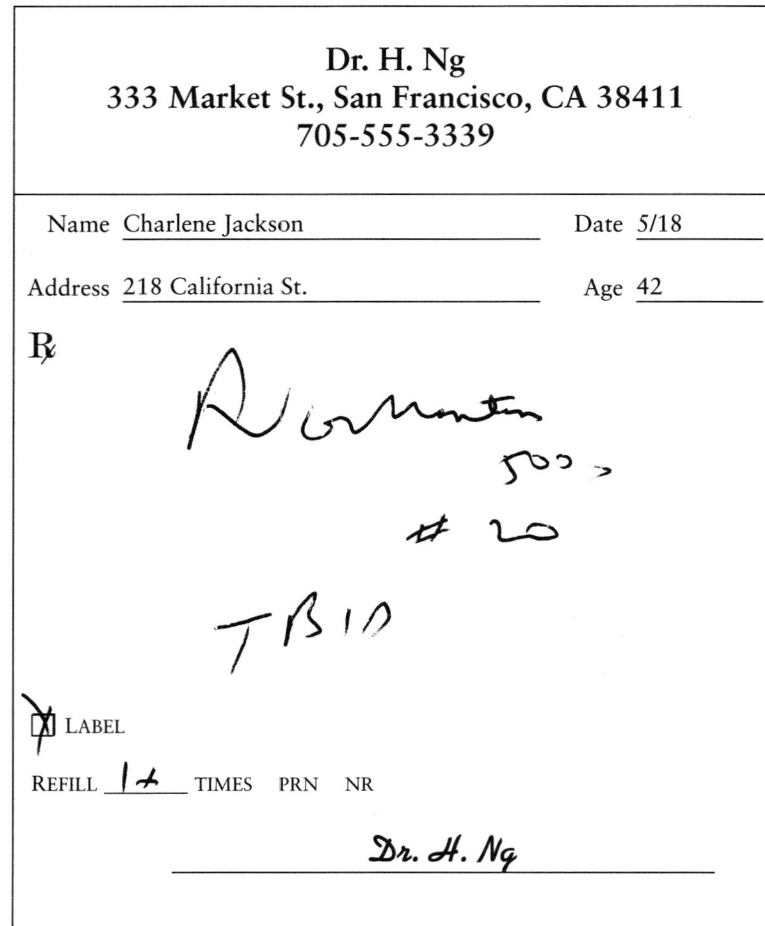
Dr. H. Ng
333 Market St., San Francisco, CA 38411
705-555-3339
Name Charlene Jackson Date 5/18
Address 218 California St. Age 42
℞ Augmentin
500
20
T BID
☒ LABEL
REFILL 1x TIMES PRN NR
Dr. H. Ng

8.22b

8.23	PT. NAME: **NATALIE FASS** AGE: **72**	GENDER: **F** DX: **GERD, IBS, HTN, OA, INSOMNIA, DEPRESSION, HIGH CHOLESTEROL**	ADDRESS: **90 SPRING ST.** ALLERGY: **PCN**	WEIGHT: **155** HX: **SOCIAL DRINKER**

MEDICATION	SIG.	PRESCRIBER	ORIG. DATE	REFILL DATE	REFILL DATE	REFILL DATE	REFILL DATE
Vytorin 10/40 mg #30	1 qd	Weinreb	8/24	9/23	10/22	11/21	12/19
Lunesta 2 mg #30	1 hs	Weinreb	11/18	12/17			
Toprol XL 50 mg #30	1/2 tab once a day	Weinreb	11/18				
Nexium 40 mg #30	1 capsule 30 min ac bkfst	Weinreb	Label only				
Furosemide 20 mg #30	1 q am	Weinreb	8/18	9/17	10/16	11/15	12/19
Lexapro 10 mg #30	1 qd	Weinreb	11/18	12/17			

Dr. Jerry Stewart, DDS
12 South Park St., Benton Falls, PA 44499
505-555-6464

Name Natalie Fass Date 12/22

Address 90 Spring St. Age 72

℞ Azithromycin 250 mg tab
Disp 6 (six)
Sig Take 2 tab one hour prior to dental visit

Refills 0

Dr. Jerry Stewart, DDS

8.23a

Dr. John Weinreb
44 South Park St., Benton Falls, PA 44499
505-555-2267

Name Natalie Fass Date 12/22

Address 90 Spring St. Age 72

℞ Celebrex
200
#30
T PAm

☐ Label

Refill 5X times PRN NR

Dr. John Weinreb

8.23b

8.24

PT. NAME: **PAM AVENTURA** AGE: **60**
GENDER: **F**
DX: **VAGINAL CANDIDIASIS, HYPOTHYROID, HTN**
ADDRESS: **12 OAK CIRCLE**
ALLERGY: **ASA**
WEIGHT: **159**
HX: **SMOKER: 45 PACK-YEARS**
HEIGHT: **5′ 7″**
BMI: **25**

MEDICATION	SIG.	PRESCRIBER	ORIG. DATE	REFILL DATE	REFILL DATE	REFILL DATE	REFILL DATE
Synthroid 25 mcg #21	1 qd	Walterman	4/1				
Synthroid 50 mcg #30	1 qd	Walterman	4/30				
Norvasc 2.5 mg #30	1 qd	Walterman	3/5	4/3	5/3		

Dr. Jay Walterman
9990 Westchester Lane, Chicago, IL 49999
222-555-9596

Name Pam Aventura Date 5/8

Address 12 Oak Circle Age 60

℞

Diflucan 150
#2
1 p. now.
1 p. in 3 weeks

Refills NR

Dr. Jay Walterman

8.24a

Dr. Jay Walterman
9990 Westchester Lane, Chicago, IL 49999
222-555-9596

Name Pam Aventura Date 5/8

Address 12 Oak Circle Age 60

℞

Lasix #30
40mg
Sig: i p.o. q d.

☐ Label

Refill 1 times

Dr. Jay Walterman

8.24b

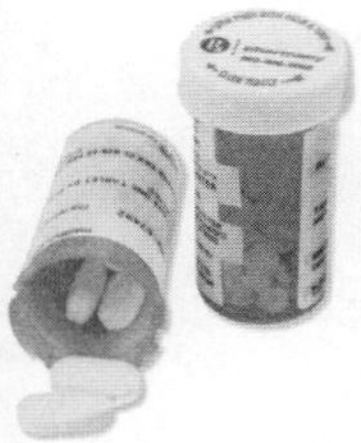

9 • MENTAL HEALTH, PART I

UPON COMPLETION OF THIS CHAPTER, THE STUDENT WILL BE ABLE TO:

- counsel patients on the importance of compliance when taking these medications.
- counsel patients on and discuss in general terms the serious side effects of these agents and the potential for habituation or dependence associated with long-term therapy.
- counsel patients on the proper order of medication administration.
- maintain appropriate records for refills on controlled substances that were dispensed.
- discuss the changes in antidepressant therapy and the time frames associated with the conversion processes.
- evaluate and rank CNS agents by class, potency, adverse effects, dose, etc.
- explain the mechanisms of action of the CNS agents based on molecular receptors and neurotransmitters.

DRUG LIST

Abilify
Ambien/Sonata/Lunesta
Amitriptyline/Desipramine/Nortriptyline/Doxepin
Anafranil
Ativan/Valium/Klonopin/Tranxene/Xanax/Niravam
BuSpar
Cymbalta
Desyrel
Effexor/Pristiq
Geodon
Halcion
Haldol
Mellaril/Thorazine
Prolixin
Prozac/Zoloft/Paxil/Celexa/Lexapro
Remeron
Restoril
Risperdal/Invega
Saphris
Seroquel
Symbyax
Zyprexa

• DRUG HOT POINTS

Abilify
Partial D_2/5-HT_{1A} agonist and 5-HT_{2A} antagonist

Ambien
Similar to benzodiazepines
More specific for sleep (binds to omega-1)
Compare with Sonata and Lunesta

Amitriptyline
High anticholinergic effects, fatal in overdose
For sleep, neuropathic pain, depression

Anafranil
TCA used for OCD

Ativan
Class mechanism (potentiate GABA effects)
Abuse potential (monitor refills)
Alcohol and driving warnings
Tablets can be used sublingually
Advantages over Valium (one-step inactivation)
Ideal for the elderly if needed
IV for status epilepticus

BuSpar
5-HT_{1A} partial agonist, normalizes 5-HT
Reduces anxiety; takes weeks for effect

Cymbalta
Serotonin and NE reuptake inhibitor (SNRI)
Antidepressant and for diabetic peripheral neuropathic pain, back pain, and OA pain

Desipramine
Less sedation than other TCAs
Less anticholinergic effects

Desyrel
Some SSRI action
Effective hypnotic; used for depressed insomniac
Less CV adverse effects
Potential for priapism in male patients

Effexor
Similar action as TCAs (SNRI)
Less anticholinergic, sedation, some HTN
Compare with Pristiq

Halcion
Fast onset, short duration
Should be limited to 30 days or less
Some anterograde amnesia has been reported

Haldol
Potent DA antagonist, high EPS
Depot formulation available; compare with Prolixin
Caution: dosing confusion (5 mg or 0.5 mg)

Klonopin
Highly lipid soluble
Higher milligram potency than Valium
Uses: epilepsy, sleep, restless legs syndrome

Mellaril
More anticholinergic effects than others
Impotence, constipation, arrhythmia
Caution over 800 mg/day: eye problems
Compare with **Thorazine**

Nortriptyline
Metabolite of amitriptyline
Less orthostasis: more appropriate for the elderly
Compare with doxepin

Prozac
Activating SSRI; dosing: qd in A.M.
Anorexia, sexual dysfunction
Active long-acting metabolite (norfluoxetine)
Inhibits CYP-450: interaction with warfarin, etc.
Compare/contrast: Zoloft/Paxil/Lexapro/Celexa. Also Prozac weekly, Sarafem

Remeron
Unique antidepressant mechanism: $alpha_2$ presynaptic, and H_1-receptor antagonist
Side effects: drowsiness, orthostasis
Dosing: HS
Effective antidepressant; can increase appetite

Restoril
Intermediate acting—used for sleep
Slow onset of action

• DRUG HOT POINTS (*continued*)

Risperdal
Atypical antipsychotic (treats both positive and negative symptoms of psychosis)
Low dose: less EPS than Haldol
Risperdal M tablets: orally disintegrating
Risperdal Consta injection every 2 weeks
Compare with Invega

Seroquel
Atypical antipsychotic: low EPS
Compare with Geodon
Compare with Saphris SL tabs

Tranxene
Quickly absorbed, intermediate acting
High abuse potential
Requires low gastric pH for active form

Valium
Lipid soluble, fast acting, long duration
Potential for abuse
High dose for skeletal muscle spasm
IV for status epilepticus

Xanax
Daytime anxiety, for sleep, for panic attack
To *ideally* D/C: taper dose ↓ by 1/4 qd Q 14 days
Driving, alcohol warnings, abuse potential
Xanax XR tablets: once daily
Compare with Niravam

Zyprexa
Atypical antipsychotic: sedation, low EPS, weight gain, DM potential
Compare with Symbyax

• QUESTIONS TO BE ANSWERED IN PREPARATION FOR CHAPTER 9 LAB

- Which dose of diazepam is appropriate for the treatment of severe skeletal muscle spasm?
- What important patient counseling should be given to a person who is starting to take Remeron?
- What is the mechanism of action of Haldol?
- How many cyclic structures are in the molecule of Elavil?
- What are the advantages of the second-generation TCAs over the first-generation TCAs?
- What is the name of the main metabolite of Valium, and what is its half-life?
- What is the name of the active metabolite of Elavil?
- What is the name of the active metabolite of imipramine?
- What serious side effect for male patients can be caused by Desyrel?
- Compare and contrast the members of the SSRI group of antidepressants.
    - Which one is most activating?
    - Which one has the most anticholinergic properties?
    - Which one has the active metabolite with the longest duration of action?
    - Which one appears to have the least interactions with other medications?
    - Which one has been known to cause the most GI problems?
    - What period of time should elapse between the use of a MAOI and these agents?
- What is the name of the metabolite of Prozac, and what is its half-life?
- Which antipsychotic agent has the highest anticholinergic effects?
- Which antipsychotic agent has the highest EPS effects?
- Which combination product containing olanzapine and fluoxetine is indicated for the treatment of depressive episodes associated with bipolar disorder?
- Which benzodiazepine products are most appropriate for elderly patients?
- How does Pristiq compare with venlafaxine?
- Which SSRI is available in a 90-mg weekly capsule?
- What are the comparative strengths (dosing equivalencies) of the typical antipsychotic agents?
- What are the comparative strengths (dosing equivalencies) of each of the benzodiazepines?
- Which pharmacologic actions characterize an "atypical" antipsychotic agent?
- Compare and contrast the "atypical" antipsychotic agents to the "typical" ones.
- What is the proposed therapeutic mechanism of action for the benzodiazepines?
- Compare and contrast the hypnotic mechanism of action of zolpidem with that of temazepam.
- Pharmacologically, how does Sonata differ from Ambien?
- At what dose is Xanax used in the treatment of panic attack?
- Which phenothiazine antipsychotic agent has a warning about 800 mg/day maximum dose to avoid eye problems?
- Which oral tablet form (PO) benzodiazepine has the shortest duration of action?
- Explain the reason why haloperidol or thioridazine is not appropriate for a patient with Parkinson's disease.
- Your client has cirrhosis of the liver. He requires a benzodiazepine for anxiety and sleep. Why would Serax or Ativan be more appropriate than Valium or Tranxene?
- A person has been taking Xanax 0.25 mg tid for the past year. The physician wants to D/C the medication. What is an effective schedule to accomplish this?
- Describe the proposed mechanism of action of buspirone.
- Which "typical" antipsychotic (neuroleptic) drug is used to treat psychosis, urticaria, and intractable hiccup?
- Which TCA has SSRI pharmacologic characteristics?
- Your client is taking Anafranil for OCD. Describe the disorder.
- What is an advantage of Niravam over Xanax tablets?

• MENTAL HEALTH, PART I, MEDICATION THERAPY MANAGEMENT QUESTIONS AND COMMENTS

- Would you like to have a discussion about ways to make your medication for nerves work better? There might be some lifestyle issues to talk about. This would also help your sleep problems.
- I notice that you have been seeing different doctors for your sleeping pills. Would you like to have a discussion with me for a few minutes to discuss the problems with this?
- Your mother seems to be doing well with her medication to treat anxiety. It is helping to control her blood pressure; however, she mentioned that she takes alcoholic beverages. Let's have a meeting with the three of us to discuss the high risks of this problem.
- You have been receiving your medication for sleep, and you mentioned that you have been buying herbal pills for nerves elsewhere. Let's have a private discussion to talk about the dangers of this.
- Your wife said that your new antidepressant has caused serious personal problems with intimate relations between you and her. Can we discuss ways for you and her to see a trained practitioner? Alternatively, I can call your physician to recommend another class of antidepressants that would have less risk of this disturbing adverse effect.
- I notice that you have been taking diazepam for quite a while. You are in the age group in which another similar product called lorazepam might be more appropriate. You mentioned that sometimes you experience drowsiness and "hangover" from diazepam. Let's have a discussion and call your physician.
- Your grandmother is receiving a prescription for amitriptyline, and she has reported dry mouth, dizziness, and constipation. Would you mind if we all meet together and discuss the possibility that we could approach the physician and recommend an equivalent dose of a similar product called nortriptyline? It is more suitable than amitriptyline for seniors.
- Because your wife has received a new prescription for an antidepressant in the "SSRI" category, it is important that we meet to discuss certain nonprescription herbals and other medications that should not be taken concurrently. The major herbal product to avoid is St. John's wort. It could cause distressing adverse effects if it were taken by a patient who is also taking an "SSRI."
- I understand that you are upset about hearing voices from your deceased grandmother. Your physician has prescribed a new medication that should make the voices stop. Would you mind having a private meeting with me to discuss the best way to take your medication? We could also discuss methods that work well to limit the side effects of the medication.
- I understand that you are a retired physician. You are questioning the fact that your wife's physician prescribed both a "typical" and an "atypical" neuroleptic drug for her. It is sometimes done for various reasons. If you have time, would you like to discuss the pharmacology of these two classes of drugs? Let's invite your wife so she does not feel left out of the conversation. We can talk in plain language. She would feel good about our trying to help her.
- I understand that the new doctor prescribed risperidone for your mother. It is a small dose. It should limit the visions that she has experienced with low risk of adverse effects. Let's make a meeting with the three of us to discuss how to take the medication and which OTC medications to use and which should be avoided.
- Your husband has stated that since he received his antianxiety medication, he has had serious "hangover" and depression when he takes his allergy medication called diphenhydramine. We should have a meeting to discuss the problems with these two medications.
- Your patient has been taking an "atypical" neuroleptic drug and has gained 4 kg or about 9 pounds of weight last year. It is important to discuss diet control and food selection. Your patient should see a physician to check his or her blood sugar and long-term effects of the new medication. Let's meet to discuss this problem and look at the drug's literature to find a solution.

9.1

PT. NAME: **LISA MILLER**	GENDER: **F**	ADDRESS: **522 ELEPHANT DR.**	WEIGHT: **122**	HEIGHT: **5′ 2″**	BMI: **22**
AGE: **48**	DX: **COPD, BACK PAIN, URI, ANXIETY**	ALLERGY: **PCN**	HX: **ETOH**		

MEDICATION	SIG.	PRESCRIBER	ORIG. DATE	REFILL DATE	REFILL DATE	REFILL DATE	REFILL DATE
Percocet 5/325 mg #60	I q 6 h	Griffin	9/27				
Soma 350 mg #60	I bid	Griffin	9/1	10/1			
Cipro 500 mg #20	I bid	Griffin	8/25				
Theophylline SR 200 mg #120	I bid prn	Griffin	8/23				

Dr. Doug Griffin
7611 147th Terrace, Monterey, CA 38411
705-555-6644

Name Lisa Miller Date 10/2

Address 522 Elephant Dr. Age 48

℞

Xanax 0.25 #30
i hs prn sleep

Refills 0

Dr. Doug Griffin

DEA# AG1234563

9.1a

Dr. Jesse Holdman
4545 144th St., Monterey, CA 38411
705-555-2323

Name Lisa Miller Date 10/2

Address 522 Elephant Dr. Age 48

℞

Lunesta 3 mg
#10
Sig: i T QHS PRN sleep

SUBSTITUTION ALLOWED ______

PRIOR APPROVAL REQUIRED ______

NUMBER OF REFILLS ALLOWED ______

Dr. Jesse Holdman

DEA# AH1234563

9.1b

9.2	PT. NAME: **ROBERTA COOK**	GENDER: **F**	ADDRESS: **333 DEXTER AVE.**	WEIGHT: **145**	BMI: **23**
	AGE: **58**	DX: **HTN, CHF, HEART RHYTHM DISTURBANCE, DEPRESSION, INSOMNIA**	ALLERGY: **NKA**	HX: **SMOKER, SOCIAL DRINKER**	

MEDICATION	SIG.	PRESCRIBER	ORIG. DATE	REFILL DATE	REFILL DATE	REFILL DATE	REFILL DATE
Furosemide 20 mg #30	I q am	Sauls	6/30	7/28	8/30		
Digoxin 0.125 mg #30	I q am	Sauls	6/30	7/28	8/31		
Cordarone 200 mg #30	I q am	Sauls	7/1	8/2	8/31		

Dr. Alfred Sauls
151212 S High Rd., Chicago, IL 23875
954-555-1300

Name Roberta Cook Date 9/4

Address 333 Dexter Ave. Age 58

℞

Celexa 40mg
i tab i po daily
NO 30

Refills 0

Dr. Alfred Sauls

DEA# AS1234563

9.2a

Dr. Alfred Sauls
151212 S High Rd., Chicago, IL 23875
954-555-1300

Name Roberta Cook Date 9/4

Address 333 Dexter Ave. Age 58

℞

Ambien 10 #60
i q hs

Refills 0

Dr. Alfred Sauls

DEA# AS1234563

9.2b

9.3

PT. NAME: **MARY MCCOY**	GENDER: **F**	ADDRESS: **71 CAPITOL AVE.**	WEIGHT: **152**	BMI: **22**
AGE: **62**	DX: **OSTEOPOROSIS, CHOLESTEROL, ANGINA**	ALLERGY: **PCN**	HX: **SMOKER, SEDENTARY LIFESTYLE**	

MEDICATION	SIG.	PRESCRIBER	ORIG. DATE	REFILL DATE	REFILL DATE	REFILL DATE	REFILL DATE
Lactulose 946 mL	Take ud	Weiss	1/25	2/21	3/21	5/20	
Fosamax 70 mg #4	1 q wk	Weiss	1/25	2/21	3/21	4/21	
Pravachol 40 mg #30	1 qd	Weiss	1/25	2/21	3/21	4/21	
Tylenol caplets 500 mg #C	1 prn pain	OTC	2/10	4/1			

Dr. Barry Weiss
901 Sheridan St., Austin, TX 90902
874-555-9000

Name Mary McCoy Date 5/21

Address 71 Capitol Ave Age 62

℞

Elavil 25 mg
#30
Sig: i caps ~~…~~ 9:00 pm daily

Renew #100 & PRN
if requested

Refills 0

Dr. Barry Weiss

9.3a

Dr. Bart Matthews
2121 2 Ave., Austin, TX 90902
874-555-7641

Name Mary McCoy Date 5/22

Address 71 Capitol Ave Age 62

℞

Augmented 500 mg
Sig i BID c̄ meal
#14

Refills N.R.

Dr. Bart Matthews

9.3b

9.4

PT. NAME: **TIMOTHY BLOCK**	GENDER: **M**	ADDRESS: **555 ORIOLE WAY**	WEIGHT: **140**	BMI: **22**
AGE: **39**	DX: **CROHN'S DISEASE, NERVES, DEPRESSION**	ALLERGY: **PCN**	HX: **CLERK IN CONVENIENCE STORE**	

MEDICATION	SIG.	PRESCRIBER	ORIG. DATE	REFILL DATE	REFILL DATE	REFILL DATE	REFILL DATE
Asacol 400 mg #1080	2 tid	Smith	5/1	8/21			
Prednisone 5 mg #90	1 qd	Smith	4/17	7/4	10/2		

Dr. Anne L.W. Smith
451 W Camden St., Baltimore, MD 21201
410-555-0000

Name Timothy Block Date 11/3

Address 555 Oriole Way Age 39

℞

VALIUM 2MG
DISP: #50
SIG: 1/2 PO TID

REFILL 1 ☐ 2 ☐ 3 ☐ 4 ☐ NR ☐
LABEL ☐
MEDICALLY NECESSARY ☐
DEA # ____________

Dr. Anne Smith

9.4a

Dr. Al Brown
800 Oriole Drive, Baltimore, MD 21201
410-555-3326

Name Timothy Block Date 11/1

Address 555 Oriole Way Age 39

℞

Lexapro 20mg
tab i po daily
No. 30

Label X
Refill 1 times

Dr. Al Brown

9.4b

9.5	PT. NAME: **SUSAN HANSEN** AGE: **43**	GENDER: **F** DX: **DEPRESSION, IBS, SKIN RASH, DIARRHEA, INSOMNIA**	ADDRESS: **224 ALBERTY CIR.** ALLERGY: **NKA**	WEIGHT: **183**	HEIGHT: **5′ 8″**	BMI: **28**

MEDICATION	SIG.	PRESCRIBER	ORIG. DATE	REFILL DATE	REFILL DATE	REFILL DATE	REFILL DATE
Lorazepam 0.5 mg #30	1/2 hs prn sleep	Thomas	6/30	7/31			
Lotrisone cream 45 g	Apply prn rash	Thomas	5/12	7/15			

Erin Thomas, MD
988 North Ridge, New York, NY 88364
813-555-7554

Name Susan Hansen Date 8/30

Address 224 Alberty Cir. Age 43

℞

Prozac 20mg #60

ii AM, i NOON pc

Desyrel 50mg #30 thirty

ii-iii hs pc

Refills 0

Dr. Erin Thomas

9.5a

Erin Thomas, MD
988 North Ridge, New York, NY 88364
813-555-7554

Name Susan Hansen Date 8/30

Address 224 Alberty Cir. Age 43

℞

Lomotil #30

ii po prn diarrhea

Refills 0

Dr. Erin Thomas

9.5b

9.6

PT. NAME: **ANDREA JOHNSON**	GENDER: **F**	ADDRESS: **4779 HURRICANE DR.**	WEIGHT: **149**	BMI: **27**
AGE: **68**	DX: **ANXIETY, HRT, HYPOTHYROID, IBS, INSOMNIA**	ALLERGY: **ASA**	HX: **SALESCLERK IN DEPARTMENT STORE**	

MEDICATION	SIG.	PRESCRIBER	ORIG. DATE	REFILL DATE	REFILL DATE	REFILL DATE	REFILL DATE
Synthroid 0.15 mg #90	1 qd	Isaacs	4/13	11/29			
Prempro 0.625/2.5 mg #56	1 qd	Garvey	9/14				
Levsin 0.125 mg SL #20	1 prn cramps	Isaacs	7/14	9/15	11/20		
Guaifenesin Cough Syrup 4 oz	5 mL (1 tsp) prn with water	OTC	8/4				

Dr. Howard Isaacs
1115 Turnaround Lane, Detroit, MI 64789
343-555-7000

Name Andrea Johnson Date 12/6

Address 4779 Hurricane Dr. Age 68

℞

Ativan 0.5mg
#21 (Twenty-one)
Sig: use only as directed

Refills 0

Dr. Howard Isaacs

DEA# AI1234563

9.6a

Dr. Howard Isaacs
1115 Turnaround Lane, Detroit, MI 64789
343-555-7000

Name Andrea Johnson Date 12/6

Address 4779 Hurricane Dr. Age 68

℞

Ambien 10mg #45
Sig: Take i tab PO HS PRN

DO NOT REFILL ☑

REFILL _______ TIMES

Dr. Howard Isaacs

DEA# AI1234563

9.6b

9.7	PT. NAME: **EMMA JOHNSON**	GENDER: **F**	ADDRESS: **4952 IBIS LANE**	WEIGHT: **205**	BMI: **29**
	AGE: **72**	DX: **URINARY INCONTINENCE, CONSTIPATION, HTN, OA, GERD**	ALLERGY: **SULFA**	HX: **RETIRED TEACHER**	

MEDICATION	SIG.	PRESCRIBER	ORIG. DATE	REFILL DATE	REFILL DATE	REFILL DATE	REFILL DATE
Niravam 1 mg #30	1 tab qd	Worthing	7/5	9/12			
Lactulose 32 oz	15 mL qd	Worthing	9/2				
Voltaren XR 100 mg #30	1 qd	Worthing	8/20				
HCTZ 25 mg #90	1 qd	Worthing	1/4	4/5	7/6		
Tucks Suppositories #24	1 pr hs prn	Worthing	8/4				

Jane Engle, MD
500 N Wood St., Chicago, IL 49494
813-555-0001

Name Emma Johnson Date 9/18

Address 4952 Ibis Lane Age 72

℞

Imipramine 25 mg
#28
Sig: i HS

Refills 0

Dr. Jane Engle

9.7a

Jane Engle, MD
500 N Wood St., Chicago, IL 49494
813-555-0001

Name Emma Johnson Date 9/18

Address 4952 Ibis Lane Age 72

℞

Prilosec 20 mg
#30
Sig: i PO q AM

Refills 0

Dr. Jane Engle

9.7b

9.8 PT. NAME: **BRIAN HOOVER** AGE: **36** GENDER: **M** DX: **ANXIETY, DEPRESSION, GI PROBLEMS, BACK PAIN, SKIN FUNGUS INFECTION** ADDRESS: **758 EAGLE RUN** ALLERGY: **PCN** WEIGHT: **188** BMI: **26**

MEDICATION	SIG.	PRESCRIBER	ORIG. DATE	REFILL DATE	REFILL DATE	REFILL DATE	REFILL DATE
Diflucan 100 mg #30	I qd	Thomas	7/29				
Elavil 25 mg #30	I hs	Thomas	6/29				
Doxepin 10 mg #30	I hs	Thomas	7/29				
Ativan 1 mg #90	I tid	Thomas	7/29				
Naproxen 500 mg #30	I bid	Thomas	8/12				

Dr. Erin Thomas
988 North Ridge, New York, NY 88364
813-555-7554

Name Brian Hoover Date 8/15

Address 758 Eagle Run Age 36

℞

Desyrel Dividose 150 mg
Disp #30
Sig: 1/3 tab @ am &
1/3 tab @ HS

Refills 1

Dr. Erin Thomas

9.8a

Dr. Erin Thomas
988 North Ridge, New York, NY 88364
813-555-7554

Name Brian Hoover Date 8/15

Address 758 Eagle Run Age 36

℞

Cytotec 200 mcg tab
Sig i tab po 2xd
#60

☐ LABEL

REFILL 1 TIMES

Dr. Erin Thomas

9.8b

9.9

PT. NAME: **LISA MARTIN** | GENDER: **F** | ADDRESS: **4505 OLIVE DR.** | WEIGHT: **120** | HEIGHT: **5′ 7″** | BMI: **19**

AGE: **30** | DX: **"NERVES" AND MUSCLE SPASM** | ALLERGY: **PCN** | HX: **DANCER AND MODEL; PAYS FOR PURCHASE WITH $100 BILLS**

MEDICATION	SIG.	PRESCRIBER	ORIG. DATE	REFILL DATE	REFILL DATE	REFILL DATE	REFILL DATE
Valium 10 mg #50	I bid	Godfrey	3/12	4/10	5/15	6/20	
Vicodin #30	I bid	Godfrey	3/15	3/30	4/17	5/12	6/9
Valium 10 mg #50	I bid	Godfrey	1/4	1/26	2/18	3/8	
Carisoprodol 350 mg #50	I q 6–8 h prn	Godfrey	1/4	1/26	2/18	3/8	4/29
Delsym Susp. 5 oz (6 bottles)	prn for cough	OTC	3/5	4/6	5/9	6/20	

Dr. Arnold Godfrey
111 W Madison St., Seattle, WA 59955
705-555-1111

Name Lisa Martin Date 6/30

Address 4505 Olive Dr. Age 30

℞

Xanax (1 mg) #100
Sig: i bid–tid prn
tension/stress

Refills 0

Dr. Arnold Godfrey

DEA# AG1234563

9.9a

Dr. Arnold Godfrey
111 W Madison St., Seattle, WA 59955
705-555-1111

Name Lisa Martin Date 6/30

Address 4505 Olive Dr. Age 30

℞

Soma-350 #100
Sig: i q 6–8 h prn
muscle spasm

Refills 0

Dr. Arnold Godfrey

9.9b

9.10

PT. NAME: **ERICA JONES** AGE: **72** GENDER: **F** DX: **"NERVES—FEEL LOUSY," OSTEOPOROSIS, ACNE VULGARIS, INSOMNIA, DEPRESSION** ADDRESS: **5587 GREEN ST.** ALLERGY: **DAIRY PRODUCTS** WEIGHT: **139** HX: **SMOKER** HEIGHT: **5′ 6″** BMI: **22**

MEDICATION	SIG.	PRESCRIBER	ORIG. DATE	REFILL DATE	REFILL DATE	REFILL DATE	REFILL DATE
Renova Cream 0.05% 30 g	Apply hs	Jackson	7/12	9/30			
Actonel 35 mg #4	1 weekly	Harrison	7/12	8/11	9/10		
Tums #150	3 qd	OTC	5/5	6/10	7/20	9/3	

Dr. Alfred Soto
10 S High Rd., Chicago, IL 23875
954-555-2222

Name Erica Jones Date 10/20

Address 5587 Green St. Age 72

℞

VALIUM 2mg #120 Sig T QID PRN

RESTORIL 15mg #30 Sig T hs

Do Not Refill

Dr. Alfred Soto

DEA# AS1234563

9.10a

Dr. Alfred Soto
10 S High Rd., Chicago, IL 23875
954-555-2222

Name Erica Jones Date 10/20

Address 5587 Green St. Age 72

℞

PROZAC 20mg #60 Sig TT AM

Do Not Refill

Dr. Alfred Soto

9.10b

9.11

PT. NAME: **JASON MARTINS**
AGE: **68**
GENDER: **M**
DX: **GOUT, HTN, DEPRESSED, NERVOUS, HIGH CHOLESTEROL**
ADDRESS: **550 SW 8TH ST.**
ALLERGY: **NKA**
WEIGHT: **180**
HX: **RETIRED SALESMAN**
BMI: **29**

MEDICATION	SIG.	PRESCRIBER	ORIG. DATE	REFILL DATE	REFILL DATE	REFILL DATE	REFILL DATE
Zocor 20 mg #60	1 bid	Raskin	2/25	3/30	5/5	6/5	7/12
Zyloprim 300 mg #90	1 q am	Raskin	4/1	7/2	11/22		
Hytrin 2 mg #30	1 hs	Raskin	7/20	9/26			

Dr. Herbert Raskin
400 Tamiami Trail, Miami, FL 44718
463-555-8009

Name Jason Martins Date 12/2

Address 550 SW 8th St. Age 68

℞

Paxil
20mg
qd
#60

Label

Refill ______ times PRN NR

Dr. Herbert Raskin

9.11a

Dr. Herbert Raskin
400 Tamiami Trail, Miami, FL 44718
463-555-8009

Name Jason Martins Date 12/2

Address 550 SW 8th St. Age 68

℞

ALPVAZOLAM 0.25
Sig: T P.O. HS
#100

☑ Label

Refill 2 times PRN NR

Dr. Herbert Raskin

9.11b

9.12

PT. NAME: **JENNIFER ROSA** | AGE: **38** | GENDER: **F** | DX: **"NERVES," IBS, BACK PAIN, INSOMNIA** | ADDRESS: **1578 IBIS CT.** | ALLERGY: **PCN** | WEIGHT: **118** | HX: **SCHOOLTEACHER** | HEIGHT: **5′ 1″** | BMI: **23**

MEDICATION	SIG.	PRESCRIBER	ORIG. DATE	REFILL DATE	REFILL DATE	REFILL DATE	REFILL DATE
Bentyl 10 mg #60	1 q 6 h prn abdominal pain	Salk	9/22	11/20			
NuLYTELY Solution 4000 mL	Take ud	Berke	9/15				
Tylenol No. 3 #60	1 q 4 h prn	Salk	6/13	9/7	10/20		

Dr. Melvin Salk
12155 S High Rd., Chicago, IL 23875
954-555-1333

Name Jennifer Rosa Date 12/1

Address 1578 Ibis Ct. Age 38

℞

Elavil 25mg

HS

#30

Refills 2

Dr. Melvin Salk

9.12a

Dr. Melvin Salk
12155 S High Rd., Chicago, IL 23875
954-555-1333

Name Jennifer Rosa Date 12/1

Address 1578 Ibis Ct. Age 38

℞

Desipramine 25mg tabs

2 tabs QD

#50

Refills: Call

Dr. Melvin Salk

9.12b

9.13 PT. NAME: **RUTH PETERSON** AGE: **58** GENDER: **F** DX: **"NERVES," HTN, "ARTHRITIS," IBS** ADDRESS: **84 GREEN AVE. W** ALLERGY: **NKA** WEIGHT: **148** BMI: **25**

MEDICATION	SIG.	PRESCRIBER	ORIG. DATE	REFILL DATE	REFILL DATE	REFILL DATE	REFILL DATE
Zyrtec 10 mg #90	1 qd	Talan	3/5	6/29			
Norvasc 10 mg #30	1 qd	Talan	4/11	5/10	6/13	7/13	
Anacin Tabs #100	1–2 qid prn	OTC	2/5	3/12	4/9	5/8	6/20

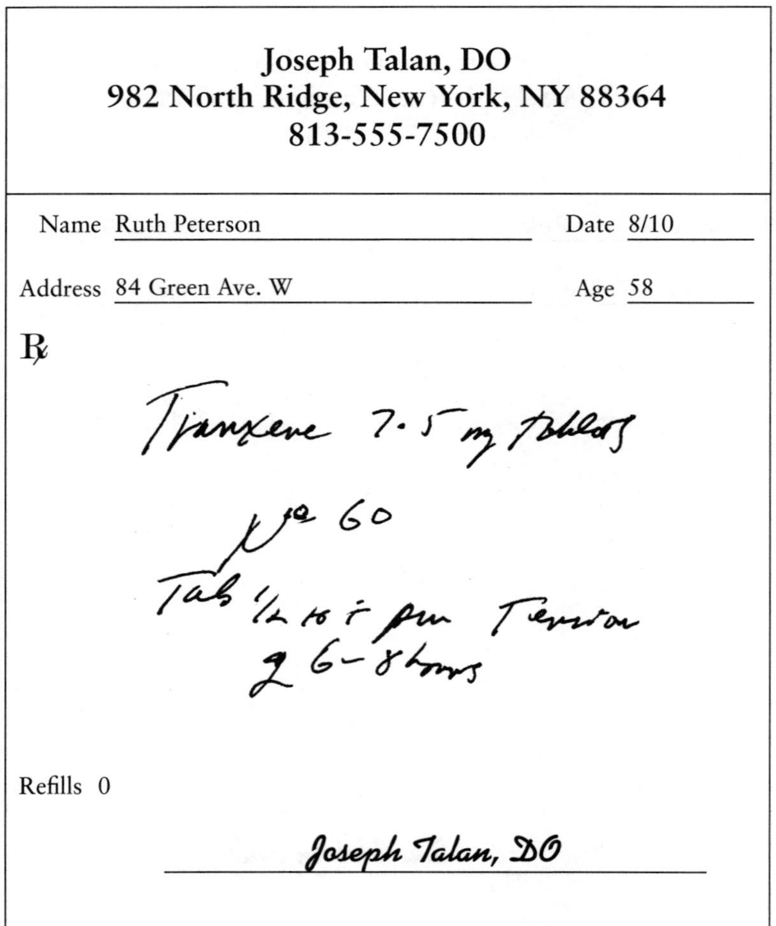

Joseph Talan, DO
982 North Ridge, New York, NY 88364
813-555-7500

Name Ruth Peterson Date 8/10
Address 84 Green Ave. W Age 58

℞

Tranxene 7.5 mg tablets
No 60
Tab ½ to i prn Tension
q 6–8 hours

Refills 0

Joseph Talan, DO

9.13a

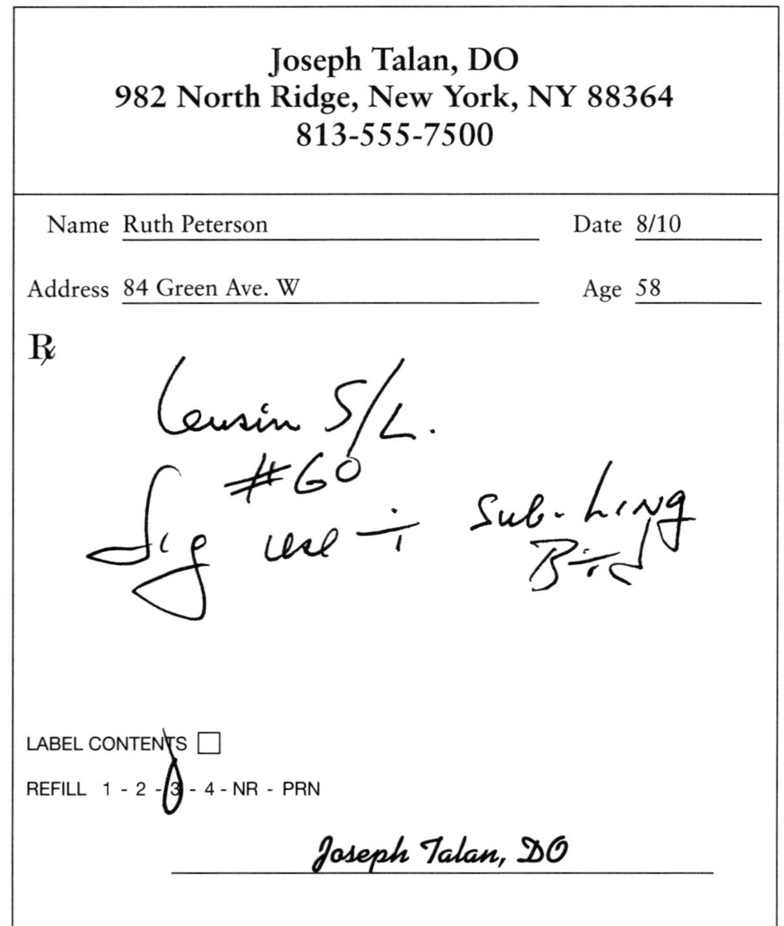

Joseph Talan, DO
982 North Ridge, New York, NY 88364
813-555-7500

Name Ruth Peterson Date 8/10
Address 84 Green Ave. W Age 58

℞

Levsin S/L.
#60
Sig use i Sub-Ling
BID

LABEL CONTENTS ☐
REFILL 1 - 2 - (3) - 4 - NR - PRN

Joseph Talan, DO

9.13b

9.14

PT. NAME: **DR. MAMIE BLOCK** GENDER: **F** ADDRESS: **354 PENNSYLVANIA AVE.** WEIGHT: **138** BMI: **25**

AGE: **48** DX: **OA, INSOMNIA, CONSTIPATION, DEPRESSION** ALLERGY: **ASA, STRAWBERRIES** HX: **GENERAL DENTIST**

MEDICATION	SIG.	PRESCRIBER	ORIG. DATE	REFILL DATE	REFILL DATE	REFILL DATE	REFILL DATE
Ultram 50 mg #20	I q 4–6 h—NMT 5 in 24 h	Ossi	2/11	4/12			
Cefadroxil 500 mg #9	I on nt. before surgery & I qd	Bressler	2/4				
Sonata 10 mg #10	I hs prn	Ossi	2/11	4/2			
Colace 100 mg #60	I qd prn	OTC	1/5	3/9			

Dr. Frank Ossi
7999 147th Terrace, Monterey, CA 38411
705-555-1259

Name Mamie Block, DDS Date 4/15

Address 354 Pennsylvania Ave. Age 48

℞

Halcion 0.25mg # 30
S ī po hs

Refill ______ times

Dr. Frank Ossi

DEA# AO1234563

9.14a

Dr. Frank Ossi
7999 147th Terrace, Monterey, CA 38411
705-555-1259

Name Mamie Block, DDS Date 4/15

Address 354 Pennsylvania Ave. Age 48

℞

Zoloft 50mg po
as instructed

#100

Refill one times

Dr. Frank Ossi

9.14b

9.15

PT. NAME: **FLORENCE GRIFF** GENDER: **F** ADDRESS: **564 CAPITOL AVE.** WEIGHT: **243** HEIGHT: **6′** BMI: **33**
AGE: **47** DX: **DEPRESSION, HEARTBURN, IBS, INSOMNIA, TOPICAL FUNGUS** ALLERGY: **IODINE, PCN** HX: **ACCOUNTANT**

MEDICATION	SIG.	PRESCRIBER	ORIG. DATE	REFILL DATE	REFILL DATE	REFILL DATE	REFILL DATE
Diprolene AF Cream 15 g	Apply bid to rash	Weiss	1/15	4/30			
Prilosec 20 mg #30	1 qd	Weiss	6/20	7/30			
Bentyl 10 mg #C	1 prn cramps	Weiss	1/20	4/30	6/20		

Dr. Barry Weiss
901 Sheridan St., Austin, TX 90902
874-555-9000

Name Florence Griff Date 8/20

Address 564 Capitol Ave. Age 47

℞

Zoloft 100 mg. # 75 Seventy five
Tablets
1/2 tab p.o.

Refills 1

Dr. Barry Weiss

9.15a

Dr. Barry Weiss
901 Sheridan St., Austin, TX 90902
874-555-9000

Name Florence Griff Date 8/20

Address 564 Capitol Ave. Age 47

℞

Sinequan 50 mg. # 60
2 cap. at HS.

Refills 1

Dr. Barry Weiss

9.15b

9.16	PT. NAME: **GEORGIA HOFFMAN** AGE: **61**	GENDER: **F** DX: **DEPRESSED, ANXIOUS, COPD, HIGH LDL CHOLESTEROL, OSTEOPOROSIS**	ADDRESS: **321 WEST RD.** ALLERGY: **ASA, EGGS**	WEIGHT: **150** HX: **ATOPIC DERMATITIS AS A CHILD**	BMI: **29**

MEDICATION	SIG.	PRESCRIBER	ORIG. DATE	REFILL DATE	REFILL DATE	REFILL DATE	REFILL DATE
Zocor 40 mg #30	I hs	Richards	3/31	4/20			
Medrol Dosepak #21	Use ud	Richards	3/8				
Theophylline SR 200 mg #60	I bid	Richards	2/21	4/20			
Advair Diskus 250/50 mcg #60	I inhalation bid	Richards	2/21				
Valium 5 mg #CXX	I bid prn nerves	Richards	1/15	3/18			

Dr. Vanessa Padron
500 Circle Rd., Omaha, NE 44718
463-555-8222

Name Georgia Hoffman Date 4/21

Address 321 West Rd. Age 61

℞

BUSPAR 10 mg
DISP: #50
SIG: ī PO BID

Refills 1

Dr. Vanessa Padron

9.16a

Dr. Vanessa Padron
500 Circle Rd., Omaha, NE 44718
463-555-8222

Name Georgia Hoffman Date 4/21

Address 321 West Rd. Age 61

℞

ZOLOFT 50 mg.
#30
Sig: ī p.o. Q.D.

Refills 1

Dr. Vanessa Padron

9.16b

9.17

PT. NAME: **GLADYS CHANDLER** | GENDER: **F** | ADDRESS: **566 EAST CT.** | WEIGHT: **128** | BMI: **25**

AGE: **64** | DX: **"DEPRESSED," HTN, ANXIETY, MUSCLE CRAMPS, OSTEOPOROSIS** | ALLERGY: **CHOCOLATE** | HX: **PHYSICIAN'S WIFE (DR. CHANDLER)**

MEDICATION	SIG.	PRESCRIBER	ORIG. DATE	REFILL DATE	REFILL DATE	REFILL DATE	REFILL DATE
Plendil 5 mg #30	1 qd	Sauls	2/1	3/29	4/29		
Catapres TTS-2 patch #4	Apply q wk	Sauls	2/5	3/4	4/1		
Fosamax 70 mg #4	1 q wk	Sauls	2/8	3/9	4/4		
Dalmane 30 mg #90	1 hs prn	Chandler	1/3	4/12			

Dr. Alfred Sauls
151212 S High Rd., Chicago, IL 23875
954-555-1300

Name Gladys Chandler Date 5/17

Address 566 East Ct. Age 64

℞

Desipramine 25 mg
30
i Qhs x i wk then
ii Qhs

☑ Label

Refill 2 times PRN NR

Dr. Alfred Sauls

9.17a

Dr. Sam Chandler
300 White Ave., Chicago, IL 23875
954-555-9909

Name Gladys Chandler Date 5/15

Address 566 East Ct. Age 64

℞

Norflex
#30

as directed

Refill 2 times

Dr. Sam Chandler

9.17b

9.18

PT. NAME: **HENRIETTA JONES**	GENDER: **F**	ADDRESS: **23 SOUTH ST.**	WEIGHT: **130**	BMI: **22**
AGE: **58**	DX: **PAIN, DEPRESSION, BACK PAIN, MUSCLE SPASM**	ALLERGY: **NKA**	HX: **UNSTABLE PERSON, DEMANDING, ARGUMENTATIVE**	

MEDICATION	SIG.	PRESCRIBER	ORIG. DATE	REFILL DATE	REFILL DATE	REFILL DATE	REFILL DATE
Elavil 50 mg #30	l hs	Gramling	5/18	6/24			
Restoril 7.5 mg #30	l hs	Gramling	4/6	5/8	6/12		
Vicoprofen #30	l q 8 h	Gramling	5/12	6/12			

Dr. Lawrence Gramling
922 Gator St., Austin, TX 90902
874-555-0101

Name Henrietta Jones Date 6/28

Address 23 South St. Age 58

℞

	Amt.	Refill
1 Klonopin 1mg Sig: ī po QHS	#30 THIRTY	three
2 Paxil 20mg Sig: ī po QAM	#30 THIRTY	three

Dr. Lawrence Gramling

DEA# AG1234563

9.18a

Dr. Rodney Jacobs
220 University Dr., Austin, TX 90902
874-555-9955

Name Henrietta Jones Date 6/25

Address 23 South St. Age 58

℞

Soma 350 mg
#30 (thirty)
ī tid [illegible]

Refill n/r times

Dr. Rodney Jacobs

9.18b

9.19 PT. NAME: **JOHN NELSON** GENDER: **M** ADDRESS: **145 NORTH AVE.** WEIGHT: **124** BMI: **21**
AGE: **87** DX: **PAIN, AGITATION, CARDIOMYOPATHY, CONSTIPATION** ALLERGY: **NKA** HX: **HOSPICE PATIENT (TERMINALLY ILL) LIVING AT HOME**

MEDICATION	SIG.	PRESCRIBER	ORIG. DATE	REFILL DATE	REFILL DATE	REFILL DATE	REFILL DATE
Ativan 1 mg #30	1 sl bid prn agitation	Suskind	3/22	4/28	5/18		
Digoxin 0.125 mg #30	1 qod for heart	Suskind	3/22	5/20			
Lasix 20 mg #15	1 qd for fluid & BP	Suskind	3/22	4/20	5/19		
Fleet Enema, saline 113 mL	prn for BM	Suskind	3/22	4/2	4/12	5/10	5/20
Lisinopril 10 mg #50	1 qd for BP	Suskind	3/22	5/12			
Duragesic 25 mcg/hr patch #15	Apply q 72 h for pain	Suskind	4/22				

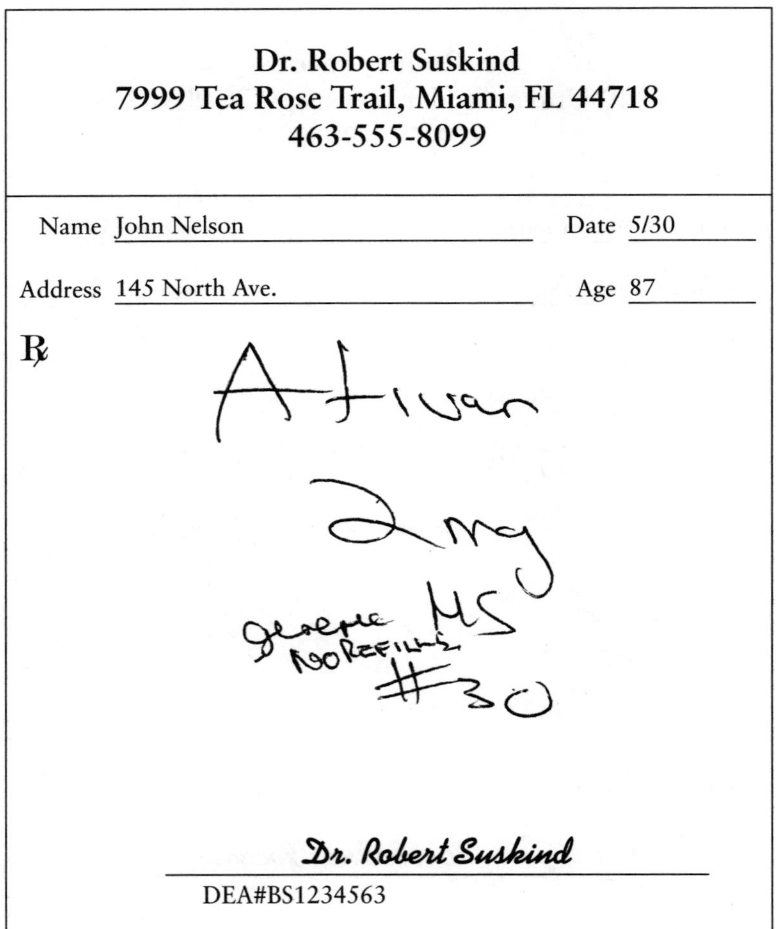
Dr. Robert Suskind
7999 Tea Rose Trail, Miami, FL 44718
463-555-8099

Name John Nelson Date 5/30
Address 145 North Ave. Age 87

℞ Ativan
2 mg
generic HS
NO REFILLS
#30

Dr. Robert Suskind
DEA#BS1234563

9.19a

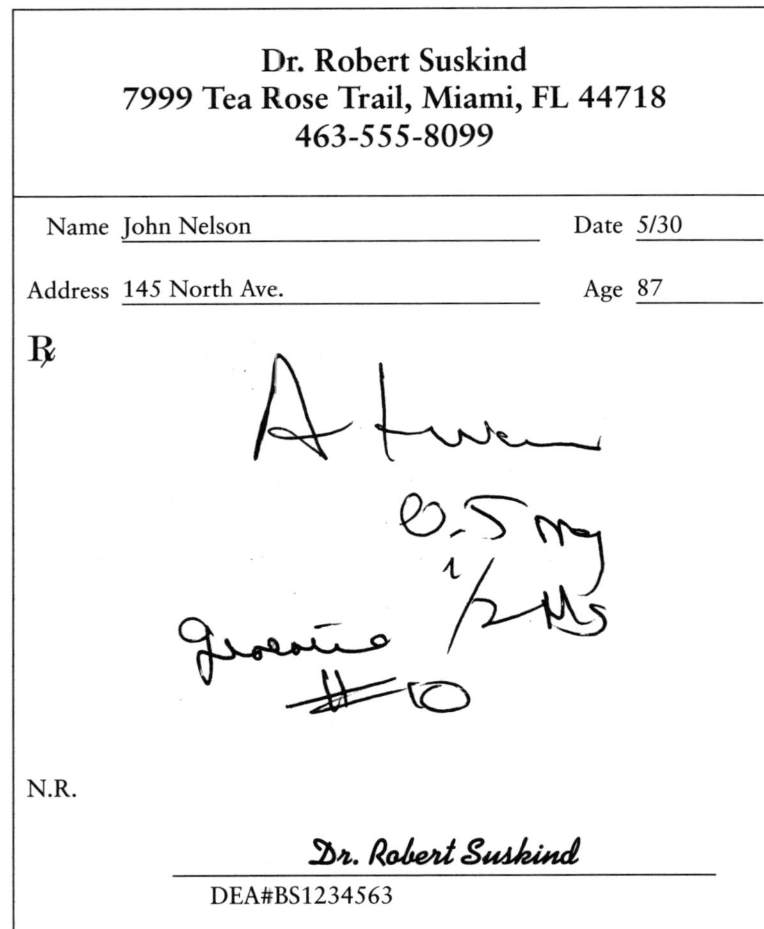
Dr. Robert Suskind
7999 Tea Rose Trail, Miami, FL 44718
463-555-8099

Name John Nelson Date 5/30
Address 145 North Ave. Age 87

℞ Ativan
0.5 mg
1/2 HS
generic
#10

N.R.

Dr. Robert Suskind
DEA#BS1234563

9.19b

9.20

PT. NAME: **HARVEY BROWN**	GENDER: **M**	ADDRESS: **785 IBIS LANE**	WEIGHT: **175**	BMI: **26**
AGE: **29**	DX: **"NERVES," PAIN, INSOMNIA, MINOR INJURY FROM VEHICLE ACCIDENT (3/20), INFECTION**	ALLERGY: **ERYTHROMYCIN, PCN**	HX: **HIGH SCHOOL FOOTBALL COACH**	

MEDICATION	SIG.	PRESCRIBER	ORIG. DATE	REFILL DATE	REFILL DATE	REFILL DATE	REFILL DATE
Tylenol PM #60	I hs for sleep	OTC	2/5	4/6			
Cipro 500 mg #30	I bid	Glucroft	4/10				
Percocet 5/325 mg #40	I bid prn	Glucroft	3/20				

Dr. Bart Glucroft
700 147th Terrace, Monterey, CA 38411
705-555-0001

Name Harvey Brown Date 5/3

Address 785 Ibis Lane Age 29

℞

Desorel 50mg
#100
1 tab Bid

☑ Label

Refill 4 times

Dr. Bart Glucroft

9.20a

Dr. James Mirow
38 128th Terrace, Monterey, CA 38411
705-555-9832

Name Harvey Brown Date 5/4

Address 785 Ibis Lane Age 29

℞

Ceftin
Sig: 250mg po BID
Disp: 20#

P.S. I am aware of pt's allergies

☑ LABEL

REFILL x ø TIMES PRN NR

Dr. James Mirow

9.20b

9.21

PT. NAME: **CAROL BRADDOCK** GENDER: **F** ADDRESS: **1135 EAST GRANDVIEW BLVD.** WEIGHT: **141** BMI: **21**

AGE: **69** DX: **INSOMNIA, NEURALGIA, URI, MIGRAINES, PSYCHOSIS** ALLERGY: **PCN** HX: **YEARS OF HEADACHES, PAIN, SMOKING**

MEDICATION	SIG.	PRESCRIBER	ORIG. DATE	REFILL DATE	REFILL DATE	REFILL DATE	REFILL DATE
Temazepam 15 mg #30	1 hs prn	O'Connell	3/2	4/1	5/3		
Ambien 10 mg #30	1 hs prn	O'Connell	6/1	7/2			
Nicotrol NS Spray 4 × 10 mL	Use ud	Johnson	7/9	8/3			
Neurontin 400 mg #30	1 bid	O'Connell	8/4				
Seroquel 25 mg #60	1 bid	O'Connell	5/9	6/3			
Seroquel 50 mg #60	1 bid	O'Connell	7/1	8/1			

Dr. Jennifer O'Connell
28 Cooke St, Morgantown, WV 49466
219-555-3333

Name Carol Braddock Date 8/9

Address 1135 East Grandview Blvd. Age 69

℞

Lunesta 2mg

#30

[illegible]

Refills 1X

Dr. Jennifer O'Connell

DEA#BO1234563

9.21a

Dr. Jennifer O'Connell
28 Cooke St, Morgantown, WV 49466
219-555-3333

Name Carol Braddock Date 8/9

Address 1135 East Grandview Blvd. Age 69

℞

Zomig 2.5

i PO QD prn

twenty

N.R.

Dr. Jennifer O'Connell

9.21b

9.22

PT. NAME: **ANNA PATAK**	GENDER: **F**	ADDRESS: **88 CREST ST.**	WEIGHT: **129**	BMI: **23**
AGE: **67**	DX: **HYPOTHYROID, HTN, ANGINA, POST MI, INSOMNIA, CHOLESTEROL**	ALLERGY: **PCN**	HX: **SMOKES, SOCIAL DRINKER**	

MEDICATION	SIG.	PRESCRIBER	ORIG. DATE	REFILL DATE	REFILL DATE	REFILL DATE	REFILL DATE
Plavix 75 mg #30	1 qd in am	Fogel	1/7	2/8	3/7	4/2	5/1
Norvasc 10 mg #30	1 qd	Fogel	1/7	2/8	3/7	4/2	5/1
Synthroid 50 mcg #30	1 in am ac bkfst	Fogel	1/7	2/8	3/7	4/2	5/1
Lisinopril 2.5 mg #30	1 qd	Fogel	1/7				
Lisinopril 5 mg #30	1 qd	Fogel	2/6	3/8	4/8	5/11	
Lipitor 10 mg #30	1 hs	Fogel	1/7	2/8	3/22	4/20	

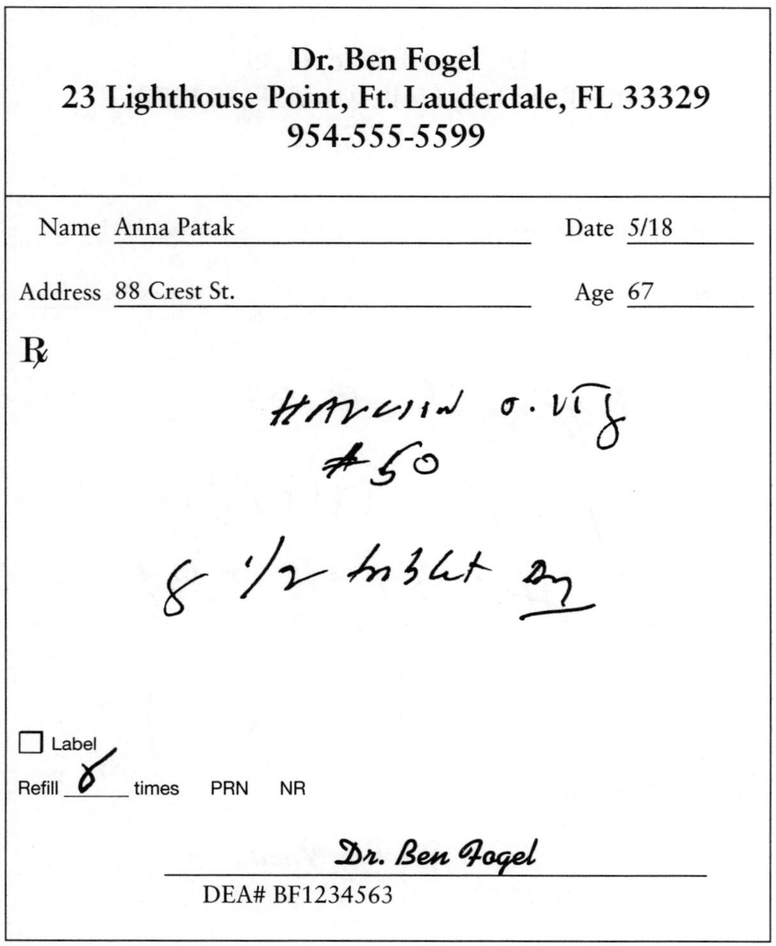
Dr. Ben Fogel
23 Lighthouse Point, Ft. Lauderdale, FL 33329
954-555-5599
Name Anna Patak Date 5/18
Address 88 Crest St. Age 67
℞
#50
Label
Refill ____ times PRN NR
Dr. Ben Fogel
DEA# BF1234563

9.22a

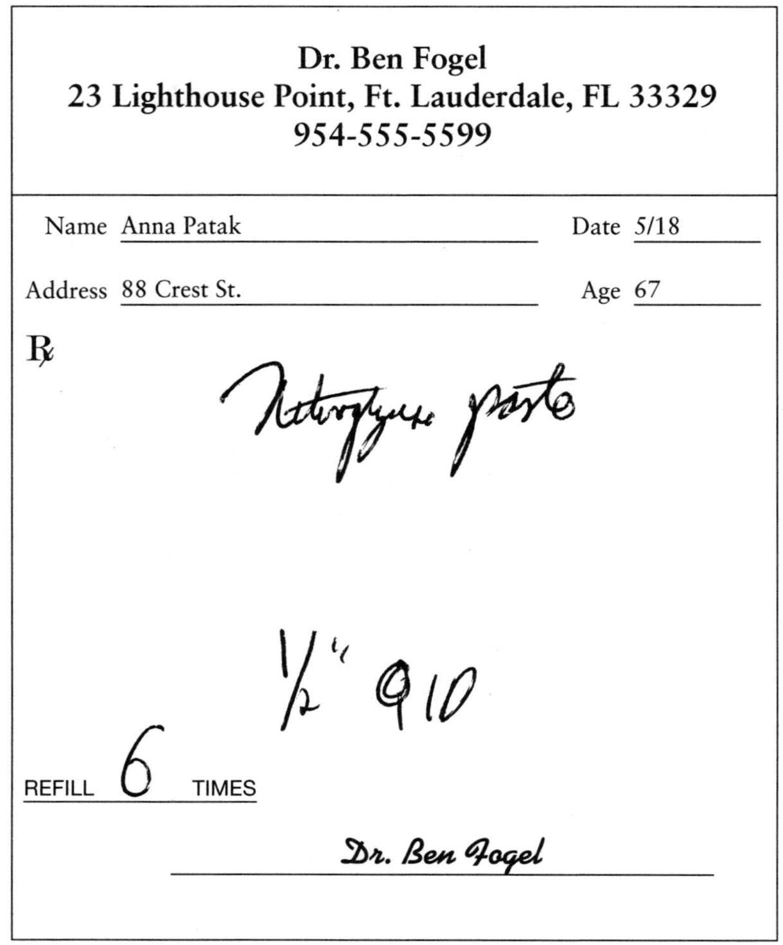
Dr. Ben Fogel
23 Lighthouse Point, Ft. Lauderdale, FL 33329
954-555-5599
Name Anna Patak Date 5/18
Address 88 Crest St. Age 67
℞
1/2" q10
REFILL 6 TIMES
Dr. Ben Fogel

9.22b

9.23

PT. NAME: **GLORIA DASILVA** GENDER: **F** ADDRESS: **142 NE 5TH ST.** WEIGHT: **128** BMI: **22**

AGE: **62** DX: **HYPERTHYROID, NERVOUS, COPD, DEPRESSED, INSOMNIA, HTN, TOOTH PAIN** ALLERGY: **ASA**

MEDICATION	SIG.	PRESCRIBER	ORIG. DATE	REFILL DATE	REFILL DATE	REFILL DATE	REFILL DATE
Furosemide 20 mg #30	1 in am	Dalen	7/3	8/1	9/4	10/30	
Lisinopril 5 mg #30	1 qd	Dalen	7/3	8/1	9/4	10/5	
Atrovent HFA Aerosol 12.9 g	Use tid ud	Dalen	7/3	8/1	9/4	10/5	
Methimazole 10 mg #60	1 bid	Dalen	9/19	10/18			
Alprazolam 0.25 mg #90	1 tid	Dalen	9/19	10/18			

Dr. Goar Dalen
33 Park Dr., Hollywood, FL 33322
954-555-1239

Name Gloria DaSilva Date 11/3

Address 142 NE 5 St. Age 62

℞

DISP

Remeron 30 mg # 30
1/2 HS x 1 week, then
1 HS –

Refill two Times/PRN/NR

Dr. Goar Dalen

9.23a

Dr. Ron Fucile, DDS
100 Park Dr., Hollywood, FL 33322
954-555-5522

Name Gloria DaSilva Date 11/4

Address 142 NE 5 St. Age 62

℞

Tylenol #3
i – ii q HS prn
#30 (thirty)

LABEL

REFILL (1) 2 3 4 N-R PRN MAX

Dr. Ron Fucile

DEA# BF1234563

9.23b

9.24

PT. NAME: **RYAN NOLE**	GENDER: **M**	ADDRESS: **70 BERKMAN AVE.**	WEIGHT: **155**	BMI: **27**
AGE: **72**	DX: **HTN, TYPE 2 DM, NERVES, COUGH**	ALLERGY: **PCN, ASA**	HX: **SMOKE, SOCIAL DRINKER**	

MEDICATION	SIG.	PRESCRIBER	ORIG. DATE	REFILL DATE	REFILL DATE	REFILL DATE	REFILL DATE
Promethazine with Codeine 4 oz	5 mL tid	Fox	3/1	4/2	5/22		
Glyburide 5 mg #30	1 q am ac bkfst	Fox	3/20	4/18	5/19	6/20	
Diovan 80 mg #30	1 qd	Fox	3/20	4/18	5/19		
Lorazepam 1 mg #30	1 bid prn nerves	Fox	2/7	2/18	2/28	3/25	4/30
Lopressor 50 mg #30	1/2 tab bid	Fox	6/4				

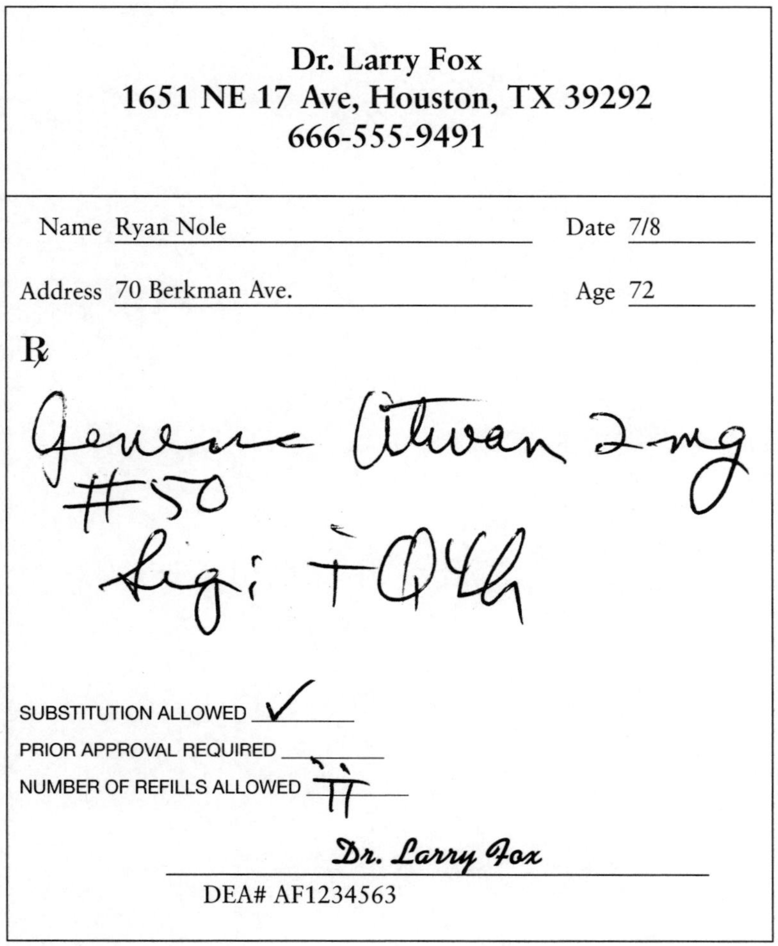

Dr. Larry Fox
1651 NE 17 Ave, Houston, TX 39292
666-555-9491

Name Ryan Nole Date 7/8

Address 70 Berkman Ave. Age 72

℞

Generic Ativan 2 mg
#50
Sig: i Q4h

SUBSTITUTION ALLOWED ✓

PRIOR APPROVAL REQUIRED

NUMBER OF REFILLS ALLOWED ii

Dr. Larry Fox

DEA# AF1234563

9.24a

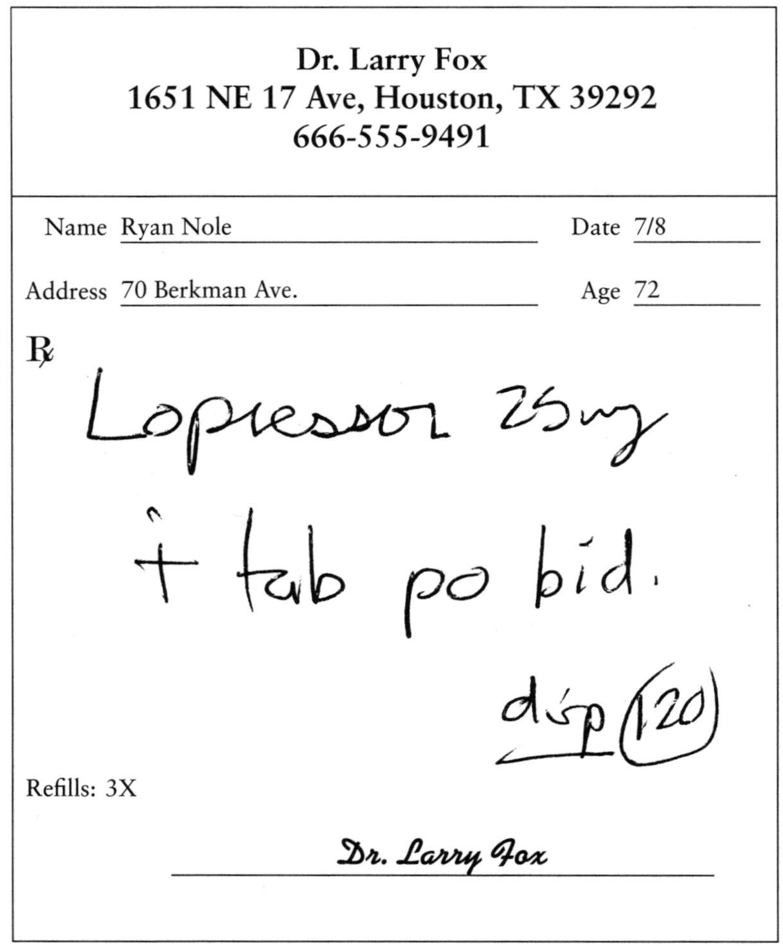

Dr. Larry Fox
1651 NE 17 Ave, Houston, TX 39292
666-555-9491

Name Ryan Nole Date 7/8

Address 70 Berkman Ave. Age 72

℞

Lopressor 25 mg
i tab po bid.

disp (120)

Refills: 3X

Dr. Larry Fox

9.24b

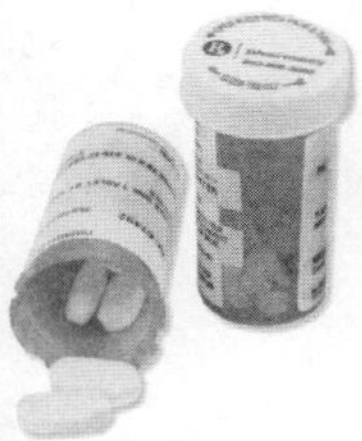

• MENTAL HEALTH, PART 2 10

UPON COMPLETION OF THIS CHAPTER, THE STUDENT WILL BE ABLE TO:

- counsel patients on the particular cautions associated with Tegretol therapy.
- discuss appropriate measures to ensure maintaining proper therapeutic levels of lithium.
- explain the role of carbidopa in Sinemet in the treatment of Parkinson's disease.
- discuss strategies with patients and caregivers concerning the treatment of Parkinson's disease.
- explain the mechanism of action of benztropine in the treatment of drug-induced EPS and in the treatment of Parkinson's disease.
- inform patients about foods and OTC drugs to avoid while taking MAO inhibitors.
- describe the unique aspects of the pharmacokinetics of phenytoin and carbamazepine.
- counsel patients and caregivers on the problems with using certain OTC medications, such as antihistamines with anticholinergic properties, in patients who have Alzheimer's disease.

DRUG LIST

Aricept/Exelon/Razadyne
Azilect
Bupropion
Cogentin
Comtan
Dilantin
Eldepryl
Keppra
Lamictal
Lithium
Lyrica
Mirapex/Requip/Parlodel
Namenda
Neurontin
Parnate/Nardil
Phenobarbital
Primidone
Sinemet
Stalevo
Symmetrel
Tegretol/Trileptal
Topamax
Valproic Acid/Depakote

• DRUG HOT POINTS

Aricept/Exelon/Razadyne
Alzheimer's disease: ↑ ACh by inhibiting ACh esterase
5, 10, 23 mg once daily at HS or in A.M.
Compare with Exelon (BID dosing)
Compare with Razadyne: regular and ER
Compare with Exelon patch

Bupropion
↑ Dopamine and NE: antidepressant (Wellbutrin) & smoking cessation (Zyban)
Warning, high doses: risk of seizures
Less risk of sexual adverse effects than the SSRI group

Cogentin
Anticholinergic—potential for side effects
Restores DA/ACh balance
Adjunct in Parkinson's disease
Controls EPS from neuroleptic drugs
Use only if EPS occurs because of side effects

Comtan
COMT inhibitor: (↑ L-dopa)
Each dose given with Sinemet dose
Compare with Stalevo

Dilantin
Kapseals, infatabs, suspension, IV
Do not substitute prompt for extended form
Strict adherence to directions
Take with food to protect stomach
Interaction with PO calcium products
Lateral nystagmus, gingival hyperplasia
Nonlinear, saturation kinetics
Used to treat seizures, neuropathic pain, diabetic neuropathy, etc.
Compare with Topamax, Keppra, Lamictal
Compare with Cerebyx (fosphenytoin)

Eldepryl
Selective MAO inhibitor type B
BID dosing, last dose at lunch
Stimulating metabolite
Adjunct to Sinemet
Interactions with tyramine-containing foods and drugs
Compare with Azilect

Lithium
Effective for bipolar disorder
Thiazide diuretic interaction
Intake of salt (NaCl) should be consistent
Avoid dehydration, take with food
Liquid, regular tablets and capsules, CR tablets

Mirapex/Requip/Parlodel
Dopamine receptor agonists
Mirapex and Requip: more selective
Caution when driving and taking Mirapex
The dose should be titrated up
Parlodel—also used to treat acromegaly

Namenda
Indicated for the treatment of moderate to severe dementia of the Alzheimer type
NMDA receptor antagonist

Neurontin
Used for epilepsy & neuropathic pain
Compare with Lyrica

Parnate
Nonselective MAO inhibitor for atypical depression
Avoid certain foods (aged cheese, Chianti or red wine, broad beans, fava beans, etc.)
Serious interactions: meperidine, TCAs, dextromethorphan, SSRIs, OTC products
At least 14 days (5 weeks for Prozac) wait to start MAO inhibitors after stopping SSRIs and TCAs
Compare with Nardil (phenelzine)

Phenobarbital
Used for epilepsy, agitation
Inducer of CYP-450 enzymes
Driving and alcohol warnings (C-IV)—controlled
Compare with primidone

• DRUG HOT POINTS (*continued*)

Sinemet
Levodopa (DA precursor) crosses blood–brain barrier
When combined with 70 to 100 mg/day of carbidopa, this inhibits peripheral metabolism of L-dopa (↑ effect, ↓ dose, & side effects)
Take with food (not protein)
Regular and long-acting tablets (CR)
Doses must be individualized
Strict compliance is very important for best results
Observe for GI bleed, psychosis

Symmetrel
Adjunct with other medications
Possibly releases dopamine from intact DA terminals in substantia nigra. Also used for prevention and treatment of influenza A virus.

Tegretol
Used for epilepsy & nerve pain
Reduces synaptic nerve responses
Must continue regular physician visits
Caution: mouth sores, sore throat (↓ WBC)
Induces CYP-450 enzymes
Compare with Trileptal

Valproic Acid
Used to treat epilepsy, manic episodes (bipolar), and migraines
Caution: monitor for hepatotoxicity
Depakote (divalproex sodium)
Delayed release and ER tablets

• QUESTIONS TO BE ANSWERED IN PREPARATION FOR CHAPTER 10 LAB

- If a patient is stabilized on Eskalith and he decides to stop eating table salt and other salty foods, what would be the pharmacologic outcome?
- If a patient is stabilized on lithium and ingests a large portion of salted popcorn, what would be the outcome?
- Explain the reason for the counseling advice to take the last daily dose of Eldepryl at lunchtime.
- Name a major metabolite of selegiline that may account for its stimulatory effect.
- Describe the contents of the boxed warning for Tegretol.
- What is the milligram strength of the chewable tablet form of Tegretol?
- A patient is stabilized on Sinemet and Mirapex. Explain the outcome or problem that would occur if the patient takes a prescription for Thorazine, for agitation, concurrently.
- What is the strength of Eskalith CR tablets?
- Explain the pharmacologic mechanism of action for Sinemet. Specifically, what is the drug doing?
- Which foods and nonprescription drugs should be avoided by persons who take either Nardil or Parnate?
- Describe the differences between Dilantin 50-mg tablets and the 100-mg Kapseals.
- To which class of controlled drugs does Lyrica (pregabalin) belong?
- Describe the difference in dosing regimens between Depakote delayed-release tablets and Depakote ER tablets.
- Describe the potential adverse effects of Lamictal.
- Explain the reason why fosphenytoin injection has advantages over phenytoin injection.
- Compare and contrast the GI absorption characteristics of Neurontin (gabapentin) with those of Lyrica (pregabalin).
- Describe the dosing strategies for Aricept 5-, 10-, and 23-mg tablets.
- To double the levels of phenytoin, would it be correct to double the daily dose of Dilantin Kapseals?
- What is the difference in the mechanism of action between Sinemet and Requip?
- Why is it recommended that Cogentin be prescribed only after EPS appears in a patient who is taking Haldol?
- To which class of drug does Cogentin belong?
- Select an appropriate dosing range for Neurontin in the treatment of painful neuropathy.
- Which side effect commonly appears early in treatment with Neurontin?
- Why is carbidopa included with levodopa in Sinemet?
- What is the optimum daily intake of the carbidopa component of Sinemet to achieve its effect?
- Describe the reason for using Comtan with Sinemet.
- Which neurotransmitter is involved with the therapeutic action of bupropion?
- To which class of controlled drugs does phenobarbital belong?
- Compare and contrast Eldepryl and Azilect.
- Describe the severe skin rash that has been reported with the use of Lamictal (lamotrigine).
- Which Alzheimer's disease medication is available in a once-daily, topically applied patch?

• MENTAL HEALTH, PART 2, MEDICATION THERAPY MANAGEMENT QUESTIONS AND COMMENTS

- I notice that your father's prescription for Exelon capsules has not been filled on time. You have said that he has experienced vivid dreams and heartburn. Let's discuss another option. With your permission, I can contact the prescriber and recommend the same medication in a patch to be applied to the skin once a day. Then, you or the caregiver would remove the old patch each day and apply a new one. The previous day's patch must be removed before applying the new one. This would reduce the following: the burden of pill taking, the risks of heartburn, and of vivid dreams.
- Your physician has prescribed Parnate for you. Can we meet to discuss certain foods and nonprescription drugs that must be avoided while taking this drug? I can supply you with printed material from the computer. If your physician has done this, then our meeting will reinforce this critically important caution.
- In our meetings, you have made it clear that your husband's medication for Parkinson's disease, Sinemet, wears off during the night. You mention that when he arises in the morning, it is difficult for him to get around normally until he takes his morning tablet and it becomes effective. This takes time and it is very discouraging for him.

  Let's try this: Keep his morning dose next to his bed and also a glass of water. Set the alarm 1 hour before he normally gets up. When the alarm goes off, help him sit up and take his Sinemet. Then he can go back to sleep. When he gets up an hour or so later, the medication will be working. At that point, he will be able to get around and function well because the medication will have had time to work during his last hour of sleep.
- Since our last meeting, I notice that your posture has become rigid, your voice has lost some of its former quality, and your handwriting has become much smaller. These meetings that we have had discussing your medications are important. You have visited our pharmacy almost every week and you see your doctor only once a year. My recommendation is that we make an appointment for you with a neurologist to examine you.
- I am pleased that you have agreed to meet with me on a regular basis to discuss your patient's medication therapy management. I notice that she has gone to a different doctor who has prescribed Reglan, or metoclopramide, for her stomach problems. Because we have her complete medication history in our pharmacy, it is critical that we contact both this doctor as well as her neurologist who has treated her with medications for Parkinson's disease. Reglan has a high risk of making her Parkinson's disease condition worse and decrease the effectiveness of her other medications. We can discuss an alternative medication for her stomach.
- I would like to thank you for these medication therapy management sessions. Our team approach to your patient has worked well for her.
- I am pleased that you have agreed to meet with me on a regular basis to discuss your patient's medication therapy management. I notice that she has gone to a different doctor who has prescribed Bentyl, or dicyclomine, for her stomach problems. Because we have her complete medication history in our pharmacy, it is critical that we contact both this doctor as well as her neurologist who has treated her with medications for Alzheimer's disease. Bentyl has a high risk of making her condition worse. We can discuss an alternative medication for her stomach.
- I would like to thank you for these medication therapy management sessions. Our team approach to your patient has worked well for her.
- Thank you for allowing us to meet to discuss your prescription for lithium. You have mentioned in our medication therapy management sessions that you take Alka-Seltzer, original, in the blue box, for digestion problems. Unfortunately, this product contains almost 4000 mg of sodium bicarbonate plus aspirin in each 2-tablet dose. The excess sodium would increase the risk of failure of the therapeutic action of lithium. Let's discuss your stomach problems, and if needed, let's allow your physician to do a complete checkup of your digestive system. At that point, we can discuss products that would not interact with lithium.

• MENTAL HEALTH, PART 2, MEDICATION THERAPY MANAGEMENT QUESTIONS AND COMMENTS *(continued)*

- I notice that in our meetings to discuss your Parkinson's disease medications, that you have had new exaggerated movements of your head and body. Is it possible that you have taken more of the medication than was prescribed? Let's discuss this and consult with your physician to fine-tune your medications.
- In our medication therapy management sessions, you have reported that your seizure medication Dilantin (phenytoin) has not worked well, and recently, you have had episodes of seizures. Let's go over all of your medications, from all stores and sources, as well as items such as dietary intake of certain calcium-containing foods or other calcium sources that might block the medicine's absorption and have an impact on your condition. Please inform your doctor about this.
- It is good that we meet frequently. I notice that you have a serious skin rash that was not there the last time we met. Your new medication for seizures, Lamictal (lamotrigine), carries a warning about skin problems as a side effect. Let's make an urgent appointment for you to meet with your physician right now.
- Your father's medication is called Cogentin, or benztropine. It is used to reduce the muscle movements that he has been experiencing as a side effect of his medications. At all our medication meetings, let us know of any other items that he takes, even over-the-counter. For instance, another product that should be avoided in combination with Cogentin is Benadryl, or diphenhydramine. It is available in many forms. It would add to the side effects of Cogentin. It is very important that we continue having our medication therapy management meetings.
- Your mother's new medication is called Tegretol, or carbamazepine. It works to relax or stabilize her nerves and reduce nerve pain. She has admitted that she sometimes takes a drink of an alcoholic beverage. She also goes to different doctors for other medications. Would you mind if we call her doctors to inform them that she takes this product? Some of the other medications might stop working if taken together with Tegretol. In addition, alcohol must not be taken with this medication.
- In our previous meetings, we discussed that your prescription for Wellbutrin is helpful for your condition. You have just mentioned that you are buying a new medication from another prescriber for Zyban from another pharmacy. This is a serious problem. Another name for the same drug is bupropion. It would not be safe to take all of these because they contain the same medication. A high dose of bupropion has a risk of serious adverse effects.
- Let's call each one of your doctors to discuss the proper method of treating your conditions.
- Your patient is taking a prescription called valproic acid. Did the physician mention that aspirin has a risk of interacting with this medication and should not be taken without consulting him or her?
- It is important that you mentioned that you have been crushing your patient's medication. This medication is called Depakote ER. It must not be crushed. Let's discuss this with the prescriber to find an alternate formulation that can be easily swallowed.

Thank you for allowing us to be together in this important medication therapy management meeting.

10.1

PT. NAME: **SHARON DAVIS** AGE: **38** GENDER: **F** ADDRESS: **14 HALL ST.** DX: **DEPRESSION, INSOMNIA, BACTERIAL INFECTION** WEIGHT: **140** ALLERGY: **CODEINE** HEIGHT: **5′ 6″** HX: **UNHAPPY HOME LIFE** BMI: **23**

MEDICATION	SIG.	PRESCRIBER	ORIG. DATE	REFILL DATE	REFILL DATE	REFILL DATE	REFILL DATE
Restoril 15 mg #30	1 hs prn	Griffin	5/4	6/15	7/12		
Wellbutrin 75 mg #30	1 bid	Griffin	5/4				

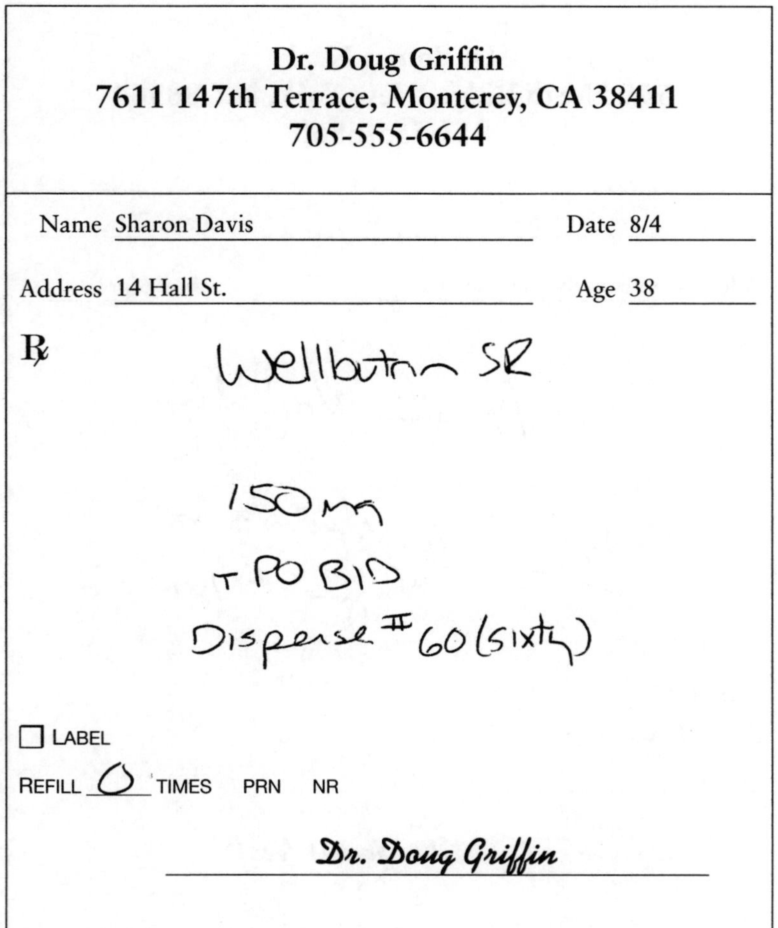
Dr. Doug Griffin
7611 147th Terrace, Monterey, CA 38411
705-555-6644

Name Sharon Davis Date 8/4

Address 14 Hall St. Age 38

℞ Wellbutrin SR

150 mg

i PO BID

Dispense # 60 (sixty)

☐ LABEL

REFILL 0 TIMES PRN NR

Dr. Doug Griffin

10.1a

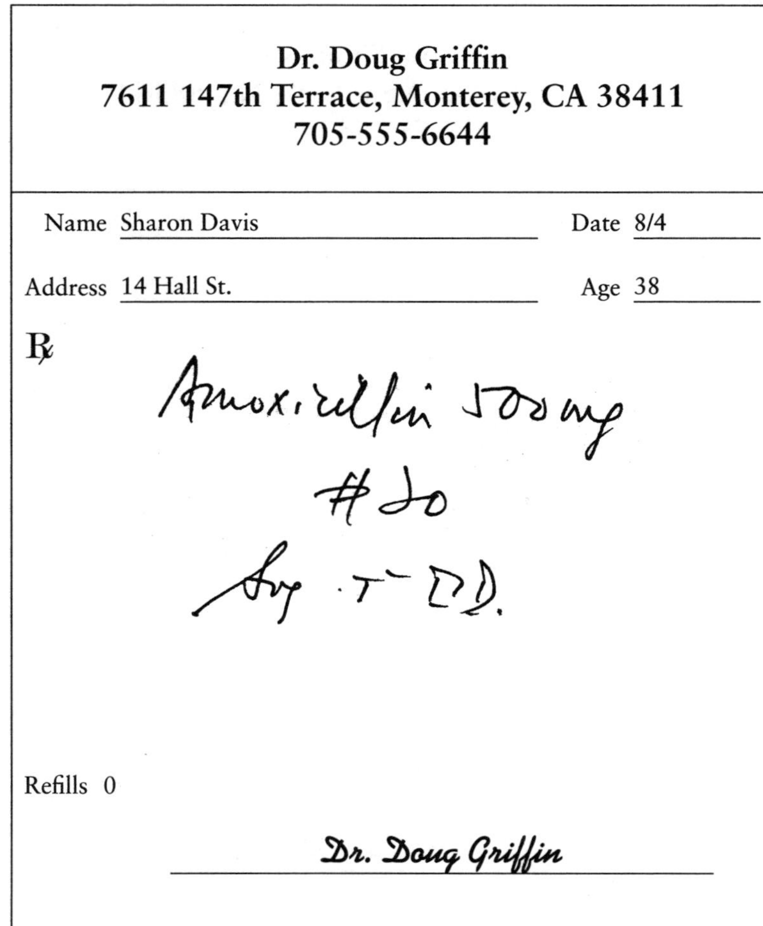
Dr. Doug Griffin
7611 147th Terrace, Monterey, CA 38411
705-555-6644

Name Sharon Davis Date 8/4

Address 14 Hall St. Age 38

℞ Amoxicillin 500 mg

#20

Sig: i TID.

Refills 0

Dr. Doug Griffin

10.1b

10.2 PT. NAME: **MARGARET GREEN** AGE: **62** GENDER: **F** ADDRESS: **6 PENNSYLVANIA AVE. NW** DX: **OSTEOPOROSIS, HYPOTHYROID, VAGINAL DRYNESS, INSOMNIA, DEPRESSION** WEIGHT: **120** ALLERGY: **NKA** HEIGHT: **5′ 2″** BMI: **22**

MEDICATION	SIG.	PRESCRIBER	ORIG. DATE	REFILL DATE	REFILL DATE	REFILL DATE	REFILL DATE
Synthroid 0.175 mg #30	I qd	Thomas	4/4	5/2	6/1	6/29	
Fosamax 70 mg #4	I qw	Thomas	6/5	7/20			

Dr. Erin Thomas
988 North Ridge, New York, NY 88364
813-555-7554

Name Margaret Green Date 7/25

Address 6 Pensylvania Ave. NW Age 62

℞

Desyrel 50 mg
Disp #40
Sig: one BID + ii HS

Refills 2

Dr. Erin Thomas

10.2a

Dr. James Neal
555 North Ridge, New York, NY 88364
813-555-6868

Name Margaret Green Date 7/23

Address 6 Pennsylvania Ave. NW Age 62

℞

Premarin Vaginal Cream

Sig: 1/2 applicator in vagina 2x/Wk

LABEL ☑

REFILL . none . TIMES

DEA NO . . . .

Dr. James Neal

10.2b

10.3

PT. NAME: **MARTHA WALKER**	GENDER: **F**	ADDRESS: **564 CAPITOL AVE.**	WEIGHT: **133**	BMI: **22**
AGE: **39**	DX: **BIPOLAR DISORDER (BD), BACK PAINS, URTICARIA, SKIN FUNGUS**	ALLERGY: **ASA**	HX: **SECRETARY**	

MEDICATION	SIG.	PRESCRIBER	ORIG. DATE	REFILL DATE	REFILL DATE	REFILL DATE	REFILL DATE
Cyclobenzaprine 10 mg #30	1–2 tabs 2 h before hs	Griffin	11/16				
Phenergan 25 mg tabs #10	1 q 6 h prn	Griffin	11/5				
Fleet Enema, saline 113 mL #3	1 pr prn BM	OTC	11/10	11/23			

Dr. John Salls
99 Old Logging Rd., Stamford, CT 33000
705-555-0003

Name Martha Walker Date 11/30

Address 564 Capitol Ave. Age 39

℞

Lith carbonate 300
2 ÷ BID
#120

REFILL X1 TIMES

Dr. John Salls

10.3a

Dr. James Riffey
929 NE 2nd Ave., Stamford, CT 44040
705-555-9990

Name Martha Walker Date 11/29

Address 564 Capitol Ave. Age 39

℞

Nizoral #4 200
ii pills after supper
w/ Cola drink

Dr. James Riffey

10.3b

10.4

PT. NAME: **MATT JOHNSON** AGE: **72** GENDER: **M** DX: **ANGINA, HTN, DELUSIONAL, CONSTIPATION** ADDRESS: **321 WEST RD.** ALLERGY: **NKA** WEIGHT: **138** HX: **HEARS VOICES** BMI: **23**

MEDICATION	SIG.	PRESCRIBER	ORIG. DATE	REFILL DATE	REFILL DATE	REFILL DATE	REFILL DATE
K-Dur 20 mEq #30	I qd	Sanders	10/20	11/16			
Prinivil 10 mg #30	I qd	Sanders	10/20	11/16			
Imdur 60 mg #30	I qd	Sanders	10/20	11/16			
Lozol 2.5 mg #30	I qd	Sanders	10/20	11/16			

Dr. Harold Ng
7878 S High Rd., Chicago, IL 23875
954-555-5234

Name Matt Johnson Date 11/29

Address 321 West Rd. Age 72

℞

Seroquel 25 mg
#60
Sig i q 6 PM & ii qhs.

Refills 1

Dr. Harold Ng

10.4a

Dr. Joanne Sanders
7000 S High Rd., Chicago, IL 23875
954-555-1119

Name Matt Johnson Date 11/27

Address 321 West Rd. Age 72

℞

Enulose Syrup.
Sig: 15 mL in AM
& 15 mL in PM.
Qs 500 mL

☐ Label

Refill 0 times PRN NR

Dr. Joanne Sanders

10.4b

10.5

PT. NAME: **ANNA HARRIS** | AGE: **63** | GENDER: **F** | DX: **GLAUCOMA, IBS, DANDRUFF, PARANOID** | ADDRESS: **566 EAST CT.** | ALLERGY: **NKA** | WEIGHT: **150** | HX: **AGITATED AT BEDTIME, SUSPICIOUS** | BMI: **27**

MEDICATION	SIG.	PRESCRIBER	ORIG. DATE	REFILL DATE	REFILL DATE	REFILL DATE	REFILL DATE
Bentyl 10 mg #30	I cap tid ac	Croft	9/26	10/25			
Cosopt 10 mL	I gtt os bid	Smith	7/28				
Xalatan 0.005% 2.5 mL	I gtt os hs	Smith	7/28				
Pepcid 20 mg #30	I bid prn	Croft	6/1	7/28	8/17	9/11	10/22

Dr. Barry Weiss
901 Sheridan St., Austin, TX 90902
874-555-9000

Name Anna Harris Date 10/29

Address 566 East Ct. Age 63

℞

Zyprexa 10mg
i PO QHS
#30

Refills 2

Dr. Barry Weiss

10.5a

Dr. Jack Croft
909 Sheridan St., Austin, TX 90902
874-555-9009

Name Anna Harris Date 10/29

Address 566 East Ct. Age 63

℞

Nizoral shampoo
use TIW
x 5 MINUTES

4 oz

☒ Label

Refill 0 times

Dr. Jack Croft

10.5b

10.6 PT. NAME: **MITCHELL ADAMS** GENDER: **M** ADDRESS: **23 SOUTH ST.** WEIGHT: **141** BMI: **23**
AGE: **78** DX: **PARKINSON'S DISEASE, HEARTBURN, DEPRESSION** ALLERGY: **PCN** HX: **HAS BECOME IMMOBILE**

MEDICATION	SIG.	PRESCRIBER	ORIG. DATE	REFILL DATE	REFILL DATE	REFILL DATE	REFILL DATE
Sinemet 25/100 mg #120	1 tid	Robins	3/6	4/4	4/15		
Comtan 200 mg #90	1 tid	Robins	3/6	3/21	4/5		
Klonopin 0.5 mg #30	1–2 hs prn	Robins	1/3	3/11	3/29	4/23	
Reglan 10 mg #50	1 tid ac for heartburn	Johnson	3/10	4/20			
St. John's wort #C	1 tid	OTC	2/5	3/8	4/12		

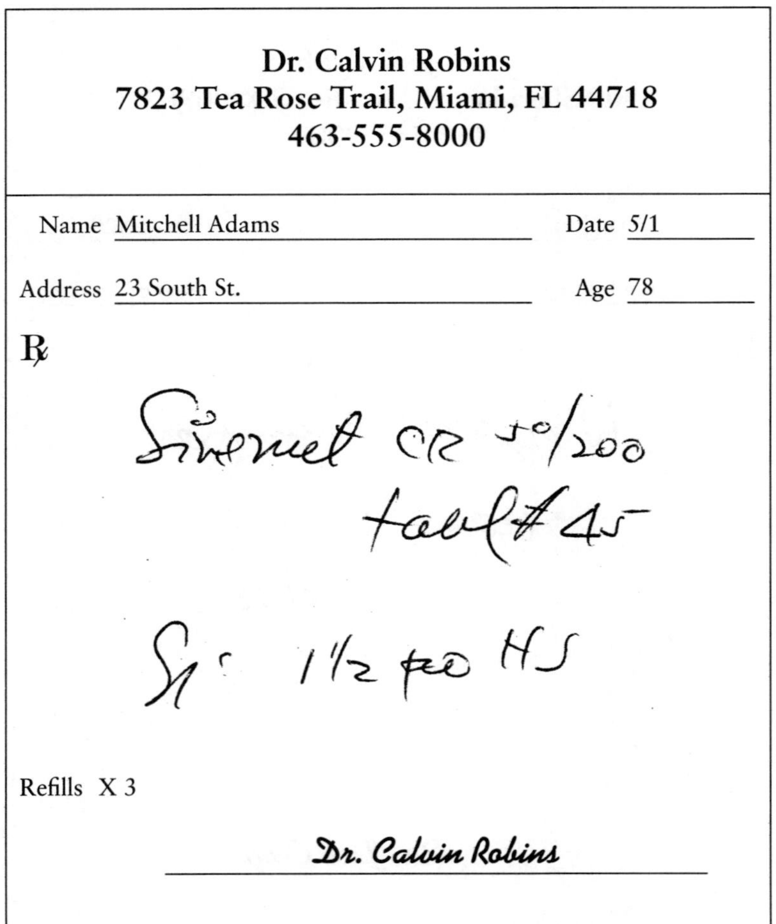
Dr. Calvin Robins
7823 Tea Rose Trail, Miami, FL 44718
463-555-8000

Name Mitchell Adams Date 5/1
Address 23 South St. Age 78

℞
Sinemet CR 50/200
tab #45
Sig: 1½ po HS

Refills X 3

Dr. Calvin Robins

10.6a

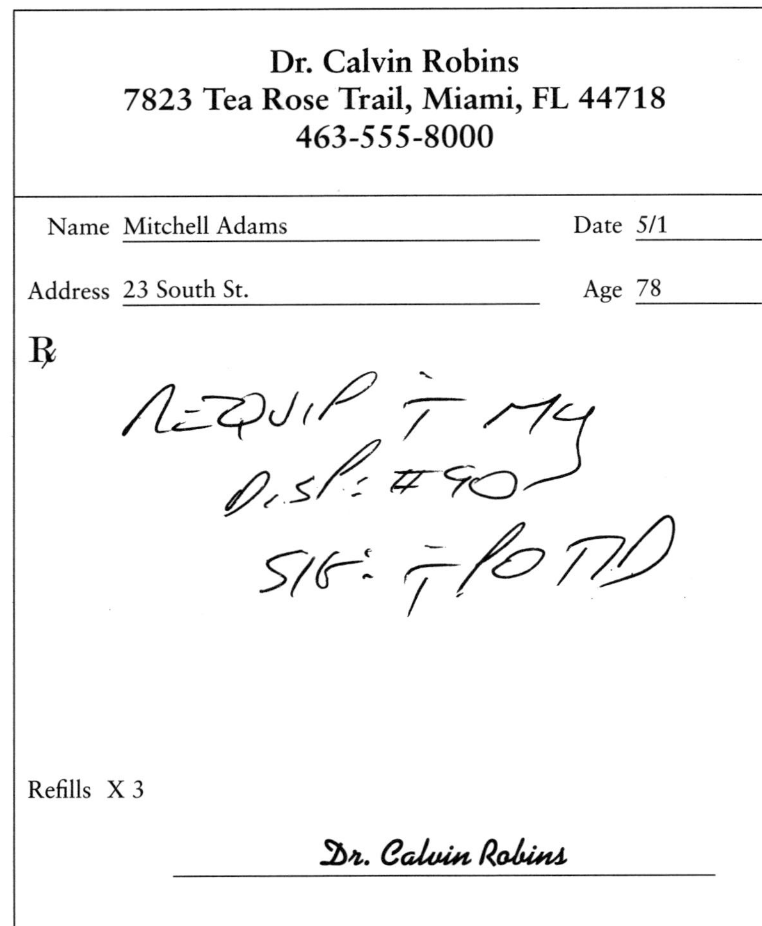
Dr. Calvin Robins
7823 Tea Rose Trail, Miami, FL 44718
463-555-8000

Name Mitchell Adams Date 5/1
Address 23 South St. Age 78

℞
Requip ī mg
0.5 #90
Sig: ī po TID

Refills X 3

Dr. Calvin Robins

10.6b

10.7	PT. NAME: **LON WAGNER**	GENDER: **M**	ADDRESS: **654 EAGLE RUN**	WEIGHT: **165**	BMI: **26**
	AGE: **79**	DX: **PARKINSON'S DISEASE, HTN, CONSTIPATION**	ALLERGY: **NKA**		

MEDICATION	SIG.	PRESCRIBER	ORIG. DATE	REFILL DATE	REFILL DATE	REFILL DATE	REFILL DATE
Eldepryl 5 mg #60	1 bid	Sauls	4/28	5/29			
Amantadine 100 mg #90	1 tid	Sauls	4/28	5/29			
Fleet Enema, saline 113 mL #6	1 prn BM	OTC	3/6	4/8	5/1	5/14	
HCTZ 25 mg #45	1 qod	Johnson	1/22	4/20			

Dr. Alfred Sauls
151212 S High Rd., Chicago, IL 23875
954-555-1300

Name Lon Wagner Date 6/30

Address 654 Eagle Run Age 79

℞

Sinemet 50/200 CR
three and 1/2 tabs a day
in divided doses
#100

Refills 5

Dr. Alfred Sauls

10.7a

Dr. Alfred Sauls
151212 S High Rd., Chicago, IL 23875
954-555-1300

Name Lon Wagner Date 6/30

Address 654 Eagle Run Age 79

℞

Sinemet 25-100
#100
ii + 1 D

Refills 5

Dr. Alfred Sauls

10.7b

10.8

PT. NAME: **NEAL KENNEDY**	GENDER: **M**	ADDRESS: **7541 NORTH AVE.**	WEIGHT: **149**	BMI: **24**
AGE: **46**	DX: **RELEASED FROM PSYCHIATRIC UNIT AT HOSPITAL**	ALLERGY: **NOT ON FILE**	HX: **PETTY CRIMES, UNDER PSYCHIATRIC CARE**	

MEDICATION	SIG.	PRESCRIBER	ORIG. DATE	REFILL DATE	REFILL DATE	REFILL DATE	REFILL DATE
Ask patient or caregiver for medication history.							

Dr. Harvey Isaacs
76 107th Terrace, Monterey, CA 38411
705-555-1234

Name Neal Kennedy Date 7/25

Address 7541 North Ave. Age 46

℞

Cogentin 1mg # 100
S: i po q4h
prn
EPS

Refill Ø times

Dr. Harvey Isaacs

10.8a

Dr. Harvey Isaacs
76 107th Terrace, Monterey, CA 38411
705-555-1234

Name Neal Kennedy Date 7/25

Address 7541 North Ave. Age 46

℞

Haldol 10mg # 100
S: i po tid
?

Refill One times

Dr. Harvey Isaacs

10.8b

10.9

PT. NAME: **JONATHAN LOPEZ** GENDER: **M** ADDRESS: **61 GREEN ST.** WEIGHT: **180** BMI: **25**
AGE: **40** DX: **BIPOLAR, NEURALGIA, FOOT FUNGUS (*CANDIDA ALBICANS, TRICHOPHYTON RUBRUM*; MIXED INFECTION)** ALLERGY: **NKA**

MEDICATION	SIG.	PRESCRIBER	ORIG. DATE	REFILL DATE	REFILL DATE	REFILL DATE	REFILL DATE
Antivert 12.5 mg #30	I bid for vertigo	Stevens	2/23	10/10			
Econazole 1% Cream 85 g	Apply bid to feet	Stevens	7/20				

Dr. Calvin Robins
7823 Tea Rose Trail, Miami, FL 44718
463-555-8000

Name Jonathan Lopez Date 10/20

Address 61 Green St. Age 40

℞

$LiCO_3$ 300 g
S: ii tab. po. BID
Disp #120

Refills 5

Dr. Calvin Robins

10.9a

Dr. Calvin Robins
7823 Tea Rose Trail, Miami, FL 44718
463-555-8000

Name Jonathan Lopez Date 10/20

Address 61 Green St. Age 40

℞

Tegretol 200 mg
#120

Sig ii B.I.D

Refills 5

Dr. Calvin Robins

10.9b

10.10

PT. NAME: **MELINDA OLSON** AGE: **39** GENDER: **F** DX: **GERD, DEPRESSION, BACK PAIN, UTI** ADDRESS: **500 SE 2ND ST.** ALLERGY: **PCN** WEIGHT: **128** HX: **SMOKER, ETOH** BMI: **20**

MEDICATION	SIG.	PRESCRIBER	ORIG. DATE	REFILL DATE	REFILL DATE	REFILL DATE	REFILL DATE
Cipro 500 mg #20	1 bid	Zoeller	8/25				
Ultracet 37.5/325 mg #50	1 q 4–6 h prn pain	Zoeller	9/1				
Soma 350 mg #60	1 bid	Zoeller	9/1				

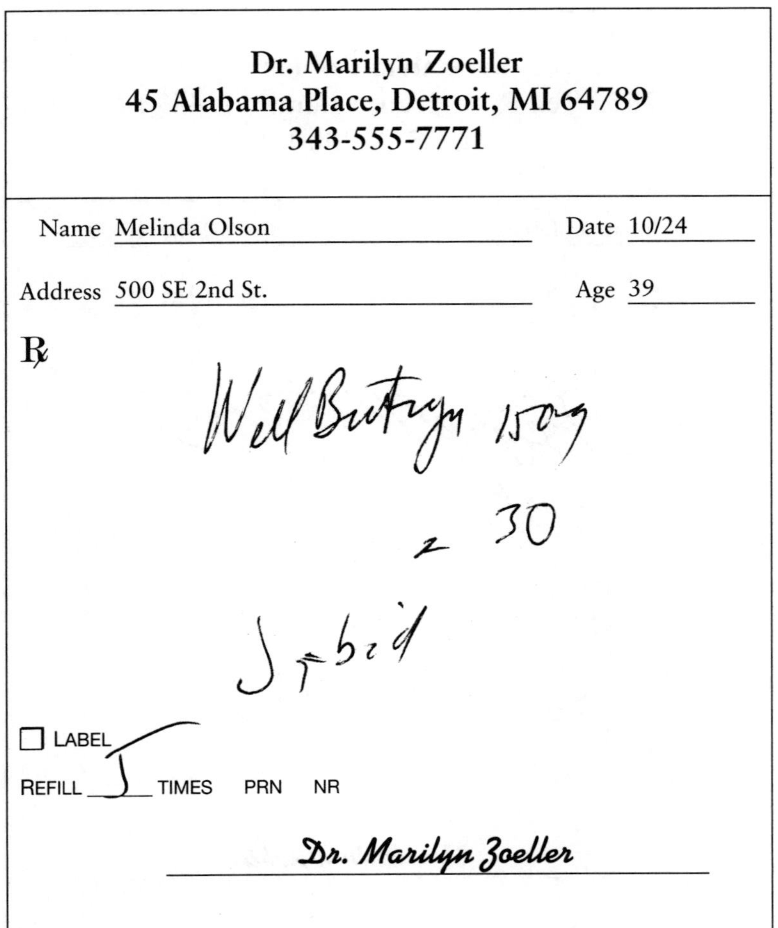
Dr. Marilyn Zoeller
45 Alabama Place, Detroit, MI 64789
343-555-7771

Name Melinda Olson Date 10/24

Address 500 SE 2nd St. Age 39

℞

Well Butryn 150g

30

i po bid

☐ LABEL

REFILL 1 TIMES PRN NR

Dr. Marilyn Zoeller

10.10a

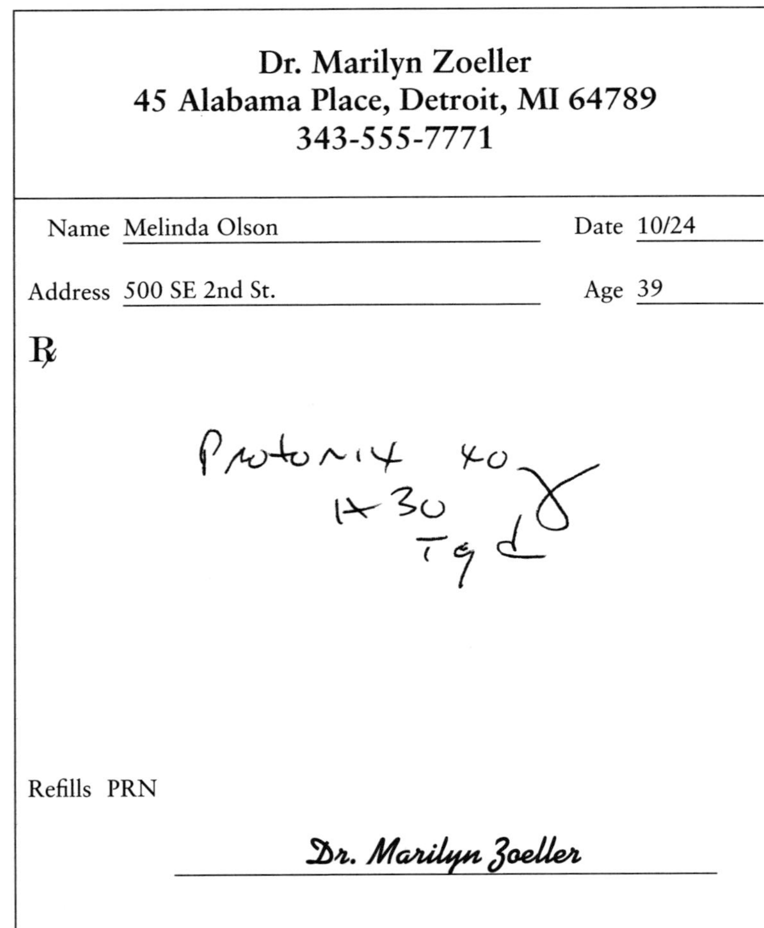
Dr. Marilyn Zoeller
45 Alabama Place, Detroit, MI 64789
343-555-7771

Name Melinda Olson Date 10/24

Address 500 SE 2nd St. Age 39

℞

Protonix 40 mg

#30

T qd

Refills PRN

Dr. Marilyn Zoeller

10.10b

10.11

PT. NAME: **GEORGE MILLER** GENDER: **M** ADDRESS: **5633 FLAMINGO CT.** WEIGHT: **160** HEIGHT: **5′ 7″**
AGE: **63** DX: **IBS, "NERVES," PSYCHOSIS, NEURALGIA** ALLERGY: **NKA** HX: **DIVORCED FIVE TIMES**

MEDICATION	SIG.	PRESCRIBER	ORIG. DATE	REFILL DATE	REFILL DATE	REFILL DATE	REFILL DATE
Pepcid 20 mg #30	I bid	Jones	5/12	6/1			
Bentyl 10 mg #C	I prn stomach pain	Jones	3/15	4/30	6/2		

Dr. Howard Isaacs
1115 Turnaround Lane, Detroit, MI 64789
343-555-7000

Name George Miller Date 6/10

Address 5633 Flamingo Ct. Age 63

℞

Risperdal 0.125 7
#30 i HS

Refills 0

Dr. Howard Isaacs

10.11a

Dr. Howard Isaacs
1115 Turnaround Lane, Detroit, MI 64789
343-555-7000

Name George Miller Date 6/10

Address 5633 Flamingo Ct. Age 63

℞

Neurontin 300mg
i po TID
#100

REFILL 1 - 2 - 3 - (NR) - PRN

Dr. Howard Isaacs

10.11b

10.12

PT. NAME: **RHONDA COOK** GENDER: **F** ADDRESS: **854 MASON ST.** WEIGHT: **126** HEIGHT: **5′ 6″** BMI: **20**

AGE: **30** DX: **SEIZURES, AGITATED** ALLERGY: **NKA** HX: **"UNHAPPY WITH MOST OF HER LIFE," UNABLE TO FIND WORK**

MEDICATION	SIG.	PRESCRIBER	ORIG. DATE	REFILL DATE	REFILL DATE	REFILL DATE	REFILL DATE
Lactulose 473 mL	1 tbs qd ud	Stevens	3/12	4/6	5/3		
Ortho-Novum 7/7/7 #28	ud, 1 qd	Stevens	1/25	2/24	3/22	4/22	5/19

Dr. Ingrid Abassi
901 Sutter St., San Francisco, CA 94109
874-555-1110

Name Rhonda Cook Date 5/20

Address 854 Mason St. Age 30

℞

Carbamazepine 200 mg
Disp # 100
Sig: ii hs

LABEL

Refill 3 times

Dr. I. Abassi

10.12a

Dr. Ingrid Abassi
901 Sutter St., San Francisco, CA 94109
874-555-1110

Name Rhonda Cook Date 5/20

Address 854 Mason St. Age 30

℞

Vistaril -
hydroxyzine
50 mg
Disp # 100
Sig: as directed

LABEL

Refill 3 times

Dr. I. Abassi

10.12b

10.13

PT. NAME: **JANE MCCOY** GENDER: **F** ADDRESS: **53 EAGLE BLVD.** WEIGHT: **130** HEIGHT: **5′ 7″**
AGE: **42** DX: **DEPRESSION, PAIN, ANXIETY, SEIZURES, DRY SCALY SKIN** ALLERGY: **NKA**

MEDICATION	SIG.	PRESCRIBER	ORIG. DATE	REFILL DATE	REFILL DATE	REFILL DATE	REFILL DATE
Ativan 0.5 mg #30	1/2 tablet prn anxiety	Ramsey	3/21	4/20			
Neurontin 400 mg #30	1 qd	Ramsey	2/12	3/10	4/5		
Lac-Hydrin Lotion 12% 400 g	Apply to feet qd	Boggess	1/13	3/20			

Dr. Evelyn Ramsey
111 Tea Rose Trail, Miami, FL 44718
463-555-9871

Name Jane McCoy Date 5/4

Address 53 Eagle Blvd. Age 42

℞

Dilantin 100 mg po

Sig 2 Tabs in morning
2 Tabs in Evening

400

Refill 2 times

Dr. Evelyn Ramsey

10.13a

Dr. Evelyn Ramsey
111 Tea Rose Trail, Miami, FL 44718
463-555-9871

Name Jane McCoy Date 5/4

Address 53 Eagle Blvd. Age 42

℞

Folic acid 1 mg

50

Sig i/d

Refill ______ times

Dr. Evelyn Ramsey

10.13b

10.14

PT. NAME: **SUSAN BLACK** GENDER: **F** ADDRESS: **2940 LEXTER DR.** WEIGHT: **140** HEIGHT: **5′ 6″**

AGE: **69** DX: **HIGH CHOLESTEROL, PAIN, OSTEOPOROSIS, DEPRESSION, ANXIETY, ACNE VULGARIS** ALLERGY: **NKA**

MEDICATION	SIG.	PRESCRIBER	ORIG. DATE	REFILL DATE	REFILL DATE	REFILL DATE	REFILL DATE
Lipitor 10 mg #60	1 qd	Griffin	9/5	11/3	12/6		
Serax 30 mg #90	1 bid prn	Griffin	6/15	8/12			
Renova 0.02% Cream 60 g	Apply hs	Griffin	5/8	10/27			
Actonel 35 mg #4	1 weekly	Griffin	3/6	4/5	8/3	9/12	10/15

Dr. Doug Griffin
7611 147th Terrace, Monterey, CA 38411
705-555-6644

Name Susan Black Date 12/20

Address 2940 Lexter Dr. Age 69

℞

NEURONTIN 100 mg

iii po qhs for 1 wk,

then iii po BID

180

Refills 2

Dr. Doug Griffin

10.14a

Dr. Lori Harris
29 132 St., Monterey, CA 38411
705-555-0011

Name Susan Black Date 12/18

Address 2940 Lexter Dr. Age 69

℞

Effexor 37.5mg XL

Sig i PO QAM

(fifteen)

SUBSTITUTION ALLOWED

REFILL 1 • 2 • 3 • (NR) • PRN

Dr. Lori Harris

10.14b

10.15

PT. NAME: **CHARLES HANSEN**	GENDER: **M**	ADDRESS: **1906 ANDERSON PARKWAY**	WEIGHT: **162**	BMI: **23**
AGE: **39**	DX: **DEPRESSION, EPILEPSY, LOWER BACK STRAIN**	ALLERGY: **NKA**		

MEDICATION	SIG.	PRESCRIBER	ORIG. DATE	REFILL DATE	REFILL DATE	REFILL DATE	REFILL DATE
Dilantin 100 mg #60	1 bid	Sauls	4/11	5/4			
Dilantin Infatab 50 mg #60	1/2 tablet with Dilantin 100 mg	Sauls	4/11				
Zoloft 50 mg #30	1 qd	Sauls	3/12	4/15	5/18		

Dr. Alfred Sauls
151212 S High Rd., Chicago, IL 23875
954-555-1300

Name Charles Hansen Date 5/20

Address 1906 Anderson Parkway Age 39

℞

Effexor XR 150mg
i PO QD
#30

Refills 1

Dr. Alfred Sauls

10.15a

Dr. Hugh Toms
3380 N High Rd., Chicago, IL 23875
954-555-1117

Name Charles Hansen Date 5/22

Address 1906 Anderson Parkway Age 39

℞

Relafen 750 mg
#30 (~~xxx~~)
i tab po BID

REFILL 1 - 2 - 3 (NR) PRN

Dr. Hugh Toms

10.15b

10.16

PT. NAME: **MARY DAVIS** AGE: **73** GENDER: **F** DX: **HTN, ALZHEIMER'S DISEASE, EPILEPSY, A-Fib** ADDRESS: **31 PHILLIP LANE** ALLERGY: **NKA** WEIGHT: **128** HX: **FORGETFUL** BMI: **24**

MEDICATION	SIG.	PRESCRIBER	ORIG. DATE	REFILL DATE	REFILL DATE	REFILL DATE	REFILL DATE
Corgard 40 mg #30	1 bid	Griffin	3/14	3/20	4/12		
Corgard 80 mg #50	1 bid	Griffin	4/20				
Warfarin 2.5 mg #90	1 qd	Griffin	1/30	5/4			

Dr. Doug Griffin
7611 147th Terrace, Monterey, CA 38411
705-555-6644

Name Mary Davis Date 5/10

Address 31 Phillip Lane Age 73

℞

Aricept 5mg
#30

Sig: T po HS

Refills 2

Dr. Doug Griffin

10.16a

Dr. Joe Kay
44 121st St., Monterey, CA 38411
705-555-7733

Name Mary Davis Date 5/11

Address 31 Phillip Lane Age 73

℞

Dilantin 100mg
#100

Sig: T cap i BID

Dilantin Infatabs 50mg
#100

Sig: T tab i [illegible]

Refill Y times

Dr. Joe Kay

10.16b

10.17

PT. NAME: **CHARLES SMITH** GENDER: **M** ADDRESS: **3906 LEE PARKWAY** WEIGHT: **115** BMI: **20**
AGE: **38** DX: **DEPRESSION, INSOMNIA, PAIN, NAUSEA** ALLERGY: **SULFA, ASA** HX: **NERVOUS PERSONALITY, SMOKER, ETOH**

MEDICATION	SIG.	PRESCRIBER	ORIG. DATE	REFILL DATE	REFILL DATE	REFILL DATE	REFILL DATE
Pen V.K. 500 mg #30	2 stat, then 1 qid	Davis, DMD	3/12				
Amoxicillin 500 mg #4	4 caps 1 hr prior to appointment	Davis, DMD	4/2				
Tylenol No. 3 #20	1 q 4–6 h prn pain	Robins	1/21	4/13			

Dr. Calvin Robins
7823 Tea Rose Trail, Miami, FL 44718
463-555-8000

Name Charles Smith Date 4/20

Address 3906 Lee Parkway Age 38

℞

Remeron 15mg
T po QHS
Disp #30

Refills 1

Dr. Calvin Robins

10.17a

Dr. Mark Rumsey
6060 NE 163rd St., Miami, FL 44722
463-555-1112

Name Charles Smith Date 4/21

Address 3906 Lee Parkway Age 38

℞

Phenergan 50 mg #20
take ī prn Nausea

REFILL 1 - 2 - 3 - (NR) - PRN

Dr. Mark Rumsey

10.17b

10.18

PT. NAME: **ANDREW KELLY**
AGE: **73**
GENDER: **M**
DX: **CHF, HYPOTHYROID, BPH, NERVES, URTICARIA**
ADDRESS: **4902 ORANGE BLVD.**
ALLERGY: **NKA**
WEIGHT: **150**
HX: **HEARS VOICES**
BMI: **24**

MEDICATION	SIG.	PRESCRIBER	ORIG. DATE	REFILL DATE	REFILL DATE	REFILL DATE	REFILL DATE
Furosemide 40 mg #90	I qd	Thomas	3/8	6/20	9/20		
Lanoxin 0.25 mg #90	I q am	Thomas	3/8	6/20	9/20		
Halfprin 81 mg #90	I q am	Thomas	2/9	6/12			
Synthroid 0.175 mg #30	I qd	Thomas	6/24	7/22	8/20	9/20	

Dr. Erin Thomas
988 North Ridge, New York, NY 88364
813-555-7554

Name Andrew Kelly Date 9/25
Address 4902 Orange Blvd. Age 73

℞

FLOMAX 0.4mg qd #30
ZYPREXA 10mg po qd #30

3 REFILLS

Dr. Erin Thomas

10.18a

Dr. Ben Fay
32 North Ridge, New York, NY 88364
813-555-3000

Name Andrew Kelly Date 9/25
Address 4902 Orange Blvd. Age 73

℞

Atarax 10mg
ī PO. T.i.d
#30

LABEL AS SUCH
MEDICALLY NECESSARY YES [ ] NO [ ]
NO. OF REFILLS (0) 1 2 3

Dr. Ben Fay

10.18b

10.19

PT. NAME: **CARLA JOHNSON**	GENDER: **F**	ADDRESS: **7201 MINORS LANE**	WEIGHT: **155**	BMI: **24**
AGE: **53**	DX: **HTN, PSYCHOTIC, AGITATED**	ALLERGY: **PCN**	HX: **NERVES, HEARS "VOICES"**	

MEDICATION	SIG.	PRESCRIBER	ORIG. DATE	REFILL DATE	REFILL DATE	REFILL DATE	REFILL DATE
Dyazide #90	I qd	Weiss	3/7	6/7	9/15		
Cozaar 50 mg #90	I q am	Weiss	5/10	8/7	11/6		
Prolixin 2 mg #90	I hs	Weiss	2/12	5/18	8/30		

Dr. Barry Weiss
901 Sheridan St., Austin, TX 90902
874-555-9000

Name Carla Johnson Date 11/12

Address 7201 Minors Lane Age 53

℞

Zyprexa 2.5
Sig i qhs
#15

☑ Label

Refill x5 c̄ 30 times PRN NR

Dr. Barry Weiss

10.19a

Dr. Harold Gunter
33 Filmore St., Austin, TX 90902
874-555-6448

Name Carla Johnson Date 11/10

Address 7201 Minors Lane Age 53

℞

Maxzide-25 #30
Sig: i PO every other Day

Refills 3x

Dr. Harold Gunter

10.19b

10.20

PT. NAME: **GEORGIA HOFFMAN**
AGE: **42**
GENDER: **F**
DX: **TYPE 2 DM, DELUSIONAL, HTN**
ADDRESS: **894 MALL ST.**
ALLERGY: **NKA**
WEIGHT: **229**
HEIGHT: **5′ 8″**

MEDICATION	SIG.	PRESCRIBER	ORIG. DATE	REFILL DATE	REFILL DATE	REFILL DATE	REFILL DATE
Prinivil 10 mg #90	I qd	Sauls	6/11	9/20			
Humulin 70/30 U-100 10 mL	ud	Sauls	4/24				
BD Syringes 3/10 cc #100	ud	Sauls	4/24				

Dr. Alfred Sauls
151212 S High Rd., Chicago, IL 23875
954-555-1300

Name Georgia Hoffman Date 9/30

Address 894 Mall St. Age 42

℞

Seroquel 100mg
#60
Sig i BID.

Refills 1

Dr. Alfred Sauls

10.20a

Dr. Alfred Sauls
151212 S High Rd., Chicago, IL 23875
954-555-1300

Name Georgia Hoffman Date 9/30

Address 894 Mall St. Age 42

℞

Furosemide 40 #100
(Lasix)
Take 40 in am and
20 at 2 PM

Refills 1

Dr. Alfred Sauls

10.20b

10.21 PT. NAME: **MAE JONES** AGE: **64** GENDER: **F** DX: **DEPRESSION, MANIC, GLAUCOMA, SKIN FUNGAL INFECTION** ADDRESS: **771 CARTON WAY** ALLERGY: **ASA** WEIGHT: **193** HX: **SPEAKS VERY FAST; IMPATIENT** HEIGHT: **5′ 11″**

MEDICATION	SIG.	PRESCRIBER	ORIG. DATE	REFILL DATE	REFILL DATE	REFILL DATE	REFILL DATE
Alphagan-P 0.15% 10 mL	ud	Black	9/5	10/6	10/26		
Lotrisone Cream 15 g	Apply tid	Robins	6/22	7/28	8/20	9/15	10/26

Dr. Calvin Robins
7823 Tea Rose Trail, Miami, FL 44718
463-555-8000

Name Mae Jones Date 10/28
Address 771 Carton Way Age 64

℞

Lithium CO3 300mg
Disp #100
Sig: as directed

Refills 1

Dr. Calvin Robins

10.21a

Dr. Calvin Robins
7823 Tea Rose Trail, Miami, FL 44718
463-555-8000

Name Mae Jones Date 10/28
Address 771 Carton Way Age 64

℞

Remeron 15mg
Disp #30
Sig: ne HS

Refills 1

Dr. Calvin Robins

10.21b

10.22

PT. NAME: **LOIS BROWN** GENDER: **F** ADDRESS: **801 NE 7 ST.** WEIGHT: **149** BMI: **22**
AGE: **70** DX: **TYPE 2 DM, ALZHEIMER'S DISEASE, POST-MI, HTN, CONJUNCTIVITIS** ALLERGY: **NKA** HX: **FORGETFUL**

MEDICATION	SIG.	PRESCRIBER	ORIG. DATE	REFILL DATE	REFILL DATE	REFILL DATE	REFILL DATE
Furosemide 40 mg #30	I q am	Lander	6/4	7/5	8/3	9/2	10/4
Tobradex Op. Sol. 5 mL	I gtt ou tid	Sanders	9/4				
Razadyne 4 mg #60	I bid	Lander	8/3	9/2	10/4		
Januvia 100 mg #30	I q am	Lander	9/12	10/10	11/2		
KCl 20 mEq tabs #60	I bid with water	Lander	6/4	7/5	8/3	9/2	10/4
Metformin 500 mg #60	I bid	Lander	9/12	10/10	11/2		
Plavix 75 mg #60	I q am	Lander	6/4	7/5	8/3	9/2	10/4

Dr. Saul Lander
33 White St., Newark, NJ 89582
923-555-1238

Name Lois Brown Date 11/3

Address 801 NE 7 St Age 70

℞

Namenda 10
one po BID
#60

REFILL 1 ☑ 2 ☐ 3 ☐ 4 ☐ NR ☐
LABEL ☑
MEDICALLY NECESSARY ☐
DEA# ______

Dr. Saul Lander

10.22a

Dr. Saul Lander
33 White St., Newark, NJ 89582
923-555-1238

Name Lois Brown Date 11/3

Address 801 NE 7 St Age 70

℞

exelon 3
one po QD after ~~lunch~~ breakfast
#30

REFILL 1 ☑ 2 ☐ 3 ☐ 4 ☐ NR ☐
LABEL ☑
MEDICALLY NECESSARY ☐
DEA# ______

Dr. Saul Lander

10.22b

10.23

PT. NAME: **CARY BARNES**	GENDER: **M**	ADDRESS: **32 RIVERO ST.**	WEIGHT: **152**	BMI: **25**
AGE: **73**	DX: **PARKINSON'S DISEASE, TYPE 2 DM, HTN, DENTAL PAIN**	ALLERGY: **NKA**	HX: **SMOKER, 50 PACK-YEARS**	

MEDICATION	SIG.	PRESCRIBER	ORIG. DATE	REFILL DATE	REFILL DATE	REFILL DATE	REFILL DATE
Glipizide 5 mg #60	1 bid	Blake	1/4	2/3	4/1		
HCTZ 25 mg #30	1 q am	Blake	1/4	2/3	4/1		
Tylenol No. 3 #12	1 q 4–6 h prn pain	Miller	4/7				
Atacand 8 mg #20	1 q am	Blake	1/4	2/3	4/1		

Dr. Greg Jones
99 North Drive, DeLand, FL 33993
888-555-1269

Name Cary Barnes Date 4/20

Address 32 Rivero St. Age 73

℞

Comtan 200 mg

i po TID

#90

☐ Label

Refill - 0 - 1 - 2 - 3 - (4) - PRN

Dr. Greg Jones

10.23a

Dr. Greg Jones
99 North Drive, DeLand, FL 33993
888-555-1269

Name Cary Barnes Date 4/20

Address 32 Rivero St. Age 73

℞

Sinemet 25/100

i po QID

#120

☐ Label

Refill - 0 - 1 - 2 - 3 - (4) - PRN

Dr. Greg Jones

10.23b

10.24

PT. NAME: **AVI KAHN** GENDER: **M** ADDRESS: **400 KINGS PT. DR.** WEIGHT: **140** HEIGHT: **5′ 3″**
AGE: **67** DX: **NEURALGIA, HTN, BPH, HIGH LIPIDS, PSYCHOSIS** ALLERGY: **STRAWBERRIES** HX: **NEUROTIC**

MEDICATION	SIG.	PRESCRIBER	ORIG. DATE	REFILL DATE	REFILL DATE	REFILL DATE	REFILL DATE
Coreg 3.125 mg #60	I bid	Gray	3/4	4/2			
Coreg 6.25 mg #60	I bid	Gray	5/1	6/3	7/1		
Risperdal 1 mg #60	I bid	Veller	3/9	4/8	5/7	6/3	7/1
Zocor 10 mg #30	I hs	Gray	3/4	4/2			
Enalapril 10 mg #60	I bid	Gray	2/8	3/9	4/6	5/2	6/22
Flomax 0.4 mg #60	I qd at 8 pm	Gray	6/14	8/1			

Dr. Guy Veller
33 W. University Ave, Laramie, WY 82071
307-555-9911

Name Avi Kahn Date 8/3

Address 400 Kings Pt. Dr. Age 67

℞

Topamax 100 mg
Disp: #30
Sig: 1/2 po qhs
x 7 nights, then
i qhs

Refills 6

Dr. Guy Veller

10.24a

Dr. Guy Veller
33 W. University Ave, Laramie, WY 82071
307-555-9911

Name Avi Kahn Date 8/3

Address 400 Kings Pt. Dr. Age 67

℞

Zyprexa 5 mg
Sig: i po BID
#60
sixty

Refills 0

Dr. Guy Veller

10.24b

10.25

PT. NAME: **BEA STONE** AGE: **73**
GENDER: **F**
DX: **ANGINA, POST-MI, HYPOTHYROID, MIGRAINES, LEG CRAMPS, NERVE PAIN**
ADDRESS: **81 GRANT ST.**
ALLERGY: **SHELLFISH**
WEIGHT: **172**
HX: **SMOKER, SOCIAL DRINKER**
BMI: **30**

MEDICATION	SIG.	PRESCRIBER	ORIG. DATE	REFILL DATE	REFILL DATE	REFILL DATE	REFILL DATE
Plavix 75 mg #30	I q am	Sand	2/4	3/1	4/6	5/12	
Imdur 30 mg #30	I q am	Sand	2/4	3/1	4/6	5/12	
Ultram 50 mg #60	I tid prn pain	Sand	3/5	4/6	5/12	6/15	
Synthroid 50 mcg #30	I q am ac bkfst	Sand	3/25	4/20	5/19	6/18	7/19
Lunesta I mg #30	I hs	Sand	5/12	6/10	7/18		
Quinine Sulfate 324 mg #30	I hs prn leg cramps	Sand	4/12	5/18	6/30		

Dr. Jim Sand
100 Campus Drive, Missoula, MT 59812
406-555-3331

Name Bea Stone Date 7/20
Address 81 Grant St. Age 73

℞

Lyrica 50g
#30

Label
Refill PRN times

☐ NON-REPETATUR

Dr. Jim Sand
DEA# BS1234563

10.25a

Dr. Jim Sand
100 Campus Drive, Missoula, MT 59812
406-555-3331

Name Bea Stone Date 7/20
Address 81 Grant St. Age 73

℞

Depakote ER-500g
#60
Sig 2 q am

Refills: Call

Dr. Jim Sand

10.25b

10.26

PT. NAME: **SARAH LYMAN** GENDER: **F** ADDRESS: **82 SOUTH ST.** WEIGHT: **141** BMI: **20**

AGE: **69** DX: **MANIA, ASSOCIATED WITH BIPOLAR DISORDER, ANGINA, HTN, ANXIETY, OA** ALLERGY: **NKA** HX: **YEARS OF SMOKING**

MEDICATION	SIG.	PRESCRIBER	ORIG. DATE	REFILL DATE	REFILL DATE	REFILL DATE	REFILL DATE
Atenolol 25 mg #30	1 q am	Haines	3/2	4/1	5/6	6/1	7/8
NTG 0.2 mg/hr patch #30	Apply 1 qd, 12 hrs on, 12 hrs off	Haines	3/2	4/1	5/6	6/1	7/8
Lorazepam 0.5 mg #30	1 bid prn nerves	Haines	6/7	7/22			
St. John's wort #100	tid	OTC	3/15	4/1	5/18	6/4	7/1
Bayer aspirin 325 mg #200	tid prn	OTC	Buys in grocery store				

Dr. Joel Haines
100 Barker Dr., Cicero, IL 60515
630-555-9871

Name Sarah Lyman Date 8/4

Address 82 South St. Age 69

℞

① Depakote ER 250mg #30
Sig i qam
② Depakote ER 500mg #30
Sig i qhs

☐ LABEL

REFILL 1 TIMES PRN

Dr. Joel Haines

10.26a

Dr. Joel Haines
100 Barker Dr., Cicero, IL 60515
630-555-9871

Name Sarah Lyman Date 8/4

Address 82 South St. Age 69

℞

Klonopen 0.5mg.
(#60)
Sig: i BID.

Refills NR

Dr. Joel Haines

DEA# BH1234563

10.26b

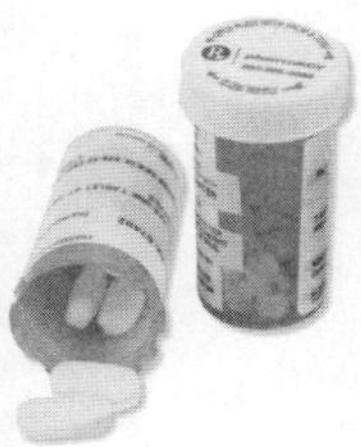

• MUSCLE RELAXANTS AND NONSTEROIDAL ANTI-INFLAMMATORY DRUGS 11

UPON COMPLETION OF THIS CHAPTER,
THE STUDENT WILL BE ABLE TO:

- inform patients about the proper administration of NSAIDs (take with food, milk, etc.).
- discuss the mechanism of action of aspirin and the other NSAIDs by their action on cyclooxygenase and the resulting effects on prostaglandin production.
- choose agents from each class of NSAIDs to recommend as alternatives in case one family of NSAIDs loses its effectiveness.
- identify and monitor patients with predisposing risk factors for NSAID-induced GI problems. Be able to discuss NSAID-induced ulceration and the various therapeutic options available as preventive therapy.
- caution people who take muscle relaxants on the possibility of serious adverse effects such as falls and difficulty driving vehicles, operating machinery, using sharp tools, etc.
- identify potential prescription drug abusers by using patient profiles.
- discuss the roles of COX-1 and COX-2 in the body's normal state and with inflammation.

DRUG LIST

Baclofen
Celebrex
Clinoril
Daypro
Disalcid
Feldene
Flexeril
Ibuprofen
Indocin
Lodine
Mobic
Naprosyn
Norflex
Relafen
Robaxin
Skelaxin
Soma
Toradol
Voltaren/Arthrotec
Zanaflex

• DRUG HOT POINTS

Baclofen
Structural analog of GABA
Indicated to treat spasticity from multiple sclerosis

Celebrex
Selectively inhibits COX-2; should protect GI
Has a sulfonamide moiety (not for people with sulfa allergies)
Counseling: no OTC analgesics with this Rx
General counseling: diet, exercise, etc.
QD to BID
OA, RA, familial adenomatous polyposis

Clinoril
Prodrug, converted to active metabolite, then to inactive metabolite in kidneys
Should spare adverse renal effects
BID dosing
Caution: adverse GI effects

Daypro
Long acting: once-a-day dosing

Diclofenac
Voltaren: enteric-coated sodium salt
Cataflam: potassium salt (not enteric coated)
Hepatotoxicity cautions
Arthrotec: combined with misoprostol, a prostaglandin analog that protects gastric mucosa
Available as a topical gel (Rx)

Disalcid
Two salicylates fused together
Less gastric irritation
Less action on platelets than ASA

Flexeril
Tricyclic related (similar to amitriptyline)
Muscle relaxation: from CNS depression
Warning: constipation, no alcohol
Should be used for no more than 14 days

Ibuprofen
After aspirin, the second NSAID
Rx: flexible doses up to 3200 mg/day
OTC (Advil, etc.): up to 1200 mg/day
Cautions: take with food, milk
NeoProfen: IV to treat PDA (preferred)

Indocin
Potent NSAID
PO dose: treatment for gout
Has been used IV to treat PDA

Lodine
Possible advantage fewer GI adverse effects

Mobic
Potent, take with food; no exposure to sun
Adverse effects: GI, renal (caution: elderly)
Compare with Feldene

Naprosyn
Dosed BID
Rx (Naprosyn, Naprelan, Anaprox)
OTC: Aleve—caution about its potency

Norflex
Related to diphenhydramine
Muscle relaxation: from CNS depression
Long-acting tablets; BID dosing
Caution: no alcohol, driving cautions

Relafen
Nonacidic prodrug
Converted to NSAID, similar to Naprosyn
Possibly less direct GI effects
Slightly selective for COX-2

Skelaxin
Muscle relaxation: from CNS depression
Take with food to protect stomach
Caution: no alcohol, driving cautions
Compare with Robaxin

Soma
Abuse potential (meprobamate = metabolite)
Muscle relaxation: from CNS depression
Caution: no alcohol, driving cautions
Caution for pharmacist: highly abused agent
Mixed with prescription and recreational drugs for abuse

Toradol
Potent NSAID
Monitor GI and renal adverse events
Short-term use: for pain (5-day limit)
Monitor other meds: ASA, NSAIDs

Zanaflex
Central-acting alpha-2 adrenergic agonist (related to clonidine)
Inhibits presynaptic motor neurons
Tablets and capsules

• QUESTIONS TO BE ANSWERED IN PREPARATION FOR CHAPTER 11 LAB

- How many milligrams of active drug are contained in each Voltaren XR tablet?
- What is the milligram strength of the largest size Naprosyn tablet?
- Which enzyme does Feldene inhibit?
- How many milligrams of active drug are in each teaspoonful of Naprosyn Suspension?
- What is the advantage of using Cataflam instead of Voltaren in treating pain and primary dysmenorrhea?
- What is the indicated use for cyclobenzaprine?
- How many milligrams of active drug are in each teaspoonful of Indocin Suspension?
- Because Relafen is a nonacidic NSAID, it should irritate the stomach very little or not at all. Explain why some patients who take Relafen still experience GI upset.
- Is Soma a DEA-controlled drug? In which state(s)?
- If a physician prescribes "naproxen sodium 275 mg," what is the brand name of the product?
- How is Voltaren gel applied to the skin?
- Explain why some proton pump inhibitors (PPIs) are indicated for patients who are prescribed NSAIDs.
- Describe the use of IV ibuprofen in the treatment of patent ductus arteriosus (PDA).
- Describe the use of IV indomethacin in the treatment of PDA.
- A patient receives Toradol injections today (all day) in the hospital for severe pain. He is then released with a prescription for Toradol tablets to be purchased in your pharmacy. The prescription is for 1 tablet TID. How many tablets should be dispensed?
- What is the name of the active metabolite of carisoprodol?
- How many milligrams of active drug are contained in each indomethacin sustained-release capsule?
- What is the brand name of the potassium salt of diclofenac?
- Describe the functions of COX-1 and COX-2.
- Which tricyclic antidepressant is structurally closely related to Flexeril?
- Which antihistamine is structurally related to Norflex?
- Which NSAID has an inactive metabolite that is produced in the kidneys and may have fewer adverse effects in the kidneys when given to patients with renal disorders?
- What is the advantage of combining misoprostol with diclofenac in Arthrotec?
- Explain why pregnant patients should *not* take NSAIDs.
- Explain the additive CNS depressant effects if a person takes unapproved high doses of baclofen and Xanax.

• MUSCLE RELAXANTS AND NSAIDS MEDICATION THERAPY MANAGEMENT QUESTIONS AND COMMENTS

- Your physician prescribed a medication called a nonsteroidal anti-inflammatory drug, or NSAID. This family of medications includes nonprescription as well as prescription products. Some nonprescription products include aspirin, ibuprofen (Advil, Motrin, etc.), naproxen sodium (Aleve, etc.), as well as many combination products.
- It should always be taken with food or milk. This will protect your stomach. Additionally, please do not take any nonprescription (OTC) drugs or products for pain or fever without checking with us first. Some OTC products contain essentially the same medication as your prescription. Taking too much of this class of medication increases the risk of bad effects on your stomach and body. In your bag, you will find a medication guide to help you take the medication effectively.
- If you take this NSAID medication for many days according to your physician's orders and you experience heartburn or stomach problems, contact your doctor for advice. However, some physicians order an OTC product called omeprazole to be taken in the mornings 1 hour before breakfast when this stomach problem occurs or to prevent this problem. If you do not eat breakfast, it can be taken 1 hour before a major meal of the day. Omeprazole acts to decrease the production of acid in the stomach. This would reduce the risk of upset stomach.
- Has your doctor explained how to use this medication? The prescription was written as PRN. That means that it should be taken only if needed. If you do not need it, wait and take the medication if the pain or inflammation comes back. Would you like to meet with us for a brief explanation of how to make a plan for using your pain pill?
- Your prescription is written for Toradol. Its generic name is ketorolac. It is a potent anti-inflammatory drug and pain killer; however, it can be taken only for 5 days total after an initial injection by the doctor. The prescription was written for more than 5 days' supply. We will dispense only the amount that is allowed to total 5 days' supply.
- After 5 days, if you need more medication, we will have to call the prescriber to reevaluate your condition and make a plan for treatment. In the bag with your prescription, I am including a medication guide for your medication that explains the situation. Please read it carefully to appreciate and respect the value and cautions for this medication.
- If you would like, we can meet quietly or by phone to look over all your medications. This review might help us find issues unrelated to your pain. Our review would include lifestyle suggestions that could help to reduce your muscle pain. We have literature that shows range-of-motion stretches as well as nutritional suggestions. Drinking appropriate amounts of water each day to hydrate your body might help your muscles and other body tissues to be firmer. This would reduce the risk of the aches and pains that you have been experiencing.
- The physician at the medical office prescribed a medication for muscle spasm called Zanaflex (tizanidine). Unfortunately, this medication might interact with another one of your medications called Catapres (clonidine). We will discuss this situation with the doctor and offer some alternative products that are useful for muscle spasm and that would have low risk for adverse effects with your other medications. While we are discussing your medications, it would be helpful if we could schedule a meeting, in person or by phone, to do an overall evaluation of your medications. Our medication therapy management meeting includes suggestions that we would offer for you to do lifestyle or dietary changes. This has had a major impact on our other patients and their health and quality of life.
- Since you have started taking your new prescription for 800 mg ibuprofen four times a day, your blood pressure has gone up dramatically. Your blood pressure medications have been controlling your blood pressure well for the last few years. Since we are doing our annual medication therapy management session, our blood pressure measurement shows a serious increase in your blood pressure. I will call your physician now to discuss this. If he or she needs to examine you now, it would be best for you to do that. Please remember that this class or family of drugs carries a risk of increasing the blood pressure, especially in seniors.

• MUSCLE RELAXANTS AND NSAIDS MEDICATION THERAPY MANAGEMENT QUESTIONS AND COMMENTS *(continued)*

- Your new prescription is for Norflex, or orphenadrine citrate. It has been prescribed to help treat muscle spasm in your back. I notice that in our medication therapy management sessions you report that you have been buying an OTC pain reliever/sleep aid in the grocery store. It is called Tylenol PM. Many people report that it is an effective product. Upon looking at your brown bag collection of medications that we are reviewing, it appears that the active relaxing ingredient in Tylenol PM is diphenhydramine. It is a close relative to the active relaxing product in Norflex. It would be risky to take both of these products during the same time frame. Please do not take the OTC product while taking Norflex. The doctor prescribed this medication to be taken twice a day. Please do not take it more frequently. To do so would increase the risk of experiencing drowsiness and potential for falls.
- Your new prescription is for back spasm. It is called Flexeril, or cyclobenzaprine. I notice that one of your other prescriptions is for another medicine called amitriptyline. We should contact both of your doctors. It appears that the doctor who prescribed Flexeril did not know about the amitriptyline that you take from your other doctor. This combination of drugs, if taken at the same time frame, would predictably cause bothersome side effects. This includes very dry mouth, constipation, and blurred vision, among other problems. We can call the doctors and suggest another product for back spasm that would have less risk of these problems.
- If you would like, we can schedule a brief meeting, in person or by phone, to look over all of your medications and OTC products. This would include all of the products, whether purchased here or elsewhere. This medication therapy management review has helped many of our patients or clients. If needed, it would also allow us to give you literature about the value of a physical or occupational therapist. These specialists have helped many of our clients with joint and muscle problems after referrals by their physicians.

11.1

PT. NAME: **THELMA HARRIS** AGE: **58**
GENDER: **F**
DX: **OA, MIGRAINES, IBS, CONSTIPATION, BACTERIAL CONJUCTIVITIS**
ADDRESS: **7100 NEW UTRECHT AVE.**
ALLERGY: **ASA**
WEIGHT: **150**
HX: **DYSFUNCTIONAL BACKGROUND**
BMI: **24**

MEDICATION	SIG.	PRESCRIBER	ORIG. DATE	REFILL DATE	REFILL DATE	REFILL DATE	REFILL DATE
Donnatal tab #90	1 prn	Wessel	4/3	6/12			
Bacitracin eye ointment 3.5 g	0.5 inch to ou bid	Zalasnicks	6/18				
Surfak 240 mg #C	1 bid for BM	OTC	2/3	3/6	4/9	5/5	6/12

Dr. Rocco Sorieri
1629 83rd St., Brooklyn, NY 88364
812-555-5567

Name Thelma Harris Date 7/20

Address 7100 New Utrecht Ave. Age 58

℞

Fiorinal tablet
#100
1 q8h prn

Refills 0

Dr. Rocco Sorieri

11.1a

Dr. Angelina Teveso
8809 21st Ave., Brooklyn, NY 88364
812-555-2929

Name Thelma Harris Date 7/20

Address 7100 New Utrecht Ave. Age 58

℞

Restoril 15 mg
#30
i hs PRN

☐ Label

Refill 1 times PRN NR

Dr. A. Teveso

DEA# AT1234563

11.1b

11.2

PT. NAME: **MARY ALAZIO** AGE: **62** GENDER: **F** DX: **HTN, DEPRESSION, CHOLESTEROL, BACK PAIN, SPASM, INSOMNIA** ADDRESS: **325 IRIS BLVD.** ALLERGY: **PCN, SULFA** WEIGHT: **180** HX: **OWNS AND RUNS AN ITALIAN RESTAURANT** HEIGHT: **5′ 2″** BMI: **33**

MEDICATION	SIG.	PRESCRIBER	ORIG. DATE	REFILL DATE	REFILL DATE	REFILL DATE	REFILL DATE
Paxil 10 mg #30	I q am	Johnson	10/26				
Tenormin 50 mg #30	I q pm	Johnson	5/12	7/11	8/3		
Zocor 20 mg #30	I hs	Johnson	7/27	8/26	9/24		
Advil PM caplets #40	I hs	OTC	3/6	5/20	7/21	8/30	9/28

Dr. Theodore Von Hoenheim
400 NE 2nd Ave., Minneapolis, MN 88484
222-555-9999

Name Mary Alazio Date 10/31

Address 325 Iris Blvd. Age 62

℞

Mobic 15 mg
Disp: #30
Sig: i QD pc

REFILL 1☐ 2☑ 3☐ 4☐ NR☐
LABEL ☐
MEDICALLY NECESSARY ☐
DEA# ______

Dr. T. Von Hoenheim

11.2a

Dr. Theodore Von Hoenheim
400 NE 2nd Ave., Minneapolis, MN 88484
222-555-9999

Name Mary Alazio Date 10/31

Address 325 Iris Blvd. Age 62

℞

Norflex i po BID
#30

Refills 5

Dr. T. Von Hoenheim

11.2b

11.3 PT. NAME: **DANA ROBINS** AGE: **38** GENDER: **F** DX: **BAD BACK, ASTHMA, ALLERGIES** ADDRESS: **452 HALL ST.** ALLERGY: **PCN** WEIGHT: **205** HX: **SEDENTARY LIFESTYLE** HEIGHT: **5′ 6″** BMI: **33**

MEDICATION	SIG.	PRESCRIBER	ORIG. DATE	REFILL DATE	REFILL DATE	REFILL DATE	REFILL DATE
Claritin 10 mg #30	1 qd	Sauls	2/14	3/24			
Symbicort 80/4.5 #120	2 inhalations bid	Sauls	1/21	3/24			
Zyrtec 10 mg #30	1 qd	Sauls	4/4				
Aleve tabs #100	1 bid	OTC	3/5	4/3	5/1		

Dr. Alfred Sauls
151212 S High Rd., Chicago, IL 23875
954-555-1300

Name Dana Robins Date 5/5

Address 452 Hall St. Age 38

℞

Relafen 750mg #60
ii po QD

Prilosec 20mg #30
i po QD

Label

Refill (1) times

Dr. Alfred Sauls

11.3a

Dr. Alfred Sauls
151212 S High Rd., Chicago, IL 23875
954-555-1300

Name Dana Robins Date 5/5

Address 452 Hall St. Age 38

℞

Prednisone 20 mg #12
i PO TID
x 4 days

☒ DO NOT REFILL

☐ REFILL ______ TIMES

Dr. Alfred Sauls

11.3b

11.4

PT. NAME: **JONATHAN GREEN** GENDER: **M** ADDRESS: **688 GREEN ST.** WEIGHT: **165** HEIGHT: **5′ 8″**
AGE: **43** DX: **DEPRESSION, MUSCLE PAIN, LUMBAR PAIN, IBS, JOCK ITCH** ALLERGY: **PCN** HX: **TRUCK DRIVER**

MEDICATION	SIG.	PRESCRIBER	ORIG. DATE	REFILL DATE	REFILL DATE	REFILL DATE	REFILL DATE
Vicodin #30	1 bid	Covington	10/16				
Librax #100	1 bid prn	Griffin	1/5	10/25			
Motrin 800 mg #60	1 bid	Griffin	7/27				
Lotrisone Cream 45 g	Apply qd using "dot method"	Sobotka	3/12	5/30			

Dr. Tim Hardigan
3344 5th Ave., Atlanta, GA 54545
766-555-9000

Name Jonathan Green Date 10/28

Address 688 Green St. Age 43

℞

Effexor XR
75 mg po BID
#60

Celebrex
200 mg po BID for acute back
#60

Dr. Tim Hardigan

11.4a

Dr. Tim Hardigan
3344 5th Ave., Atlanta, GA 54545
766-555-9000

Name Jonathan Green Date 10/28

Address 688 Green St. Age 43

℞

Flexeril 10 mg
(Flexeril)
#15

ⓢ tab i TID

Refill 1X times

Dr. Tim Hardigan

11.4b

11.5

PT. NAME: **CHRIS BAKER**	GENDER: **M**	ADDRESS: **845 FANTASTIC ST.**	WEIGHT: **192**	BMI: **28**
AGE: **29**	DX: **ACCIDENT—BACK INJURY, OTITIS EXTERNA**	ALLERGY: **PCN**	HX: **PLAYS AMATEUR ICE HOCKEY**	

MEDICATION	SIG.	PRESCRIBER	ORIG. DATE	REFILL DATE	REFILL DATE	REFILL DATE	REFILL DATE
Ofloxacin otic 0.3% 5 mL	10 gtts ad bid	Keller	9/1				

Dr. John Sobotka
555 Montgomery Rd., Mason, OH 98887
247-555-0985

Name Chris Baker Date 9/25

Address 845 Fantastic St. Age 29

℞

Flexeril 10 mg.
#30
Sig: i po TID
do not drive w/med

Refills 2

Dr. John Sobotka

11.5a

Dr. Robert Wuest
600 Central Ave., Cincinnati, OH 98887
247-555-1112

Name Chris Baker Date 9/25

Address 845 Fantastic St. Age 29

℞

Indocin 25
sig i tid

Call for Refills

Dr. Robert Wuest

11.5b

11.6

PT. NAME: **ZACHARY BAKER** AGE: **50** GENDER: **M** DX: **BACK PAIN, UTI, ANXIOUS** ADDRESS: **89 DEXTER AVE.** ALLERGY: **SULFA, ERYTHROMYCIN** WEIGHT: **240, OBESE** HX: **WORKS IN DRY CLEANING STORE** BMI: **34**

MEDICATION	SIG.	PRESCRIBER	ORIG. DATE	REFILL DATE	REFILL DATE	REFILL DATE	REFILL DATE
Vicodin #120	1 q 6 h prn	Kaler	9/19	10/17	11/16		
Alprazolam 0.5 mg #30	1 tid	Kaler	8/22	9/19	10/17		
Cephalexin 500 mg #40	1 qid	Kaler	10/17				

Dr. Tom Coving
323 Lakeshore Dr., Birmingham, AL 33232
247-555-0980

Name Zachary Baker Date 11/17

Address 89 Dexter Ave. Age 50

℞

Celebrex 200 mg
i po bid
#60

Refills NR

Dr. Tom Coving

11.6a

Dr. Tom Coving
323 Lakeshore Dr., Birmingham, AL 33232
247-555-0980

Name Zachary Baker Date 11/17

Address 89 Dexter Ave. Age 50

℞

Tylenol #3
#30
T q6H prn

Refills NR

Dr. Tom Coving

DEA# BC1234563

11.6b

11.7

PT. NAME: **WILMA SMITH** GENDER: **F** ADDRESS: **564 CAPITOL AVE.** WEIGHT: **142** HEIGHT: **5′ 8″**

AGE: **39** DX: **BACK PAIN, CONSTIPATION** ALLERGY: **PCN** HX: **CAR ACCIDENT MANY YEARS AGO; STILL HAS PAIN**

MEDICATION	SIG.	PRESCRIBER	ORIG. DATE	REFILL DATE	REFILL DATE	REFILL DATE	REFILL DATE
Percocet 5/325 mg #56	1 q 6 h prn pain	Griffin	6/20				
Soma 350 mg #90	1 pc prn	Griffin	4/12	6/18			
Cyclobenzaprine 10 mg #80	1 tid	Griffin	3/12	4/10	5/20	6/30	
Ex-Lax Chocolate Reg. Str. #24	prn hs	OTC	3/15	3/20	4/13	4/30	5/28

Dr. Doug Griffin
7611 147th Terrace, Monterey, CA 38411
705-555-6644

Name Wilma Smith Date 7/6

Address 564 Capitol Ave. Age 39

℞

Valium 5 mg #60 1 p

Relafen 500 #60 2 a day

Refills 1

Dr. Doug Griffin

11.7a

Dr. Doug Griffin
7611 147th Terrace, Monterey, CA 38411
705-555-6644

Name Wilma Smith Date 7/6

Address 564 Capitol Ave. Age 39

℞

Medrol Dose Pak

#1

Taper as per directions

Dr. Doug Griffin

11.7b

11.8

PT. NAME: **FRANK SCHNEIDER** GENDER: **M** ADDRESS: **7584 GREEN AVE.** WEIGHT: **245** HEIGHT: **6′** BMI: **33**
AGE: **62** DX: **CHF, HIGH CHOLESTEROL, HTN, INSOMNIA, OA PAIN** ALLERGY: **SULFA** HX: **RETIRED POLICE OFFICER**

MEDICATION	SIG.	PRESCRIBER	ORIG. DATE	REFILL DATE	REFILL DATE	REFILL DATE	REFILL DATE
Lanoxin 0.25 mg #30	I q am	Yountz	2/13	3/10			
Lotensin 20 mg #30	I q am	Yountz	2/13	3/10			
Crestor 5 mg #30	I hs	Yountz	2/13	3/10			
Ambien 10 mg #30	I hs	Yountz	1/4	2/12	3/20		

Dr. Andrew Yountz
888 NW 27th Ave., Miami, FL 98885
247-555-6613

Name Frank Schneider Date 3/30

Address 7584 Green Ave. Age 62

℞

Naproxen 250
#120

Sig T bid

Refills 1

Dr. Andrew Yountz

11.8a

Dr. Andrew Yountz
888 NW 27th Ave., Miami, FL 98885
247-555-6613

Name Frank Schneider Date 3/30

Address 7584 Green Ave. Age 62

℞

Sulindac 200
T po bid

60

Refills 1

Dr. Andrew Yountz

11.8b

11.9 PT. NAME: **HANK HERNANDEZ** AGE: **38** GENDER: **M** DX: **MUSCLE PAIN, ANXIETY** ADDRESS: **2940 LEXTER DR.** ALLERGY: **NKA** WEIGHT: **168** HX: **ALCOHOLISM** BMI: **24**

MEDICATION	SIG.	PRESCRIBER	ORIG. DATE	REFILL DATE	REFILL DATE	REFILL DATE	REFILL DATE
Tylenol PM #100	prn	OTC	Buys from food store				
Anacin tabs #100	prn	OTC	Buys from food store				

Dr. Barry Weiss
901 Sheridan St., Austin, TX 90902
874-555-9000

Name Hank Hernandez Date 10/17

Address 2940 Lexter Dr. Age 38

℞

Relafen 500mg
#60
[illegible] two daily

Refills 0

Dr. Barry Weiss

11.9a

Dr. Barry Weiss
901 Sheridan St., Austin, TX 90902
874-555-9000

Name Hank Hernandez Date 10/17

Address 2940 Lexter Dr. Age 38

℞

hydroxyzine #50
25 mg

Sig: 1 TID

Refills 0

Dr. Barry Weiss

11.9b

11.10 PT. NAME: **HANNAH CARLSON** AGE: **51** GENDER: **F** DX: **LUMBAR PAIN** ADDRESS: **1906 BAY PARKWAY** ALLERGY: **NKA** WEIGHT: **140** HX: **DENTIST; SMOKER, 36 PACK-YEARS** HEIGHT: **5′ 3″**

MEDICATION	SIG.	PRESCRIBER	ORIG. DATE	REFILL DATE	REFILL DATE	REFILL DATE	REFILL DATE
Anacin tabs #C	1–2 q 4–6 h	OTC	3/12	3/20			
Tylenol No. 3 #L	1–2 q 4–6 h prn pain	Young	2/5	4/3			

Dr. Abraham Andrews
2929 Manhattan Blvd.
Coney Island, Brooklyn, NY 54555
813-555-7651

Name Hannah Carlson Date 4/5

Address 1906 Bay Parkway Age 51

℞

45

Voltaren 75 mg

1 BID x 3wks
pc

☐ Label

Refill ______ times

Dr. Abraham Andrews

11.10a

Dr. Abraham Andrews
2929 Manhattan Blvd.
Coney Island, Brooklyn, NY 54555
813-555-7651

Name Hannah Carlson Date 4/5

Address 1906 Bay Parkway Age 51

℞

40

Ultram

1 Q4-6h PRN pain

☐ Label

Refill ______ times

Dr. Abraham Andrews

11.10b

11.11

PT. NAME: **JANET MARTIN** GENDER: **F** ADDRESS: **31 PHILLIP LANE** WEIGHT: **140** BMI: **26**
AGE: **60** DX: **HTN, LOW BACK PAIN, LUMBAR SPINE SCOLIOSIS** ALLERGY: **NKA** HX: **SMOKER FOR 45 YEARS**

MEDICATION	SIG.	PRESCRIBER	ORIG. DATE	REFILL DATE	REFILL DATE	REFILL DATE	REFILL DATE
Dyazide #30	1 qd	Johns	1/17	2/20	3/28		
Inderal 40 mg #90	1 tid	Johns	1/17	2/17	3/28		
Tylenol No. 3 #24	1 q 4 h prn	Johns	3/12				

Dr. Donna Johns
7000 SW 1st Ave., Santa Fe, NM 54545
766-555-9097

Name Janet Martin Date 3/30

Address 31 Phillip Lane Age 60

℞

toradol 10 mg

PO PC TID #90

Refills NR

Dr. Donna Johns

11.11a

Dr. Donna Johns
7000 SW 1st Ave., Santa Fe, NM 54545
766-555-9097

Name Janet Martin Date 3/30

Address 31 Phillip Lane Age 60

℞

Tenormin

25 mg

#60

[illegible] 4 day

☑ LABEL

REFILL 12x TIMES PRN NR

Dr. Donna Johns

11.11b

11.12

PT. NAME: **MARTHA JOHNSON** GENDER: **F** ADDRESS: **3906 LEE PARKWAY** WEIGHT: **128** HEIGHT: **5′ 8″** BMI: **20**

AGE: **62** DX: **OSTEOPOROSIS, HIGH CHOLESTEROL, SKELETAL MUSCLE PAIN AND SPASM FROM FALL** ALLERGY: **NKA**

MEDICATION	SIG.	PRESCRIBER	ORIG. DATE	REFILL DATE	REFILL DATE	REFILL DATE	REFILL DATE
Fosamax 70 mg #4	1 q wk ud	Keller	4/1				
Lipitor 10 mg #30	1 qd	Keller	2/5	3/2	4/4		
Bufferin tabs #130	1 prn	OTC	3/7	4/11			

Dr. Daniel Keller
5007 Turtle Dr., Miami, FL 98887
247-555-9876

Name Martha Johnson Date 4/12

Address 3906 Lee Parkway Age 62

℞

Naproxen 500 mg
20
ī tid c̄ meals

x fall

Dr. Daniel Keller

11.12a

Dr. Daniel Keller
5007 Turtle Dr., Miami, FL 98887
247-555-9876

Name Martha Johnson Date 4/12

Address 3906 Lee Parkway Age 62

℞

Skelaxin
1 tab B.I.D
#10

Refills 0

Dr. Daniel Keller

11.12b

11.13

PT. NAME: **JOSEPHINE MARTINS**
AGE: **42**
GENDER: **F**
DX: **ALLERGIES, OVERWEIGHT, MUSCLE PAIN AND SPASM FROM CAR ACCIDENT**
ADDRESS: **894 WEST RD.**
ALLERGY: **NKA**
WEIGHT: **243**
HX: **CONSTANTLY DIETING**
BMI: **33**

MEDICATION	SIG.	PRESCRIBER	ORIG. DATE	REFILL DATE	REFILL DATE	REFILL DATE	REFILL DATE
Phentermine 15 mg #30	1 q am	Isaacs	1/21	2/19	3/24		
Alavert ODT 10 mg #18	1 qd	Isaacs	1/12	2/14	3/20		

Dr. Howard Isaacs
1115 Turnaround Lane, Detroit, MI 64789
343-555-7000

Name Josephine Martins Date 3/30

Address 894 West Rd. Age 42

℞

SOMA
i p.o. BID PRN
øeton
#30

Refills 0

Dr. Howard Isaacs

11.13a

Dr. Howard Isaacs
1115 Turnaround Lane, Detroit, MI 64789
343-555-7000

Name Josephine Martins Date 3/30

Address 894 West Rd. Age 42

℞

Disalcid tabs 750mg
#120
ii po tid p.c.

Refills 0

Dr. Howard Isaacs

11.13b

11.14 PT. NAME: **CAROL ZIMMERMAN** AGE: **29** GENDER: **F** DX: **MUSCLE PAINS, MUSCLE SPASMS** ADDRESS: **2 TALLAHASSEE CT.** ALLERGY: **NKA** WEIGHT: **160** HX: **ARTHRITIS (RA)** BMI: **23**

MEDICATION	SIG.	PRESCRIBER	ORIG. DATE	REFILL DATE	REFILL DATE	REFILL DATE	REFILL DATE
Tylenol No. 4 #15	1 q 4–6 h prn pain	Robins	2/26	3/12			
Esgic #15	1 tid	Robins	2/26	3/12			

Dr. Calvin Robins
7823 Tea Rose Trail, Miami, FL 44718
463-555-8000

Name Carol Zimmerman Date 3/20

Address 2 Tallahassee Ct. Age 29

℞

Voltaren 100mg XR
ī po qd
#30

Refills 3

Dr. Calvin Robins

11.14a

Dr. Calvin Robins
7823 Tea Rose Trail, Miami, FL 44718
463-555-8000

Name Carol Zimmerman Date 3/20

Address 2 Tallahassee Ct. Age 29

℞

Norflex
#XXX
Sig: ī qid

Refills ×2

Dr. Calvin Robins

11.14b

11.15

PT. NAME: **JANE BURKE** GENDER: **F** ADDRESS: **6 PENNSYLVANIA AVE. NW** WEIGHT: **159** BMI: **24**
AGE: **32** DX: **CHRONIC LOW BACK PAIN, GERD** ALLERGY: **NKA** HX: **SPORTS INJURY**

MEDICATION	SIG.	PRESCRIBER	ORIG. DATE	REFILL DATE	REFILL DATE	REFILL DATE	REFILL DATE
Mobic 15 mg #30	1 q am with food	Thomas	4/12	5/10	6/9		
Zantac 150 mg #60	1 bid	Thomas	4/12	5/10	6/9		

Dr. Harry Carmichael
900 North Ridge, New York, NY 88364
813-555-0022

Name Jane Burke Date 6/22

Address 6 Pennsylvania Ave. NW Age 32

℞

Arthrotec 50 mg

Sig: i bid Disp #60

Notify your physician

Refills 2

Dr. Harry Carmichael

11.15a

Dr. Harry Carmichael
900 North Ridge, New York, NY 88364
813-555-0022

Name Jane Burke Date 6/22

Address 6 Pennsylvania Ave. NW Age 32

℞

Carafate 1 gm

#100

Sig: i tab AC & hs

Refills 2

Dr. Harry Carmichael

11.15b

11.16

PT. NAME: **ROGER HARRIS** AGE: **56**
GENDER: **M** DX: **HTN, OA, SEVERE BACK PAIN, GERD**
ADDRESS: **88 BANK ST.** ALLERGY: **ERYTHROMYCIN**
WEIGHT: **188** HX: **SALES CLERK**
HEIGHT: **6′**

MEDICATION	SIG.	PRESCRIBER	ORIG. DATE	REFILL DATE	REFILL DATE	REFILL DATE	REFILL DATE
Motrin 400 mg #20	I q 4–6 h with food prn pain	Fox	2/8	2/20			
Chlorthalidone 25 mg #30	I q am for BP	Fox	1/30	2/28			
Pepcid 20 mg #30	I bid for acid	Fox	2/15	3/1			

Dr. Al Fox
60 Campus Drive, Weatherford, OK 73096
580-555-9871

Name Roger Harris Date 3/8

Address 88 Bank St. Age 56

℞

Mevacor 20 mg qd #30
Norvasc 2.5 mg qd.. #30
Celebrex 100 mg BID #60.

Label

Refill 3 times

Dr. Al Fox

11.16a

Dr. Al Fox
60 Campus Drive, Weatherford, OK 73096
580-555-9871

Name Roger Harris Date 3/8

Address 88 Bank St. Age 56

℞

Flexeril 10 mg
1 tab po. B.i.d.
prn muscle spasm.

[illegible] 40

Refills 1X

Dr. Al Fox

11.16b

11.17

PT. NAME: **HARVEY BRINE** GENDER: **M** ADDRESS: **55 FLOWER LANE** WEIGHT: **138** HEIGHT: **5′ 11″**

AGE: **44** DX: **HERNIATED DISK, SPRAINED KNEE, ALLERGIC RHINITIS** ALLERGY: **ERYTHROMYCIN** HX: **TAXI DRIVER**

MEDICATION	SIG.	PRESCRIBER	ORIG. DATE	REFILL DATE	REFILL DATE	REFILL DATE	REFILL DATE
Knee brace #1 medium	Use ud	Warnock	6/7				
Allegra 180 mg #30	1 qd for allergy	Warnock	2/7	3/8	4/20		
Atrovent Nasal Spray 0.06% 15 mL	2 sprays per nostril tid	Warnock	2/7	3/30			
Zyrtec-D 12-hr #20	1 tab bid	Warnock	5/8	6/30	7/22		

Dr. Arnie Warnock
51 Stadium Dr., West Lafayette, IN 47907
765-555-1201

Name Harvey Brine Date 8/3

Address 55 Flower Lane Age 44

℞

Cataflam 50mg
Sig i Po BID c̄ food
#60

Refills 5

Dr. Arnie Warnock

11.17a

Dr. Arnie Warnock
51 Stadium Dr., West Lafayette, IN 47907
765-555-1201

Name Harvey Brine Date 8/3

Address 55 Flower Lane Age 44

℞

ULTRAM 50 mg
TABS #10 (TEN)
i q 4h prn pain

Refills 1x

Dr. Arnie Warnock

11.17b

11.18

PT. NAME: **DANA SIMPSON** GENDER: **F** ADDRESS: **333 SO. 9 ST.** WEIGHT: **120** BMI: **19**
AGE: **68** DX: **OSTEOPOROSIS, HTN, GERD, URINARY INCONTINENCE** ALLERGY: **PCN** HX: **INACTIVE, RETIRED, SMOKED 1 PACK/DAY FOR 30 YEARS (30 PACK-YEARS)**

MEDICATION	SIG.	PRESCRIBER	ORIG. DATE	REFILL DATE	REFILL DATE	REFILL DATE	REFILL DATE
Ultracet 37.5/325 mg #50	1 q 6 h prn pain	Matthew	10/1	10/28	11/7	12/8	12/22
Amitriptyline 10 mg #30	1 hs	Matthew	9/1	10/3	11/1	12/5	
Fosamax Plus D 70 mg-2800 IU #4	1 q wk ac bkfst	Matthew	8/1	9/2	10/1	11/1	12/3
Protonix 40 mg #30	1 qd	Matthew	11/30				

Dr. Arnold Cross
29 Foster St., Worcester, MA 01608
508-555-8871

Name Dana Simpson Date 12/29

Address 333 So. 9 St. Age 68

℞

Naproxen 500 mg

ī tab PO BID

60

☑ Label

Refill - 0 - 2 - 3 - (4) - PRN

Dr. Arnold Cross

11.18a

Dr. Arnold Cross
29 Foster St., Worcester, MA 01608
508-555-8871

Name Dana Simpson Date 12/29

Address 333 So. 9 St. Age 68

℞

Triamterene/HCTZ 37.5/25

ī tab PO qd

30

☑ Label

Refill - 0 - 2 - 3 - (4) - PRN

Dr. Arnold Cross

11.18b

11.19 PT. NAME: **SHARON MORENO** AGE: **50** GENDER: **F** DX: **HTN, UTI, COPD, TYPE 2 DM, SEVERE BACK SPASM, VAGINAL MONILIASIS, HIGH BLOOD LIPIDS** ADDRESS: **91 NW 8TH AVE.** ALLERGY: **SULFA** WEIGHT: **166** HX: **SMOKER, 52.5 PACK-YEARS** HEIGHT: **5′ 6″**

MEDICATION	SIG.	PRESCRIBER	ORIG. DATE	REFILL DATE	REFILL DATE	REFILL DATE	REFILL DATE
Fluconazole 150 mg #2	1 PO hs, rep. in 2 wks	Strasser	3/1				
Lovastatin 20 mg #30	1 qd	Strasser	1/5	2/6	3/1	4/5	5/2
Advair Diskus 250/50 mcg #60	1 inhalation bid	Strasser	1/5	2/6	3/1	4/4	5/2
Ceftin 250 mg #14	1 bid	Strasser	5/7				
Avapro 150 mg #30	1 qd	Strasser	1/5	2/6	3/1	4/5	5/2
Januvia 100 mg #30	1 qd	Strasser	4/12				

Dr. Hal Strasser
522 Main St., Ada, OH 45810
419-555-3388

Name Sharon Moreno Date 5/9

Address 91 NW 8 Ave. Age 50

℞

Baclofen 10 mg
1/2 po qHS x1 wk
then ↑ i po qHS
#35

☐ Label

Refill - 0 - 1 - 2 - (3) - 4 - PRN

Dr. Hal Strasser

11.19a

Dr. Hal Strasser
522 Main St., Ada, OH 45810
419-555-3388

Name Sharon Moreno Date 5/9

Address 91 NW 8 Ave. Age 50

℞

Tylenol #3 tab
i-ii tab po 3x d prn
#90

Refills NR

Dr. Hal Strasser

DEA# BS 1234563

11.19b

11.20 PT. NAME: **LATRICE POPE** AGE: **38** GENDER: **F** DX: **MIGRAINES, INJURY FROM CAR ACCIDENT** ADDRESS: **800 SMITH ST.** ALLERGY: **NKA** WEIGHT: **151** HX: **HIGH SCHOOL TEACHER, GOLFER** BMI: **22**

MEDICATION	SIG.	PRESCRIBER	ORIG. DATE	REFILL DATE	REFILL DATE	REFILL DATE	REFILL DATE
Imitrex Inj. 6 mg/0.5 mL #2	6 mg SQ, may repeat after 1 hr	Pastor	4/7	4/20	5/9		
Ativan 1 mg #30	1 tid prn	Pastor	3/20	4/12	5/22	6/29	

Dr. Frank Pastor
88 Mall Blvd, Savannah, GA 31406
912-555-3450

Name Latrice Pope Date 7/5

Address 800 Smith St. Age 38

℞

Zanaflex 4mg

T PO BID

disp: 70

Refills X 5

Dr. Frank Pastor

11.20a

Dr. Frank Pastor
88 Mall Blvd, Savannah, GA 31406
912-555-3450

Name Latrice Pope Date 7/5

Address 800 Smith St. Age 38

℞

Percocet

X po PRN Q8H

pain

#7

Refills NR

Dr. Frank Pastor

DEA# BP1234563

11.20b

11.21

PT. NAME: **TANIA BELTRAN** AGE: **62** GENDER: **F** DX: **OSTEOPOROSIS, BACK PAIN, ANXIETY, IBS WITH CONSTIPATION** ADDRESS: **123 BLAKE AVE.** ALLERGY: **PCN, ASA** WEIGHT: **118** HX: **WORKS PART-TIME IN DEPARTMENT STORE** HEIGHT: **5′ 4″**

MEDICATION	SIG.	PRESCRIBER	ORIG. DATE	REFILL DATE	REFILL DATE	REFILL DATE	REFILL DATE
Lorazepam 1 mg #30	1 hs prn	Clay	4/1	5/6	5/28	6/14	7/7
Amitiza 24 mcg #60	1 bid	Clay	6/22				
Alprazolam 0.5 mg #50	1 bid prn	Clay	5/9	6/8	7/7		
Ultram ER 100 mg #30	1 qd for pain	Clay	6/30				
Lyrica 25 mg #30	1 capsule tid	Clay	6/2				

Dr. James Clay
1700 E. Mabel, Tucson, AZ 85721
520-555-1291

Name Tania Beltran Date 7/18

Address 123 Blake Ave. Age 62

℞

Naproxen 375 mg
caps #100
Sig: 1 cap q 12 hrs
for arthritis

Three Refills

Dr. James Clay

11.21a

Dr. James Clay
1700 E. Mabel, Tucson, AZ 85721
520-555-1291

Name Tania Beltran Date 7/18

Address 123 Blake Ave. Age 62

℞

Fosamax 70 mg
#4
1 tab weekly

☐ Label

Refill PRN times (PRN) NR

Dr. James Clay

11.21b

11.22

PT. NAME: **ROSE GRAY** GENDER: **F** ADDRESS: **700 WINGATE DR.** WEIGHT: **133**

AGE: **41** DX: **LOW BACK PAIN AND SPASM, NERVES, ANXIETY** ALLERGY: **NKA** HX: **WAITRESS, WORKS TWO JOBS**

MEDICATION	SIG.	PRESCRIBER	ORIG. DATE	REFILL DATE	REFILL DATE	REFILL DATE	REFILL DATE
Cataflam 50 mg #30	1 tid pc	Spivey	10/6	11/7	12/19		
Neurontin 300 mg #90	1 tid	Spivey	10/6	11/7	12/19		
Ambien CR 6.25 mg #14	1 hs prn	Spivey	11/19				

Dr. Harvey Spivey
160 New Scotland, Albany, NY 12208
518-555-3948

Name Rose Gray Date 12/30

Address 700 Wingate Dr. Age 41

℞

Soma Cmpd c̄ Codeine #30
Sig i po hs prn

Refills 2

Dr. Harvey Spivey

DEA# BS1234563

11.22a

Dr. Harvey Spivey
160 New Scotland, Albany, NY 12208
518-555-3948

Name Rose Gray Date 12/30

Address 700 Wingate Dr. Age 41

℞

Voltaren 50 mg
#14
i bid c̄ meals

Refills 5

Dr. Harvey Spivey

11.22b

• CHRONIC OBSTRUCTIVE PULMONARY DISEASE AND ASTHMA 12

UPON COMPLETION OF THIS CHAPTER, THE STUDENT WILL BE ABLE TO:

- counsel patients on the proper use of inhalers.
- explain the appropriate intervals and order of administration of oral and nasal inhalers and sprays.
- demonstrate the use of spacing devices such as InspirEase and AeroChamber.
- identify solid oral dosage forms that cannot be crushed before being administered, explain the reasons for these restrictions, and list alternative dosing forms.
- list the interactions of agents that inhibit or induce the actions of theophylline.
- identify and explain the potential hazards associated with the use of OTC products containing agents that are pharmacologically similar to prescription medications (antihistamines, decongestants, and bronchodilators).
- counsel the person with COPD about controlling the therapy by using the products correctly and according to the prescriber's plan. This includes smoking cessation, weight and stress reduction, and environmental measures.
- describe the differences in pathophysiology and physical appearance between asthma, emphysema, and chronic bronchitis.

DRUG LIST

Accolate
Advair
Aerochamber
Albuterol
Atrovent HFA
Combivent Inhaled Spray
Cromolyn
Flonase
Flovent HFA
Foradil
InspirEase
Maxair
Nasonex
Omnaris
QVAR
Serevent
Singulair
Spiriva
Symbicort
Theophylline

• DRUG HOT POINTS

Accolate
Leukotriene receptor antagonist
BID dosing; interaction with warfarin

Aerochamber
Increases delivery of medication to the site of drug action
Compare with InspirEase

Albuterol
Short-acting β_2-agonist: bronchodilator
Positive chronotropic effect on heart
Stimulates skeletal muscle: fine hand tremor
PO formulation & aerosol (MDI)
Also used in treatment with side arm nebulizer (SAN)
Syrup available for children
Volmax and Proventil Repetabs: long acting
Use bronchodilator inhalation first, then the corticosteroid inhalation next
When using two puffs of albuterol, use the correct technique (shake well), remove the front cover, separate the two puffs by about 1 minute
Counsel the asthmatic patient: no aspirin or other NSAIDs
Each MDI can = 200 sprays; if using two sprays QID, each can should last 25 days
MDI: Metered Dose Inhaler
Monitor refills to check compliance

Atrovent HFA
Anticholinergic inhalation: bronchodilator
QID
Quaternary ammonium derivative: less absorption than atropine, fewer systemic effects
Less tachycardia than β_2-agonists
Oral inhalation and nasal spray
Compare with β_2-agonist in COPD and in asthma
Use corticosteroid inhaled spray after anticholinergic bronchodilator inhaled spray
Wait a few minutes between different inhaled spray products
HFA propellant replaces CFC

Combivent Inhaled Spray
Combination of albuterol and ipratropium
Two different mechanisms to produce bronchodilation
Produces greater bronchodilator effect than when either drug is used alone at its recommended dose

Cromolyn
Stabilizes mast cells
Maintenance; not for acute attack
May allow patient to decrease inhaled steroid
Solution for nebulizer

Flonase
Glucocorticoid for allergic rhinitis
Compare with Nasacort AQ, Omnaris, Nasonex

Flovent HFA
Anti-inflammatory agent
Different strengths: use the lowest dose required to reduce symptoms
Compare with Asmanex, Pulmicort, QVAR; combination products: Advair, Symbicort

Maxair
Similar to albuterol; more sprays per can
Autohaler (breath activated)

Serevent
Long-acting β_2-agonist: bronchodilator
BID administration should be q 12 h
Not indicated for acute attack of bronchospasm
Available as DISKUS
Compare with Foradil

Singulair
Leukotriene receptor antagonist (modifier)
May reduce bronchoconstrictor effects of leukotrienes
Once a day, children- and adult-strength tablets

• DRUG HOT POINTS (*continued*)

Spiriva
Anticholinergic
Once a day administration
Dry powder for inhalation in a capsule to be pierced and the powder is inhaled

Theophylline
Role in COPD: respiratory stimulant, relaxes bronchial smooth muscle
Therapeutic range: 5 to 15 mcg/mL (variable)
Toxicity at high doses (GI, CNS)
Saturation (nonlinear) elimination kinetics: hepatic CYP-450 enzymes
Do not switch from one sustained release product to another (variation in response)
Do not crush long-acting products
Generic liquids contain 20% ETOH; caution with Flagyl
Long-acting products at HS reduce overnight declines in FEV_1 and A.M. symptoms
Interactions: quinolones, macrolides, charcoal
Others: smoking, barbiturates, rifampin, etc.

• QUESTIONS TO BE ANSWERED IN PREPARATION FOR CHAPTER 12 LAB

- Focusing on β-receptors, explain the mechanism of action of sympathomimetics such as albuterol.
- Focusing on muscarinic receptors, explain the mechanism of action of anticholinergics such as Atrovent (as an HFA inhaler and a nasal spray)
- What are the names of the two therapeutic agents contained in Combivent?
- Explain the rationale for combining the two agents in Combivent.
- Describe some signs and symptoms of theophylline toxicity.
- List some drugs that inhibit and some that induce the metabolism of theophylline.
- Explain the reason for administering Flovent MDI after, not before, albuterol MDI.
- What is the mechanism of action of Serevent?
- Is Serevent indicated for use in an acute bronchospasm? Explain your answer.
- What is the generic name of Proventil?
- What is the mechanism of action of pirbuterol?
- Describe the appropriate steps for effective patient self-administration of an MDI.
- What is the mechanism of action of an ipratropium inhaler?
- What is the mechanism of action of an ipratropium nasal spray?
- What is the adverse effect if a patient with narrow-angle glaucoma and COPD uses Atrovent HFA MDI for its bronchodilator effect and inadvertently allows some of the spray to reach the surface of his eye?
- How does Advair differ from Symbicort?
- What would be problematic if a patient swallowed Spiriva capsules instead of inhaling them?
- Describe the advantages of Singulair over Accolate.
- Why would the use of Singulair result in less need for acute use of the albuterol MDI?
- Compare the potencies of the orally used corticosteroids and identify the potent ones.
- How would you counsel a person who uses medications for control of COPD and continues to smoke two packs of cigarettes a day?
- Describe your advice to an elderly person who uses Primatene Mist for control of COPD.
- Identify the adverse effects Primatene Mist could have on an elderly person with cardiovascular disease.
- Explain the mechanism of the fine hand tremor that occurs in a person who uses albuterol inhaled spray.
- Would it be appropriate for a physician to use propranolol to treat the tremor from albuterol?
- Which agent would be effective and produce fewer adverse effects than propranolol for the treatment of the fine hand tremor produced by albuterol?
- What is the rationale for the use of spacing devices such as InspirEase and Aerochamber?
- Why are chlorofluorocarbon (CFC) propellants being replaced by hydrofluoroalkane (HFA) propellants?
- Describe the cautions for long-acting β_2-agonists.
- Explain the calculations for determining pack-years for a smoker.
- Why are orally taken H_2-receptor antagonists sometimes prescribed for patients with asthma or COPD in addition to their inhaled medications?

• COPD AND ASTHMA MEDICATION THERAPY MANAGEMENT QUESTIONS AND COMMENTS

- Because this is our first medication therapy management session, I would like to thank you for agreeing to participate in your healthcare. Your first medication to discuss is a tablet called Singulair, or montelukast. It is very important to take one tablet each night without exception. Your doctor has prescribed this tablet to help your other medications work better. Please remember that Singulair does not give immediate relief. It might be required to be taken indefinitely. Do you have any questions about the medication, how it works, or any other issue about your other prescriptions? Please remember to avoid smoking or places where other people are smoking.
- I notice that you have questions about your Spiriva prescription. This medication is contained in capsules; however, it must be used in the plastic device and inhaled according to the instructions. It must not be swallowed. Let's have a short meeting to go through the steps needed for the medication to be effectively used.
- Would you like to review the correct technique for inhaling your medication for your lungs? Our meeting will be brief. We can use demonstration sprays with no medication for practice. I have noticed that many people start with good technique, but later on, the proper steps are forgotten and the medication does not work as well as in the beginning. This meeting is called medication therapy management. We conduct these medication review sessions routinely once a year and then again whenever a change in medication occurs, or if there is a medication-related problem.
- Your doctor has prescribed a medication in an inhaled spray for your breathing. Let's have a brief discussion of this medication and how to use it. I will supply you with material to use the spray correctly. Please ask questions and follow the directions on the printed material. I also have a demonstration device that we can both use as practice. It contains no medication; however, by us working together and practicing with the demonstration devices, you will be able to effectively deliver the medication to your lungs with the real prescription.
- This is our first meeting with you and your son, our patient. He is receiving a liquid to be swallowed and followed with a glass of water. It is called albuterol syrup. It is important to watch him for the first few days. It is not uncommon for young patients to feel dizzy, have mild muscle tremors, and to act aggressively. These effects tend to diminish over time. Please watch him and make sure that he does not engage in sports or athletics right after taking the syrup. Albuterol will help his breathing, but it is important for you and him to know what to expect. It is unlikely to cause harm; however, it can be distressing if the patient and/or caregiver is not expecting these side effects. Once he is ready and mature enough to use the inhalation formulations for breathing, we can have another medication therapy management meeting to demonstrate the technique for effective delivery of the medication by inhalation.
- Would you care to spend a few moments with a discussion of the proper technique for your breathing inhalation spray? I notice that you have been refilling the inhalation product more frequently than the doctor had prescribed.
- I understand that you have not felt it necessary to use the controller spray. You have been refilling only the inhaled spray to open the lungs. However, by not using both, your asthma condition will not be effectively treated. Both of these medications, the bronchodilator called albuterol and the controller called fluticasone, work together, one to open the lungs, the other to heal and reduce lung inflammation. There is a combination product that contains a long-acting form of the bronchodilator combined in one product with the controller. There are sprays, and also other forms called dry powders for inhalation. Would you like us to call the physician to set up an appointment? At that time, we can make recommendations for proper selection of a product that would be best for you. By using a product that contains both active ingredients, you will be certain to have proper treatment for your condition.

• COPD AND ASTHMA MEDICATION THERAPY MANAGEMENT QUESTIONS AND COMMENTS *(continued)*

- Thank you for asking the question about your inhalation spray for your son's breathing condition. You have mentioned that the spray does not seem to help. He has experienced frustration with the hand-breathing coordination technique. Would you mind if we call the physician to recommend a prescription for a plastic device called a spacer, or holding chamber? I can show you literature with pictures illustrating the technique for proper use of the product. These plastic devices deliver more active medication to the lungs, with less waste and practically no advanced skills. They are very effective for young as well as elderly or disabled patients. The most commonly prescribed one is called Aerochamber.
- You have mentioned that the spray that you use for breathing has a different taste and feel in the back of your throat. That probably is because of the fact that your doctor has changed your spray to another manufacturer's product. Each manufacturer uses different spray propellants, and each one has a different feel and taste in the throat and mouth. It would be good to go ahead and use the technique that we have practiced. Your medication will work well. Please let me know how the new prescription is working.
- Has your doctor explained how to use this medication? The prescription was written as PRN. That means that it should be taken only if needed. If you do not need it; wait until you do need it. Would you like to sit with us for a brief explanation of how to make a plan for using your medications?
- Your new medication, Flonase or fluticasone, for your nasal condition is similar to the one that you use for breathing. In fact, it is the same medication, only to be used in the nostrils. The one that you inhale through the mouth requires that you keep your head looking up to help the delivery of medication to the lungs. That one is called Flovent.
- With the nasal formulation, it is a liquid watery suspension spray. It requires that after shaking the bottle and clearing the nostrils, the spray is delivered to the nostrils with the head tilted slightly forward. This will allow the medication to reach the nasal area without reaching the throat or lungs.
- Does this medication therapy management session help your understanding?
- Your physician has ordered a device called a peak flow meter. This will measure your breathing ability. We have different types. Would you like to meet for a few moments to examine them and choose one that is appropriate for the patient?

12.1

PT. NAME: **MARK GREEN** GENDER: **M** ADDRESS: **1 EAGLE RUN** WEIGHT: **188** BMI: **29**
AGE: **68** DX: **HTN, EMPHYSEMA, URI** ALLERGY: **PCN** HX: **SMOKER SINCE CHILDHOOD**

MEDICATION	SIG.	PRESCRIBER	ORIG. DATE	REFILL DATE	REFILL DATE	REFILL DATE	REFILL DATE
Flovent HFA 220 mcg 12 g	Use ud	Isaacs	4/2	5/6	6/9		
ProAir HFA 8.5 g	2 puffs tid	Isaacs	3/28	4/21	5/15	6/19	
Plendil 10 mg #90	1 qd	Isaacs	5/10				
HCTZ 25 mg #20	1 qd	Isaacs	5/10				

Dr. Daniel Keller
5007 Turtle Drive, Miami, FL 98887
247-555-9876

Name Mark Green Date 7/16

Address 1 Eagle Run Age 68

℞

Ventolin Inhaler
c̄ instructions (instruction to use.)
Sig 2 puffs qid

Refills 3

Dr. Daniel Keller

12.1a

Dr. Daniel Keller
5007 Turtle Drive, Miami, FL 98887
247-555-9876

Name Mark Green Date 7/16

Address 1 Eagle Run Age 68

℞

Cipro 500 mg
P.O. BID
#14

N.R.

Dr. Daniel Keller

12.1b

12.2

PT. NAME: **MARGARET JONES**	GENDER: **F**	ADDRESS: **977 IBIS LANE**	WEIGHT: **126**	BMI: **21**
AGE: **39**	DX: **ASTHMA**	ALLERGY: **PCN**	HX: **NA**	

MEDICATION	SIG.	PRESCRIBER	ORIG. DATE	REFILL DATE	REFILL DATE	REFILL DATE	REFILL DATE
Accolate 20 mg #60	1 bid	Davis	2/17				
Symbicort 80/4.5 #120	2 inhalations bid	Johns	1/24	2/28			

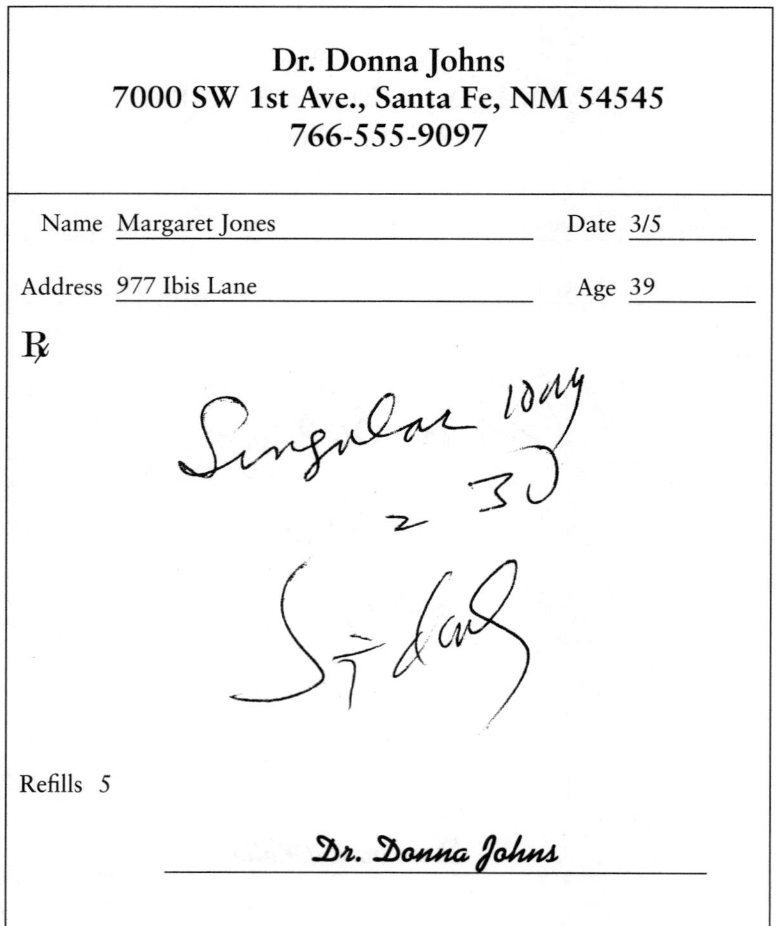

Dr. Donna Johns
7000 SW 1st Ave., Santa Fe, NM 54545
766-555-9097

Name Margaret Jones Date 3/5

Address 977 Ibis Lane Age 39

℞

Refills 5

Dr. Donna Johns

12.2a

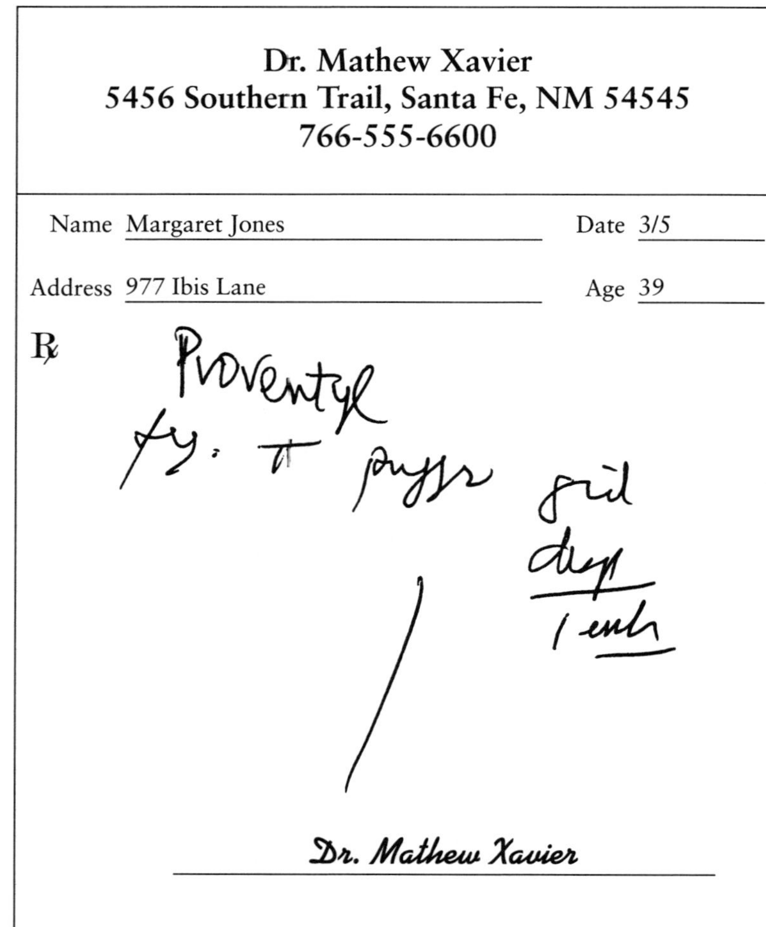

Dr. Mathew Xavier
5456 Southern Trail, Santa Fe, NM 54545
766-555-6600

Name Margaret Jones Date 3/5

Address 977 Ibis Lane Age 39

℞

Dr. Mathew Xavier

12.2b

12.3

PT. NAME: **JESSE PHILLIPS**	GENDER: **M**	ADDRESS: **684 UNIVERSITY DR.**	WEIGHT: **163**	BMI: **28**
AGE: **58**	DX: **COPD, BPH, HYPERLIPIDEMIA, HTN, ALLERGIC RHINITIS, DEPRESSION**	ALLERGY: **NKA**	HX: **SMOKER, 40 PACK-YEARS**	

MEDICATION	SIG.	PRESCRIBER	ORIG. DATE	REFILL DATE	REFILL DATE	REFILL DATE	REFILL DATE
Hytrin 5 mg #90	ud	Griffin	2/7	6/22	8/9		
HCTZ 25 mg #C	1 qd	Griffin	1/20	4/30	6/30		
Celexa 20 mg #60	1 q am	Sauls	4/17	6/22	8/2		
Lipitor 10 mg #30	1 q pm	Griffin	4/17	5/12	6/10	7/24	

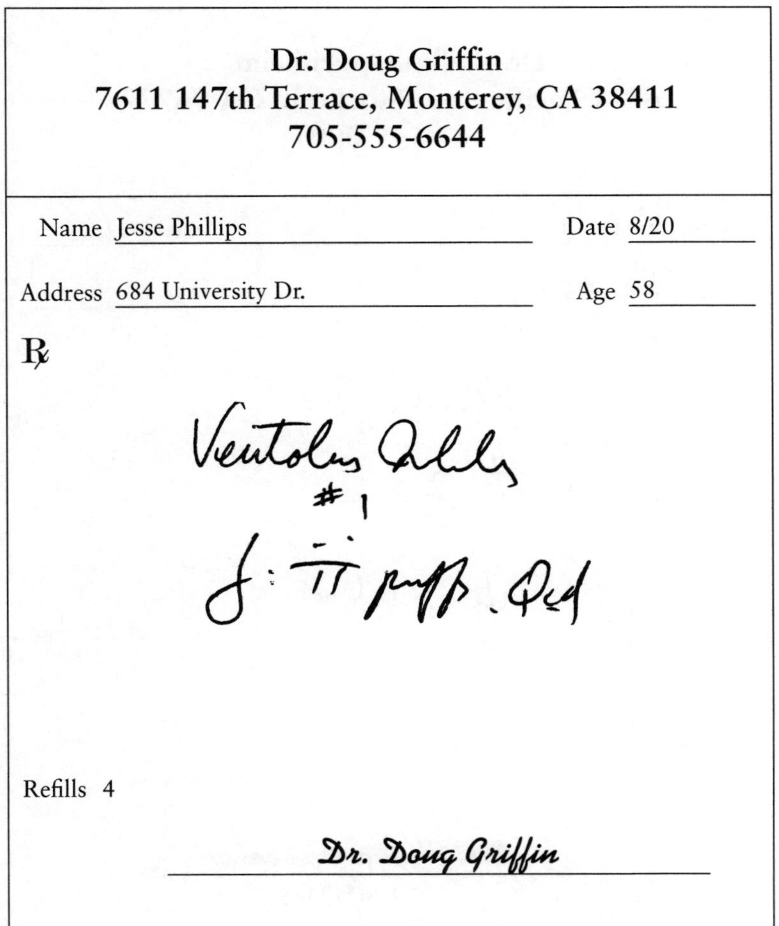
Dr. Doug Griffin
7611 147th Terrace, Monterey, CA 38411
705-555-6644

Name Jesse Phillips Date 8/20

Address 684 University Dr. Age 58

℞

Ventolin Inhaler
#1
Sig: ii puffs qid

Refills 4

Dr. Doug Griffin

12.3a

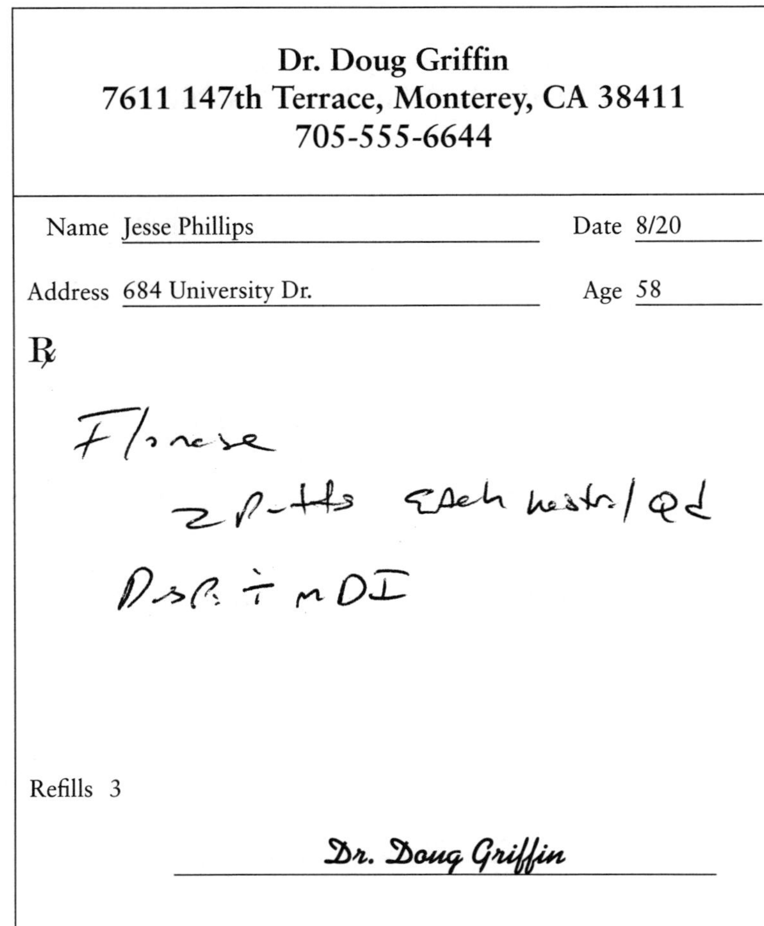
Dr. Doug Griffin
7611 147th Terrace, Monterey, CA 38411
705-555-6644

Name Jesse Phillips Date 8/20

Address 684 University Dr. Age 58

℞

Flonase
2 puffs each nostril qd
Disp: i MDI

Refills 3

Dr. Doug Griffin

12.3b

12.4

PT. NAME: **JIM LEWIS**	GENDER: **M**	ADDRESS: **1984 W 28TH ST.**	WEIGHT: **168**	BMI: **25**
AGE: **63**	DX: **HTN, COPD, ANXIETY**	ALLERGY: **SULFA**	HX: **ETOH, FORMER SMOKER**	

MEDICATION	SIG.	PRESCRIBER	ORIG. DATE	REFILL DATE	REFILL DATE	REFILL DATE	REFILL DATE
Theophylline SR 300 mg #60	1 q 12 h	Gray	6/6	7/31	9/9		
Norvasc 10 mg #30	1 qd	Gray	6/6	7/14	8/12		
Proventil HFA 6.7 g	2 puffs tid	Gray	6/19	7/19	8/24		

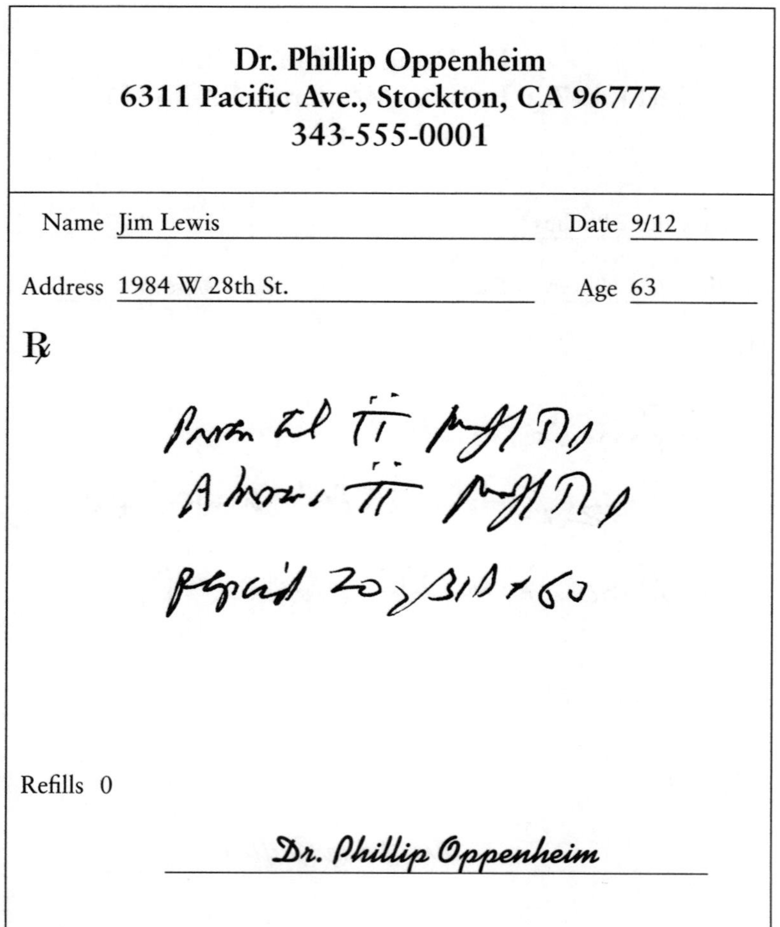

Dr. Phillip Oppenheim
6311 Pacific Ave., Stockton, CA 96777
343-555-0001

Name Jim Lewis Date 9/12

Address 1984 W 28th St. Age 63

℞

Proventil ii puffs TID
Atrovent ii puffs TID

Refills 0

Dr. Phillip Oppenheim

12.4a

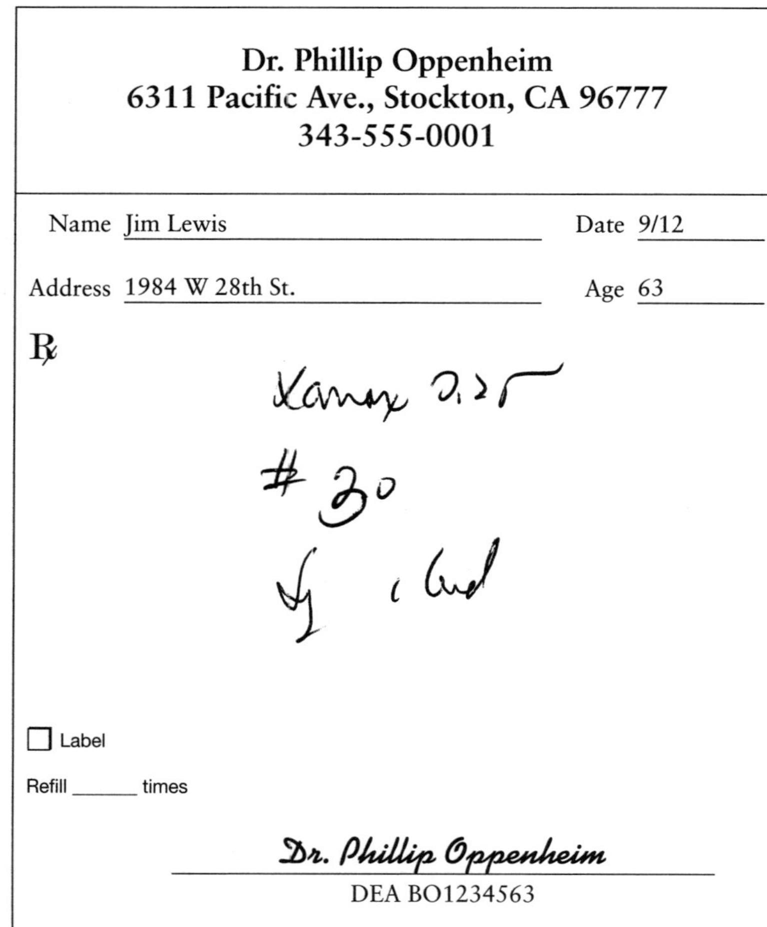

Dr. Phillip Oppenheim
6311 Pacific Ave., Stockton, CA 96777
343-555-0001

Name Jim Lewis Date 9/12

Address 1984 W 28th St. Age 63

℞

Xanax 0.25
#30

☐ Label

Refill ______ times

Dr. Phillip Oppenheim
DEA BO1234563

12.4b

12.5

PT. NAME: **BRANDON HARRIS**	GENDER: **M**	ADDRESS: **774 FIRST ST.**	WEIGHT: **49 (22.3 kg)**
AGE: **6**	DX: **ASTHMA**	ALLERGY: **PCN**	HX: **PEDIATRIC PATIENT; WHEEZES**

MEDICATION	SIG.	PRESCRIBER	ORIG. DATE	REFILL DATE	REFILL DATE	REFILL DATE	REFILL DATE
Children's Robitussin Cough and Cold CF 120 mL	2 tsp q 4 h, not to exceed 6 doses in 24 h	OTC	1/4	2/3	2/27		

Dr. Donna Johns
7000 SW 1st Ave., Santa Fe, NM 54545
766-555-9097

Name Brandon Harris Date 3/1

Address 774 First St. Age 6

℞

Ventolin syrup 8oz

[illegible]

Refills prn

Dr. Donna Johns

12.5a

Dr. Donna Johns
7000 SW 1st Ave., Santa Fe, NM 54545
766-555-9097

Name Brandon Harris Date 3/1

Address 774 First St. Age 6

℞

Poly-vi-flor 0.25mg

50cc

1cc qd

Refills prn

Dr. Donna Johns

12.5b

12.6

PT. NAME: **ANTHONY JOHNSON**
AGE: **73**
GENDER: **M**
DX: **HTN, COPD, FUNGAL SKIN RASH, SEASONAL ALLERGIES, ALLERGIC RHINITIS**
ADDRESS: **4589 BLUEJAY LANE**
ALLERGY: **SULFA**
WEIGHT: **180**
HX: **EX-SMOKER: 15-YEAR HISTORY**
BMI: **24**

MEDICATION	SIG.	PRESCRIBER	ORIG. DATE	REFILL DATE	REFILL DATE	REFILL DATE	REFILL DATE
Lotrisone Cream 15 g	Apply ud	Davis	8/30	9/22			
Advair 100/50 Diskus #60	1 puff bid	Robins	7/3				
HCTZ 25 mg #60	1 qd	Davis	4/3	6/1	8/2	9/15	
Primatene Mist 15 mL (0.5 oz)	prn	OTC	2/1	6/6	7/1		
Afrin Original Nasal Spray 1 oz (30 mL)	prn	OTC	2/1	3/9	4/22	5/6	7/1

Dr. Calvin Robins
7823 Tea Rose Trail, Miami, FL 44718
463-555-8000

Name Anthony Johnson Date 9/23

Address 4589 Bluejay Lane Age 73

℞

Albuterol 8.5g
2 puffs PRN SOB

Refills PRN

Dr. Calvin Robins

12.6a

Dr. Calvin Robins
7823 Tea Rose Trail, Miami, FL 44718
463-555-8000

Name Anthony Johnson Date 9/23

Address 4589 Bluejay Lane Age 73

℞

OMNARIS
12.5 g
2 sprays per nostril
once daily.

☑ Label

Refill 3 times PRN

Dr. Calvin Robins

12.6b

12.7 PT. NAME: **JENNY ADAMS** GENDER: **F** ADDRESS: **774 STATE ST.** WEIGHT: **149** BMI: **23**
AGE: **62** DX: **COPD, HTN, HRT, SEASONAL ALLERGIES** ALLERGY: **NKA** HX: **ETOH, SMOKED FOR 50 YEARS**

MEDICATION	SIG.	PRESCRIBER	ORIG. DATE	REFILL DATE	REFILL DATE	REFILL DATE	REFILL DATE
Prednisone 1 mg #90	1 ud	Weiss	4/23				
Premarin 0.625 #60	1 qd	Carter	3/6	5/2	7/3		
Lisinopril 5 mg #90	1 qd	Thomas	1/20	5/1			
Loratadine 10 mg #30	1 qd	Weiss	1/15	3/20	5/30		
Guaifenesin Syrup 4 oz (120 mL)	5 mL (1 tsp) qid with water prn cough	OTC	1/10	2/22	4/30		

Dr. Barry Weiss
901 Sheridan St., Austin, TX 90902
874-555-9000

Name Jenny Adams Date 7/10

Address 774 State St. Age 62

℞

UNIT DOSE ATROVENT

SIG i TID

90

Label

Refill x 6 times

Dr. Barry Weiss

12.7a

Dr. Barry Weiss
901 Sheridan St., Austin, TX 90902
874-555-9000

Name Jenny Adams Date 7/10

Address 774 State St. Age 62

℞

UNIT DOSE ALBUTEROL

SIG i TID

90

Label

Refill x 6 times

Dr. Barry Weiss

12.7b

12.8

PT. NAME: **BRIAN BLACK** | GENDER: **M** | ADDRESS: **8544 FLORIDA DR.** | WEIGHT: **139** | HEIGHT: **5′ 3″**
AGE: **46** | DX: **ASTHMA/COPD** | ALLERGY: **NKA** | HX: **SMOKER, OCCASIONAL ETOH**

MEDICATION	SIG.	PRESCRIBER	ORIG. DATE	REFILL DATE	REFILL DATE	REFILL DATE	REFILL DATE
Flovent HFA 220 mcg 12 g	Use 3 puffs bid	Weiss	10/20				
Theophylline SR 100 mg #90	1 bid	Weiss	10/20				

Dr. Barry Weiss
901 Sheridan St., Austin, TX 90902
874-555-9000

Name Brian Black Date 10/30

Address 8544 Florida Dr. Age 46

℞

Atrovent medi inhaler
#1
Sig ii puffs q 6°

☐ Label

Refill X3 times

Dr. Barry Weiss

12.8a

Dr. Barry Weiss
901 Sheridan St., Austin, TX 90902
874-555-9000

Name Brian Black Date 10/30

Address 8544 Florida Dr. Age 46

℞

Albuterol MDI
#one
as directed

Refills 4

Dr. Barry Weiss

12.8b

12.9

PT. NAME: **RONALD WILLIAMS** GENDER: **M** ADDRESS: **564 CAPITOL AVE.** WEIGHT: **175** HEIGHT: **5′ 6″**
AGE: **67** DX: **COPD, OA PAIN** ALLERGY: **NKA** HX: **RETIRED, SMOKED FOR 55 YEARS**

MEDICATION	SIG.	PRESCRIBER	ORIG. DATE	REFILL DATE	REFILL DATE	REFILL DATE	REFILL DATE
Singulair 10 mg #15	1 qd	Triplett	4/26				
Celebrex 100 mg #30	1 qd	Triplett	4/26				

Dr. Suzanne Triplett
2828 SW 44th Ave., Plantation, FL 38411
705-555-0909

Name Ronald Williams Date 5/10

Address 564 Capitol Ave. Age 67

℞

Ultram 50

#100 i po q 8h prn pain

N.R.

Dr. Suzanne Triplett

12.9a

Dr. Suzanne Triplett
2828 SW 44th Ave., Plantation, FL 38411
705-555-0909

Name Ronald Williams Date 5/10

Address 564 Capitol Ave. Age 67

℞

Flovent 220 mcg 2 puffs BID #3

Albuterol MDI 2 puffs QID PRN #3

N.R.

Dr. Suzanne Triplett

12.9b

12.10

PT. NAME: **MICHELLE LARSON** GENDER: **F** ADDRESS: **321 WEST RD.** WEIGHT: **142** HEIGHT: **5′ 4″**
AGE: **53** DX: **COPD, NASAL ALLERGY** ALLERGY: **NKA** HX: **ETOH, ½ PACK/DAY SMOKER FOR 40 YEARS**

MEDICATION	SIG.	PRESCRIBER	ORIG. DATE	REFILL DATE	REFILL DATE	REFILL DATE	REFILL DATE
Primatene tabs #60	1 tid	OTC	6/2	7/15	8/14		
Robitussin DM Syrup 4 oz	2 tsp (10 mL) tid	OTC	6/2	7/15			

Dr. Donna Johns
7000 SW 1st Ave., Santa Fe, NM 54545
766-555-9097

Name Michelle Larson Date 8/19
Address 321 West Rd. Age 53

℞ Prednisone
10 mg po q AM x 3 d #3
QVAR 40
2 puff qid #1 - Rinse mouth p̄ use
Proventil 2 puff q 4° prn #1
Atrovent 2 puff qid
Theophylline S.R. 200 mg po q12° #60
BIAXIN 500 mg po q12° #40

Dr. Donna Johns

12.10a

Dr. Donna Johns
7000 SW 1st Ave., Santa Fe, NM 54545
766-555-9097

Name Michelle Larson Date 8/19
Address 321 West Rd. Age 53

℞
FLONASE
SIG i SPRAY EACH NOSTRIL
QD

Refill 3 times

Dr. Donna Johns

12.10b

12.11

PT. NAME: **SHIRLEY ANDERSON** GENDER: **F** ADDRESS: **145 NORTH AVE.** WEIGHT: **132** HEIGHT: **5′ 6″**
AGE: **30** DX: **ASTHMA, BACTERIAL INFECTION** ALLERGY: **NKA** HX: **ASTHMA SINCE CHILDHOOD**

MEDICATION	SIG.	PRESCRIBER	ORIG. DATE	REFILL DATE	REFILL DATE	REFILL DATE	REFILL DATE
Prednisone 5 mg #90	ud	Griffin	1/31				
Singulair 10 mg #30	1 qd	Griffin	2/5	5/6	9/30	11/2	
Z-Pak	Take ud	Griffin	9/11				

Dr. Doug Griffin
7611 147th Terrace, Monterey, CA 38411
705-555-6644

Name Shirley Anderson Date 11/5

Address 145 North Ave. Age 30

℞ Serevent Diskus
#1
i puff q12hr

QVAR 80mcg MDI
#1
4 puffs q 12 hr c AeroChamber

AeroChamber Kit
#1
Use c inhalers

Refills 5

Dr. Doug Griffin

12.11a

Dr. Doug Griffin
7611 147th Terrace, Monterey, CA 38411
705-555-6644

Name Shirley Anderson Date 11/5

Address 145 North Ave. Age 30

℞ Zithromax 250g
#3
S i qd

Refills NR

Dr. Doug Griffin

12.11b

12.12

PT. NAME: **JERRY SMITH** | GENDER: **M** | ADDRESS: **92 LOG ST.** | WEIGHT: **155** | BMI: **25**

AGE: **69** | DX: **ANGINA, COPD, OA** | ALLERGY: **PCN** | HX: **SMOKER FOR 30 YEARS**

MEDICATION	SIG.	PRESCRIBER	ORIG. DATE	REFILL DATE	REFILL DATE	REFILL DATE	REFILL DATE
Vicodin #100	1 q 6 h prn pain	Blouin	6/24	7/1			
Imdur 30 mg #30	1 qd	Blouin	4/21	5/19	6/20	7/15	
Proventil HFA Inhaler 6.7 g	ud	Blouin	4/21	5/19	6/20	7/15	

Dr. Marc Blouin
325 St. Marie St., Manchester, NH 64789
343-555-7999

Name Jerry Smith Date 7/20

Address 92 Log St. Age 69

℞

Atrovent Spray

Sig: 2 puffs qid

~~after~~ Maxair

Refills 2

Dr. Marc Blouin

12.12a

Dr. Marc Blouin
325 St. Marie St., Manchester, NH 64789
343-555-7999

Name Jerry Smith Date 7/20

Address 92 Log St. Age 69

℞

Maxair auto-Inhaler

ii puffs qid

#1

Refills 2

Dr. Marc Blouin

12.12b

12.13

PT. NAME: **TERRY KELLER**	GENDER: **F**	ADDRESS: **9 EAGLE RUN**	WEIGHT: **192**	HEIGHT: **6′**
AGE: **64**	DX: **ANGINA, ASTHMA AND COPD, TYPE 2 DM**	ALLERGY: **NKA**	HX: **FORMER SMOKER AND ETOH**	

MEDICATION	SIG.	PRESCRIBER	ORIG. DATE	REFILL DATE	REFILL DATE	REFILL DATE	REFILL DATE
Biaxin 500 mg #20	I bid	Johns	2/4				
NTG 0.4 mg #C	ud prn cp	Johns	1/12	2/8			
DiaBeta 5 mg #C	I bid	Johns	1/3				
Guaifenesin Cough Syrup 4 oz	2 tsp prn cough	OTC	2/1				

Dr. Donna Johns
7000 SW 1st Ave., Santa Fe, NM 54545
766-555-9097

Name Terry Keller Date 2/12

Address 9 Eagle Run Age 64

℞

Proventil MDI
ii sprays Q6° prn
#one

Refills 3

Dr. Donna Johns

12.13a

Dr. Donna Johns
7000 SW 1st Ave., Santa Fe, NM 54545
766-555-9097

Name Terry Keller Date 2/12

Address 9 Eagle Run Age 64

℞

Pulmicort Inhaler
ii Inh. BID
#1

Refills 3

Dr. Donna Johns

12.13b

12.14

PT. NAME: **ANN RILEY**	GENDER: **F**	ADDRESS: **145 NORTH AVE.**	WEIGHT: **148**	BMI: **21**
AGE: **64**	DX: **OPEN-ANGLE GLAUCOMA, COPD, NERVES, HIGH LDL**	ALLERGY: **IODINE, ASA**	HX: **SMOKER MOST OF HER LIFE**	

MEDICATION	SIG.	PRESCRIBER	ORIG. DATE	REFILL DATE	REFILL DATE	REFILL DATE	REFILL DATE
Singulair 10 mg #50	1 qd	Keller	4/12	9/30			
Ativan 0.5 mg #50	ud	Keller	3/10	4/30	7/20		
Zocor 10 mg #90	1 qd	Keller	1/10	4/8	7/10		
Timoptic 0.5% 15 mL	1 gtt ou bid	Sanders	8/8				
Benadryl 25 mg #24	1 prn cold	OTC	8/15	10/9			

Dr. Daniel Keller
5007 Turtle Drive, Miami, FL 98887
247-555-9876

Name Ann Riley Date 10/12

Address 145 North Ave. Age 64

℞

Atrovent
2 puff qid
#1

Refills 1

Dr. Daniel Keller

12.14a

Dr. Daniel Keller
5007 Turtle Drive, Miami, FL 98887
247-555-9876

Name Ann Riley Date 10/12

Address 145 North Ave. Age 64

℞

Albuterol
2 puffs q4h
2 units.

Refills 1

Dr. Daniel Keller

12.14b

12.15

PT. NAME: **JESSICA WILLIAMS**	GENDER: **F**	ADDRESS: **61 GREEN ST.**	WEIGHT: **145**	HEIGHT: **5′ 4″**
AGE: **70**	DX: **COPD, HTN, NASAL ALLERGY**	ALLERGY: **NKA**	HX: **SMOKER, ETOH**	

MEDICATION	SIG.	PRESCRIBER	ORIG. DATE	REFILL DATE	REFILL DATE	REFILL DATE	REFILL DATE
Symbicort 80/4.5 #120	Use bid	Zoeller	4/4	5/1	6/2		
Lozol 2.5 mg #30	1 q am	Zoeller	2/25	3/19	4/21	5/18	6/20

Dr. Marilyn Zoeller
45 Alabama Place, Detroit, MI 64789
343-555-7771

Name Jessica Williams Date 7/1

Address 61 Green St. Age 70

℞

Proventil puffer
2 puffs TID ↑ puffer

Aerochamber
Use as directed.

Refills 1

Dr. Marilyn Zoeller

12.15a

Dr. Marilyn Zoeller
45 Alabama Place, Detroit, MI 64789
343-555-7771

Name Jessica Williams Date 7/1

Address 61 Green St. Age 70

℞

Zyrtec 10mg
#30
i qd

Refills PRN

Dr. Marilyn Zoeller

12.15b

12.16

PT. NAME: **BEN SMITH** GENDER: **M** ADDRESS: **3906 LEE PARKWAY** WEIGHT: **159** BMI: **22**

AGE: **42** DX: **COPD, INFECTION, ANXIETY, DIARRHEA** ALLERGY: **NKA** HX: **SMOKER SINCE GRADE SCHOOL**

MEDICATION	SIG.	PRESCRIBER	ORIG. DATE	REFILL DATE	REFILL DATE	REFILL DATE	REFILL DATE
Theophylline Elixir 1 pt	15 mL tid for cough	Xavier	4/1	4/15			
Ativan 0.5 mg #30	1 bid prn	Xavier	2/13	3/15			
Pepto Bismol Suspension 16 oz	2 tbs (30 mL) q 2 h	OTC	3/6	3/20	4/12	4/17	

Dr. Mathew Xavier
5456 Southern Trail, Santa Fe, NM 54545
766-555-6600

Name Ben Smith Date 4/20

Address 3906 Lee Parkway Age 42

℞

Advair 250/50
i Inh BID
#1

Refills 0

Dr. Mathew Xavier

12.16a

Dr. Harry Nelson
222 Southern Trail, Santa Fe, NM 54545
766-555-3434

Name Ben Smith Date 4/19

Address 3906 Lee Parkway Age 42

℞

Flagyl 250 g
i po TID
#50

NR

Dr. Harry Nelson

12.16b

12.17

PT. NAME: **AL HAUSMAN** GENDER: **M** ADDRESS: **30 N TRACY ST.** WEIGHT: **166** HEIGHT: **5′ 10″**
AGE: **68** DX: **COPD, ANGINA, GERD, BPH, HTN, NASAL ALLERGY, ANXIETY** ALLERGY: **ASA, SULFA** HX: **SMOKES ½ PACK/DAY**

MEDICATION	SIG.	PRESCRIBER	ORIG. DATE	REFILL DATE	REFILL DATE	REFILL DATE	REFILL DATE
Aciphex 20 mg #30	1 q am	Colby	11/7	12/8			
HCTZ 12.5 mg #30	1 q am	Colby	4/25	6/30	9/15	11/30	12/15
NTG 0.4 mg #25	1 sl prn	Colby	4/25	6/30	9/15	10/1	12/15
Doxazosin 2 mg #30	1 qd 8 pm	Bloom	5/30	6/29	7/20	8/15	11/30
Lorazepam 1 mg #90	1 bid prn	Colby	4/25	6/30	9/15	11/30	
Norvasc 5 mg #30	1 q am	Colby	4/25	6/30	9/15	11/30	12/15

Dr. Tim Colby
7787 University Ave, Des Moines, IA 50311
474-555-7761

Name Al Hausman Date 12/29

Address 30 N. Tracy St. Age 68

℞

① Combivent inhaler 2 puffs QID

② flonase nasal spray 1 puff QD

③ theophylline 300 mg PO BID

☐ Label

Refill 1 2 (3) 4 PRN NR

Dr. Tim Colby

12.17a

Dr. Tim Colby
7787 University Ave, Des Moines, IA 50311
474-555-7761

Name Al Hausman Date 12/29

Address 30 N. Tracy St. Age 68

℞

#100

Ativan 1 mg

Sig 1 Tab BID prn

for nerves

Refill NR times

Dr. Tim Colby

12.17b

12.18

PT. NAME: **ALLISON KREB** AGE: **45** GENDER: **F** DX: **COPD, URI** ADDRESS: **12 SKY CIRCLE DR.** ALLERGY: **PCN** WEIGHT: **166** HX: **SMOKER FOR 10 YEARS (1 PACK/DAY)** BMI: **31**

MEDICATION	SIG.	PRESCRIBER	ORIG. DATE	REFILL DATE	REFILL DATE	REFILL DATE	REFILL DATE
Xopenex Sol. 0.63 mg/3 mL #48	Use ud in SAN	Ortega	8/19				
Cromolyn Sod. Sol. 20 mg/2 mL #240	Use ud in SAN	Ortega	4/12	6/18	8/15		
Atrovent HFA Inhaler 12.9 g	Use tid	Ortega	5/1	6/3	7/8	8/1	

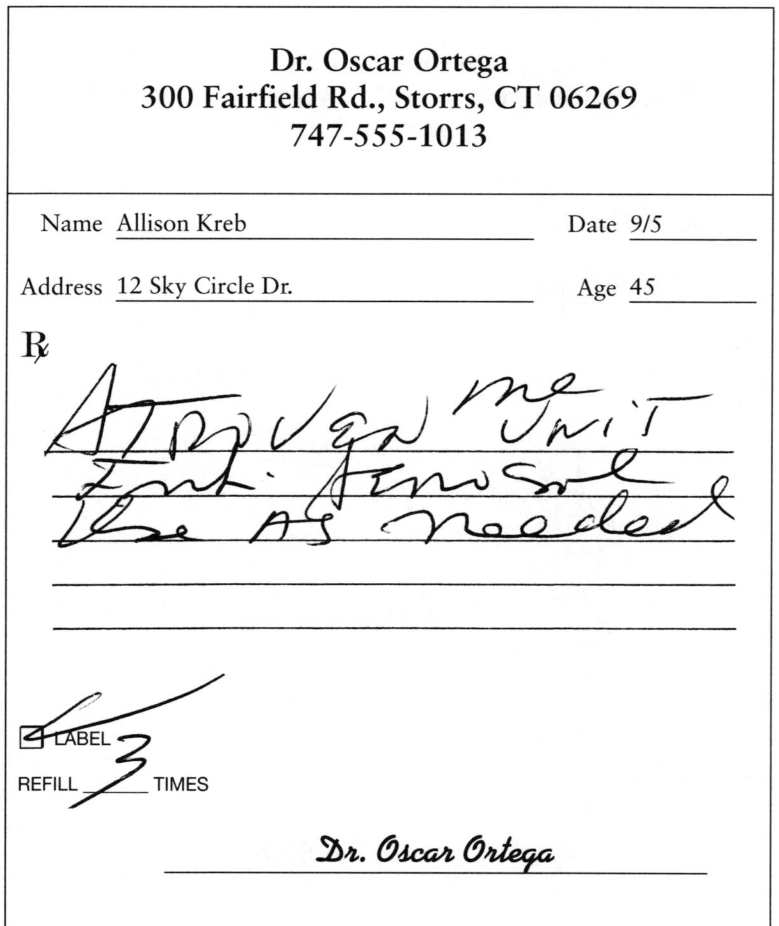

Dr. Oscar Ortega
300 Fairfield Rd., Storrs, CT 06269
747-555-1013

Name Allison Kreb Date 9/5

Address 12 Sky Circle Dr. Age 45

℞

Atrovent Unit
Inh. Aerosol
Use As needed

☑ LABEL

REFILL 3 TIMES

Dr. Oscar Ortega

12.18a

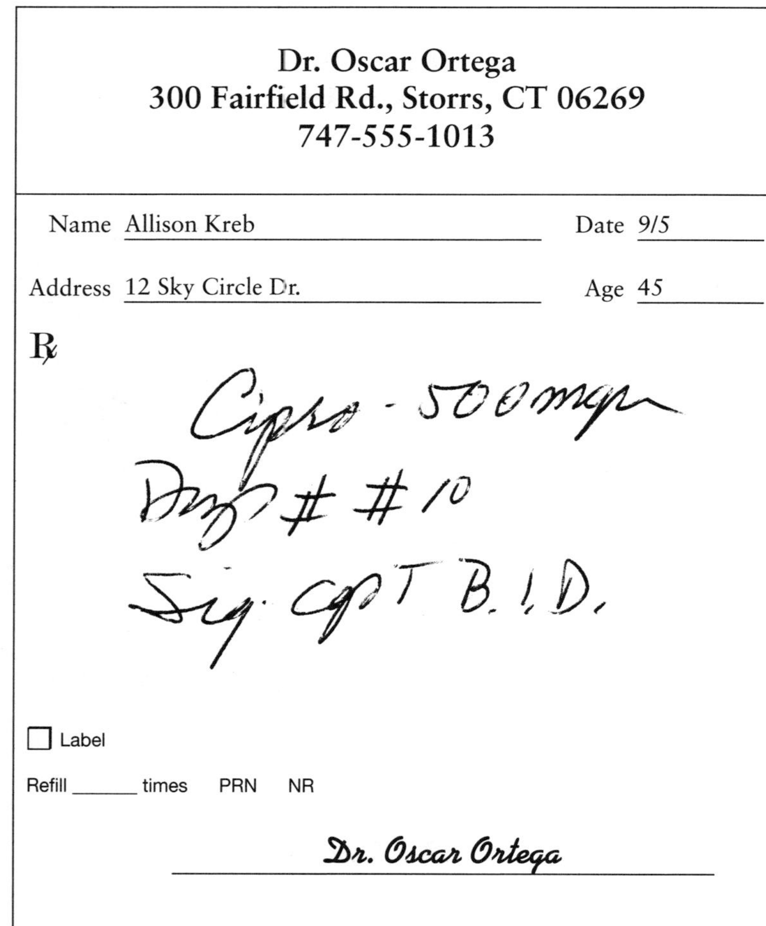

Dr. Oscar Ortega
300 Fairfield Rd., Storrs, CT 06269
747-555-1013

Name Allison Kreb Date 9/5

Address 12 Sky Circle Dr. Age 45

℞

Cipro - 500mg
Disp # #10
Sig: cap T B.I.D.

☐ Label

Refill _____ times PRN NR

Dr. Oscar Ortega

12.18b

12.19

PT. NAME: **JANET ABRAMS**	GENDER: **F**	ADDRESS: **7 NW 2ND AVE.**	WEIGHT: **136**	BMI: **20**
AGE: **50**	DX: **COPD, INSOMNIA, DEPRESSION, COUGH**	ALLERGY: **ASA**	HX: **YEARS OF SMOKING, SOCIAL DRINKER**	

MEDICATION	SIG.	PRESCRIBER	ORIG. DATE	REFILL DATE	REFILL DATE	REFILL DATE	REFILL DATE
Desyrel 50 mg #50	1 hs for sleep	Lilly	8/1	9/10	10/21		
Lunesta 2 mg #30	1 hs for sleep	Lilly	11/19				

Dr. Harold Lilly
188 South Ave, Fargo, ND 58105
885-555-2921

Name Janet Abrams Date 11/30

Address 7 N.W. 2 Ave. Age 50

℞

Proventil HFA

2 puffs QID

☐ Label

Refill ______ times (PRN) NR

Dr. Harold Lilly

12.19a

Dr. Harold Lilly
188 South Ave, Fargo, ND 58105
885-555-2921

Name Janet Abrams Date 11/30

Address 7 N.W. 2 Ave. Age 50

℞

Tussionex
120z

T BID
for cough

☒ Label

Refill ______ times PRN NR

Dr. Harold Lilly

12.19b

12.20 PT. NAME: **SAM BLUE** AGE: **73** GENDER: **M** DX: **HIGH CHOLESTEROL, NASAL ALLERGY, COPD, GERD, HTN** ADDRESS: **31 BATH AVE.** ALLERGY: **PCN, ASA** WEIGHT: **153** HX: **30-YEAR SMOKER, 1½ PACKS/DAY** BMI: **26**

MEDICATION	SIG.	PRESCRIBER	ORIG. DATE	REFILL DATE	REFILL DATE	REFILL DATE	REFILL DATE
Lisinopril 10 mg #30	1 q am	Hanson	2/8	3/22	5/31	6/30	8/1
KCl 10 mEq tabs #30	1 q am	Hanson	1/9	4/6	7/3		
HCTZ 25 mg tabs #30	1 q am	Hanson	1/9	2/8	4/12	7/30	
Nexium 20 mg #30	1 q am	Best	1/20	2/19	3/4	4/8	7/12
Nasonex Spray 17 g	2 sprays per nostril qd	Hanson	6/8	8/12			
Lipitor 10 mg #30	1 q pm	Hanson	6/12	6/30	7/29		

Dr. Eric Hanson
290 Calhoun St., Charleston, SC 29424
792-555-3220

Name Sam Blue Date 9/1

Address 31 Bath Ave. Age 73

℞

Advair 250/50
Sig i P.O. Bid
Disp #1

LABEL

REFILL 6 TIMES

☐ NON-REPETATUR

Dr. Eric Hanson

12.20a

Dr. Eric Hanson
290 Calhoun St., Charleston, SC 29424
792-555-3220

Name Sam Blue Date 9/1

Address 31 Bath Ave. Age 73

℞

theo 24 200 #100
Sig i q d

Refills 3

Dr. Eric Hanson

12.20b

12.21

PT. NAME: **NORMAN BRANDWEIN** GENDER: **M** ADDRESS: **101 CREEK DR.** WEIGHT: **188** BMI: **27**
AGE: **62** DX: **COPD, TYPE 2 DM, HIGH BLOOD LIPIDS, ALLERGIC RHINITIS** ALLERGY: **CIPRO** HX: **FAMILY HX OF TYPE 2 DM**

MEDICATION	SIG.	PRESCRIBER	ORIG. DATE	REFILL DATE	REFILL DATE	REFILL DATE	REFILL DATE
NovoLog Mix 70/30 3 mL cartridges #5	Use ud	Chalmers	4/13	6/19	10/13	12/20	
Zestril 5 mg #30	1 qd	Provost	3/16	4/18	5/20	6/16	
Zestril 5 mg #90	1 qd	Provost	7/5	10/18			
Crestor 10 mg #30	1 qd	Provost	8/22	9/18	10/19	11/22	12/18
Glucovance 5/500 mg #30	1 bid	Chalmers	2/3	3/9	4/6		
Glucovance 5/500 mg #120	1 bid	Chalmers	5/8	7/9	9/8	10/3	11/28

Dr. Marc Provost
300 Huntington Ave, Boston, MA 02115
373-555-8830

Name Norman Brandwein Date 12/22

Address 101 Creek Dr. Age 62

℞

asmanex 220

#30

use bid

Refills PRN

Dr. Marc Provost

12.21a

Dr. Marc Provost
300 Huntington Ave, Boston, MA 02115
373-555-8830

Name Norman Brandwein Date 12/22

Address 101 Creek Dr. Age 62

℞

atrovent .03% #1

2 spray each

side of nose 2X bid

☐ LABEL

REFILL 3 TIMES PRN NR

Dr. Marc Provost

12.21b

12.22

PT. NAME: **ANDREA JENSEN** GENDER: **F** ADDRESS: **32 POINT DR.** WEIGHT: **140** HEIGHT: **5′ 3″**

AGE: **58** DX: **ASTHMA, HYPOTHYROID, ANGINA, HTN, UI, COPD** ALLERGY: **PCN, ASA, CODEINE** HX: **SMOKER FOR 25 YEARS**

MEDICATION	SIG.	PRESCRIBER	ORIG. DATE	REFILL DATE	REFILL DATE	REFILL DATE	REFILL DATE
Pulmicort Respules 0.25 mg/2 mL #30	Use bid via jet nebulizer	Sharp	3/6				
Synthroid 50 mcg #30	1 am, 1 hr ac bkfst	Sharp	1/20	2/18	3/19		
Nitro-Bid Oint. 2% 60 g	Apply 0.5 inch q 6 h ud	Sharp	1/15	3/12			
Toprol XL 50 mg #30	1/2 tab q am	Sharp	2/20	3/19			
NTG 0.4 mg #25	1 sl prn angina	Sharp	1/15				
Cozaar 50 mg #30	1 q am	Sharp	1/12	2/13	3/11		
Vesicare 5 mg #30	1 q pm	Bloom	1/31	2/28	3/19		

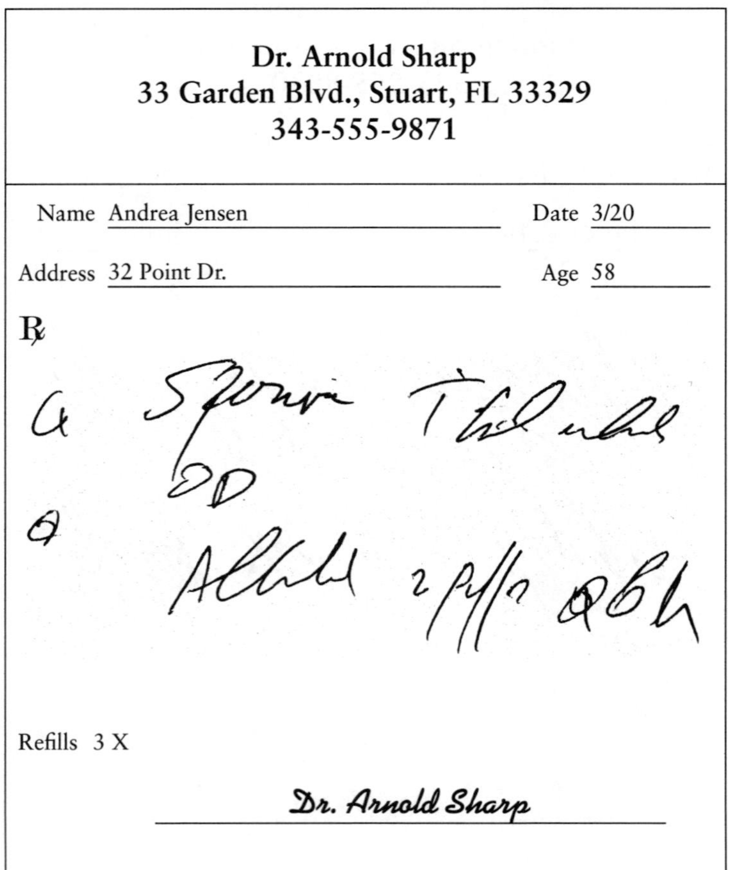

Dr. Arnold Sharp
33 Garden Blvd., Stuart, FL 33329
343-555-9871

Name Andrea Jensen Date 3/20

Address 32 Point Dr. Age 58

℞

Refills 3 X

Dr. Arnold Sharp

12.22a

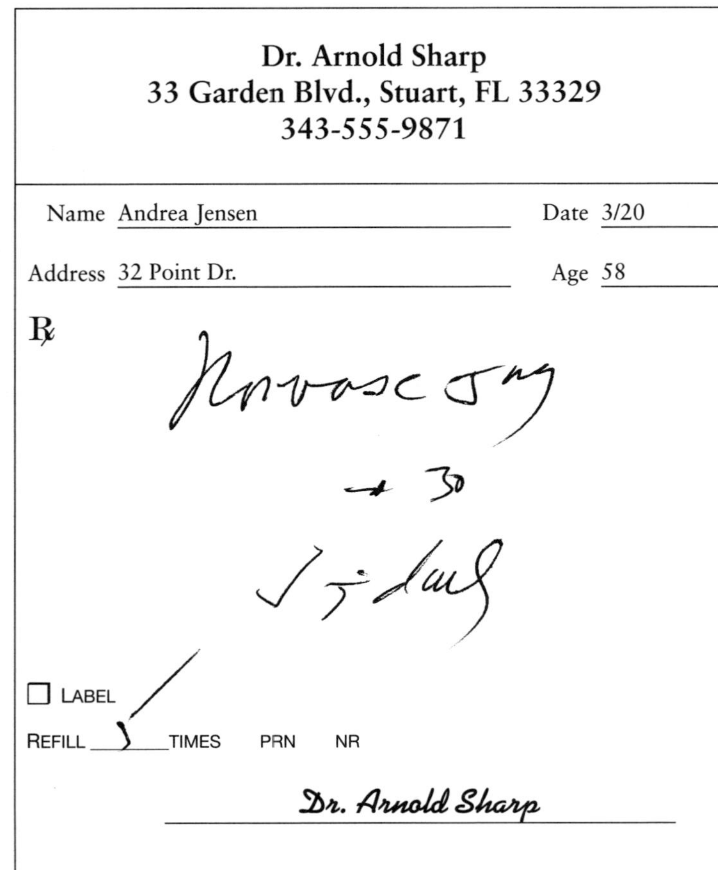

Dr. Arnold Sharp
33 Garden Blvd., Stuart, FL 33329
343-555-9871

Name Andrea Jensen Date 3/20

Address 32 Point Dr. Age 58

℞

☐ LABEL

REFILL ____ TIMES PRN NR

Dr. Arnold Sharp

12.22b

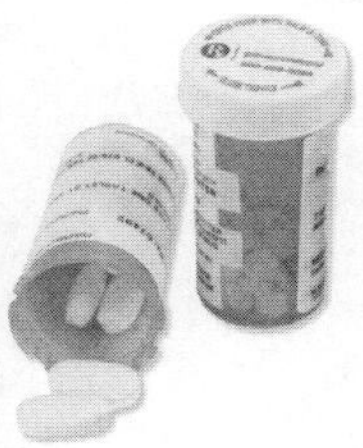

13 • OPHTHALMICS

UPON COMPLETION OF THIS CHAPTER, THE STUDENT WILL BE ABLE TO:

- describe the normal anatomy and physiology of the eye, with particular emphasis on the formation, purpose, and outflow of the aqueous humor.
- describe the differences between open-angle, narrow-angle, and normotensive glaucoma.
- describe the mechanisms of action of the commonly used agents that are used to treat glaucoma by decreasing intraocular pressure.
- advise patients on the correct administration of eye products (both liquids and ointments). This should include methods to decrease systemic absorption of ophthalmic liquids by using light finger pressure on the lacrimal sac for 1 minute following instillation to decrease drainage through the nasolacrimal duct.
- explain the mechanisms of adverse effects caused by eye preparations such as beta-blockers.
- list some precautionary methods to use when applying eye preparations to decrease the potential for spreading infection to the other eye or to others.
- counsel patients on available OTC ophthalmic products and know when to refer a client to an eye physician.
- counsel the patient who uses an ophthalmic suspension, noting the auxiliary label and the appropriate method of agitating the product.

DRUG LIST

Alphagan-P
AzaSite
Betagan/Betoptic/Timoptic/OptiPranolol
Ciloxan Ophthalmic Solution
Erythromycin Ophthalmic Ointment
Neptazane/Diamox
Nevanac
Ocuflox Ophthalmic Solution
Patanol/Pataday
Phospholine Iodide
Pilocarpine
Restasis
Sulfacetamide Ophthalmic
Tobrex/TobraDex
Trusopt/Cosopt/Azopt
Voltaren Ophthalmic Solution/Acular/Acular LS
Xalatan/Lumigan/Travatan Z/Latisse

• DRUG HOT POINTS

Alphagan-P
α_2-agonist: increases outflow & decreases production of aqueous humor (↓ IOP)

AzaSite
Azithromycin 1% Ophthalmic solution
Treats bacterial conjunctivitis

Betagan
Nonselective beta-blocker
Contraindicated in COPD

Betoptic
β_1-selective beta-blocker
Less likely than nonselective agents to cause bronchospasm
Also suspension: Betoptic-S

Ciloxan Ophthalmic Solution
Antibiotic: inhibits bacterial DNA gyrase
Indicated for treatment of superficial ocular infections involving the cornea or conjunctiva caused by strains of microbes susceptible to antibiotics
Wash hands before and after use
Compare with Ocuflox

Neptazane (methazolamide)
Inhibits production of aqueous humor by inhibiting carbonic anhydrase
Compare with Diamox (acetazolamide)

Patanol
Inhibits histamine release from mast cells
Selective H_1 antagonist
Compare with Pataday

Phospholine Iodide
Indirect-acting cholinergic agonist
Needs to be mixed before dispensing

Pilocarpine
Increases outflow by contraction of the ciliary muscle and pupil, which opens the trabecular meshwork—this facilitates drainage
Adverse effects: brow ache, diarrhea, difficulty driving at night
Dosed BID, TID, or QID
Pilopine HS 4% gel for HS use

Restasis
Cyclosporine: immunosuppressive (immunomodulator)
Reduces ocular inflammation
Increases tear production when caused by ocular inflammation

Sulfacetamide Ophthalmic
Caution: sulfa allergies
Wash hands before and after use
Compare with Erythromycin

Timoptic
Nonselective: contraindicated in COPD
Dosed QD or BID
Counsel patient on OTCs that may have anticholinergic side effects (antihistamines, cough syrups, sleep aid products, etc.)
24-hour formulation: Timoptic XE (shake before using)
Compare with OptiPranolol

TobraDex
Anti-inflammatory plus antimicrobial
Wash hands before and after use

Tobrex
Aminoglycoside
Do not use beyond prescribed date
Wash hands before and after use

Trusopt
Inhibits production of aqueous humor by inhibiting carbonic anhydrase
Also in combination with timolol (Cosopt)
Compare with Azopt, which may have less stinging on administration

Voltaren Ophthalmic Solution
NSAID
Inhibits COX, decreases inflammation
Indicated use: treatment of postoperative inflammation following cataract extraction
Some burning and stinging upon instillation
Compare with Acular and Acular LS
Compare with Nevanac

Xalatan
Prostaglandin analog (PGA)
Increases outflow through uveoscleral route
One drop a day dose
Color change of iris
Refrigerate
Less potential for systemic adverse effects than beta-blockers
Compare with Lumigan and Travatan Z
Compare with Latisse

• QUESTIONS TO BE ANSWERED IN PREPARATION FOR CHAPTER 13 LAB

- Describe the similarities and differences between open-angle and narrow-angle glaucoma.
- Explain the mechanism of action of Xalatan in the treatment of glaucoma.
- What is the dosing regimen for latanoprost ophthalmic drops?
- What is the meaning of the letter "Z" in Travatan Z?
- Describe the specific mechanism of action of Neptazane in the treatment of glaucoma.
- How do Trusopt drops help in the treatment of glaucoma?
- Describe the technique and purpose of nasolacrimal occlusion (NLO).
- A person is taking bronchodilator therapy. He has recently been diagnosed with open-angle glaucoma and he presents a new prescription for timolol ophthalmic drops. Describe the potentially harmful effect that may occur and which beta-1 selective beta-blocker ophthalmic preparation would be more appropriate.
- If timolol ophthalmic drops are administered without NLO, explain how an unsafe drop in pulse and blood pressure is a risk if the patient also takes metoprolol tablets by mouth.
- Which glaucoma eye drop is a β_1-selective beta-blocker?
- Describe the mechanism of action of pilocarpine, mentioning the specific part of the eye that is involved in its action, and also identify the autonomic receptors involved.
- Your client uses pilocarpine eye drops and complains of brow ache. How would you identify the cause of this problem?
- Explain the reason for the occasional diarrhea that occurs during the use of pilocarpine ophthalmic preparations.
- What is the percentage of pilocarpine in Pilopine HS gel?
- What is the usual dosing regimen of Neptazane?
- Explain the mechanism whereby an OTC "cold pill" may precipitate blindness in a person using an ophthalmic preparation for the control of increased IOP from narrow-angle glaucoma.
- What is the mechanism of action of Phospholine Iodide?
- Describe the mechanism of action of Alphagan-P.
- How long should a person wait between applications of different ophthalmic preparations in the treatment of glaucoma?
- Explain the reason for the contraindication of the topical ophthalmic use of an anticholinergic agent, such as atropine sulfate, in a person with narrow-angle glaucoma.
- Describe the proper method for using eye preparations.
- Show the flow of aqueous humor from its formation point through the eye and its drainage through the trabecular meshwork and the canal of Schlemm.
- What are the indicated uses for the two ingredients contained in TobraDex?
- Nevanac is a pro-drug. Explain its action as an NSAID and how it reduces pain and inflammation associated with cataract surgery.
- Why is it necessary to invert the unit dose vial a few times before using Restasis?
- AzaSite is indicated to treat bacterial conjunctivitis. Which organisms are susceptible to it?
- What is the indication for Latisse?

• OPHTHALMOLOGY MEDICATION THERAPY MANAGEMENT QUESTIONS AND COMMENTS

- Welcome to our pharmacy. I see that this is your first visit. You have a prescription for a medication that treats glaucoma or increased pressure in the eye. Would you like to review all of your medications with us? It would be a valuable experience for you to have information about all of your medications. We would contact your physicians, request copies of your labs, and obtain a current list of all of your prescriptions for the last year as well as your nonprescription products, or OTCs. This would also include products that appear not to be drugs, such as herbal products; however, many of them do have effects on your other medications.
- The importance of OTCs is that a form of glaucoma (narrow-angle) requires that the patient avoid many types of drugs, prescription or not. Examples are Sudafed (pseudoephedrine), Benadryl (diphenhydramine), and many other combination products for allergy, sleep, and pain/sleep products.
- Your eye doctor has prescribed a medication called timolol eye drops. This is a medication in drop form to be applied to the eye twice a day. We are looking at your active medication profile, or history of all your active drugs. You also take another product for high blood pressure called metoprolol. It is important that we contact both or all of your doctors and do an in-depth analysis or review of your drug history. Part of this consultation would be for us to check your pulse and blood pressure. Our medication therapy management service goes beyond the normal community pharmacy interaction. At this time, however, I would like to call both of your doctors to clear up an important point. Both the new eye drop and your current blood pressure pill belong to the same class of medication; that is, they are both beta-blockers. There are choices that need to be made by both doctors. If you must stay on the blood pressure pill, then we must have an important conversation with the eye doctor. If the timolol drops are the only ones that are medically necessary for you, then the application of the drops becomes very important. There is a technique known as nasolacrimal occlusion (NLO) that should be used for all eye drops. First, wash your hands, apply the eye drops, close the eyelids, and apply light pressure with one finger to the area in the corner of the eye, just at the bridge of the nose. Hold it for 1 minute to prevent the medication from draining out of the eye into the nasal membranes. If that were to occur, the medication would not be fully effective in the eye, and the draining of the medication would allow it to be absorbed into the bloodstream through the nasal membranes. At that point, the effects of both the eye drop and the blood pressure medication would add together and potentially cause a serious drop in blood pressure.
- Alternatively, the eye doctor might choose to order an alternate medication such as Xalatan or latanoprost. This glaucoma drop has no effect on metoprolol's action.
- Although your eye doctor has ordered four medications for your eyes, they all are important. Would you like to meet for a short medication therapy management session, in person or by phone, to discuss the importance of each medication? By knowing how your medications work and how they help each other to work, it is more likely that you will use them in the appropriate manner.
- Knowledge of the mechanism of action of medications is a powerful tool for patients. By meeting with our clinical pharmacist once a year for a routine medication review and for any additional medications, this will refresh your knowledge of your condition and how the medications work.
- Your new prescription appears to be used for cataract surgery that is scheduled in a few days. Did you inform your eye doctor that you are also taking another medication from another physician called Flomax or tamsulosin? If not, let's use the phone, or send an e-mail or text message to his or her office and wait for him or her to contact us. Flomax is the capsule that you take to increase the flow of urine. You have been using it because of a condition called benign prostatic hyperplasia or BPH. This is commonly called enlarged prostate with urinary obstruction.
- Unfortunately, when a person taking this type of medication has cataract surgery, the eye surgery becomes complicated.

• OPHTHALMOLOGY MEDICATION THERAPY MANAGEMENT QUESTIONS AND COMMENTS (*continued*)

- If Flomax is not stopped many days before cataract surgery, the iris of the eye would not be able to be dilated properly for the surgery. Let's call the eye doctor to discuss this and recommend that the Flomax be temporarily stopped well in advance of the eye surgery.
- Thanks for agreeing to join in with our program called medication therapy management. Part of our service is to do an in-depth analysis of each medication. We compare your medications from each prescriber. Then we search for problems where one medication might interfere with another. Commonly, we discover that one of your medical problems might be adversely affected by a medication written by a different prescriber who might not be aware of your total medical history.
- An example is the one that we are facing today with your new prescription from your eye doctor. Betagan, or levobunolol drops, was prescribed for your eye pressure called glaucoma. Levobunolol is called a nonselective beta-blocker. I notice that you have been seeing another doctor who has prescribed a product called Advair as well as a rescue inhaler called albuterol. These medications are useful for patients with breathing disorders such as asthma, along with other conditions: emphysema or chronic bronchitis (sometimes, the letters COPD are used to describe these last two conditions). Sometimes, Spiriva or Atrovent is used.
- In this case, levobunolol drops are contraindicated. They may have access to the bloodstream through the nasolacrimal duct.
- The eye drops have high risk of causing the lungs to constrict and make breathing difficult for patients with breathing disorders. We must call your eye doctor to recommend a switch to a different eye product such as Xalatan, Lumigan, or Travatan Z. They would have no adverse effect on your breathing condition.
- I notice that your prescription for an eye antibiotic drop has the instructions checked on a box that indicates the following: "os." That means the left eye. I can see that you have a dressing on your right eye. Please verify that the eye to be treated is the right eye in order for us to contact the prescriber to clarify the order. This is one of the reasons why it is important for us to see and talk with our patients before we fill any medical order or prescription.
- Since we have been doing our medication therapy management sessions, it has become clear that when we sit with you to talk, your eyes appear irritated and watery tears are dripping. These tears are not normal tears. Your eyes are basically dry. This causes irritation to the tissues and the eyes experience a form of watery tearing.
- Upon examining your medication history, it appears that some of your medications have effects called anticholinergic, or drying effects. Would you mind if I contact your doctors to explain the problem and offer suggestions for alternate medications that would have less or none of these anticholinergic effects while accomplishing the same therapeutic action? This service is an important part of medication therapy management.

13.1

PT. NAME: **KURT THOMAS** AGE: **68** GENDER: **M** DX: **BPH, GLAUCOMA, HTN** ADDRESS: **522 BLOSSOM DR.** ALLERGY: **DAIRY PRODUCTS, ERYTHROMYCIN** WEIGHT: **152** HX: **RETIRED PHARMACIST; REQUESTS SPECIAL DISCOUNTED PRICE** HEIGHT: **5′ 8″**

MEDICATION	SIG.	PRESCRIBER	ORIG. DATE	REFILL DATE	REFILL DATE	REFILL DATE	REFILL DATE
Uroxatral 10 mg #30	I hs	Nash	6/1	7/3			
HCTZ 12.5 mg #30	I am	Carver	2/3	3/2	4/10	5/18	6/24

Dr. David Keene
77 Cape May Drive, Marlboro, NJ 98876
247-555-6664

Name Kurt Thomas Date 7/17

Address 522 Blossom Dr. Age 68

℞

oph Sol: Trusopt 2%
Sig i gtt OU Tid

Refills 4

Dr. David Keene

13.1a

Dr. David Keene
77 Cape May Drive, Marlboro, NJ 98876
247-555-6664

Name Kurt Thomas Date 7/17

Address 522 Blossom Dr. Age 68

℞

oph Tab:
Neptazane 50mg
Sig i tab P.O.
bid c meals #78

Refills 4

Dr. David Keene

13.1b

13.2

PT. NAME: **JILL JOHNSON** | GENDER: **F** | ADDRESS: **333 DREXEL AVE.** | WEIGHT: **132** | BMI: **24**

AGE: **64** | DX: **GLAUCOMA, HTN, COPD, ASTHMA, NERVES, INSOMNIA, UI** | ALLERGY: **PCN** | HX: **WAITRESS, SMOKER, ETOH**

MEDICATION	SIG.	PRESCRIBER	ORIG. DATE	REFILL DATE	REFILL DATE	REFILL DATE	REFILL DATE
HCTZ 25 mg #L	I qod	Thomas	2/12	5/18			
Minitran 0.2 mg/hr #30	Apply qd ud	Thomas	2/12	3/15	4/9	5/7	6/7
Theophylline SR 200 mg #180	I bid	Sauls	4/12				
Atrovent HFA Inhaler 12.9 g	I spray prn SOB	Sauls	4/12				
Singulair 10 mg #50	I q hs	Sauls	4/12				

Dr. Bascom Palmer
44 Los Feliz Blvd., Los Angeles, CA 55888
705-555-7777

Name Jill Johnson Date 6/9

Address 333 Drexel Ave. Age 64

℞ Timoptic [illegible] 0.25%
Disp [illegible]
S [illegible] gtt OS BID

LABEL ALL MEDICATIONS

RENEW 3

DEA NO. ____________

SUBSTITUTION PERMITTED ____________

Dr. B. Palmer

13.2a

Dr. Joseph Rey
88 Rodney Drive, Los Angeles, CA 55888
705-555-4444

Name Jill Johnson Date 6/8

Address 333 Drexel Ave. Age 64

℞ Amitriptylline 25mg
#30
i P.O. QHS

Dr. Joseph Rey

13.2b

13.3	PT. NAME: **KATHERINE HARVEY**	GENDER: **F**	ADDRESS: **71 CAPITOL AVE.**	WEIGHT: **130**	BMI: **22**
	AGE: **72**	DX: **COPD, HTN, INCREASED IOP**	ALLERGY: **PCN**	HX: **LIVES IN AN ALF**	

MEDICATION	SIG.	PRESCRIBER	ORIG. DATE	REFILL DATE	REFILL DATE	REFILL DATE	REFILL DATE
Theophylline SR 300 mg #180	I bid	Jones	4/12				
Advair 250/50 Diskus #60	I puff bid	Jones	4/12	7/20			
Prednisone 5 mg #90	I q am	Jones	4/12	4/30			
HCTZ 25 mg #90	I q am	Smith	2/12	5/20			

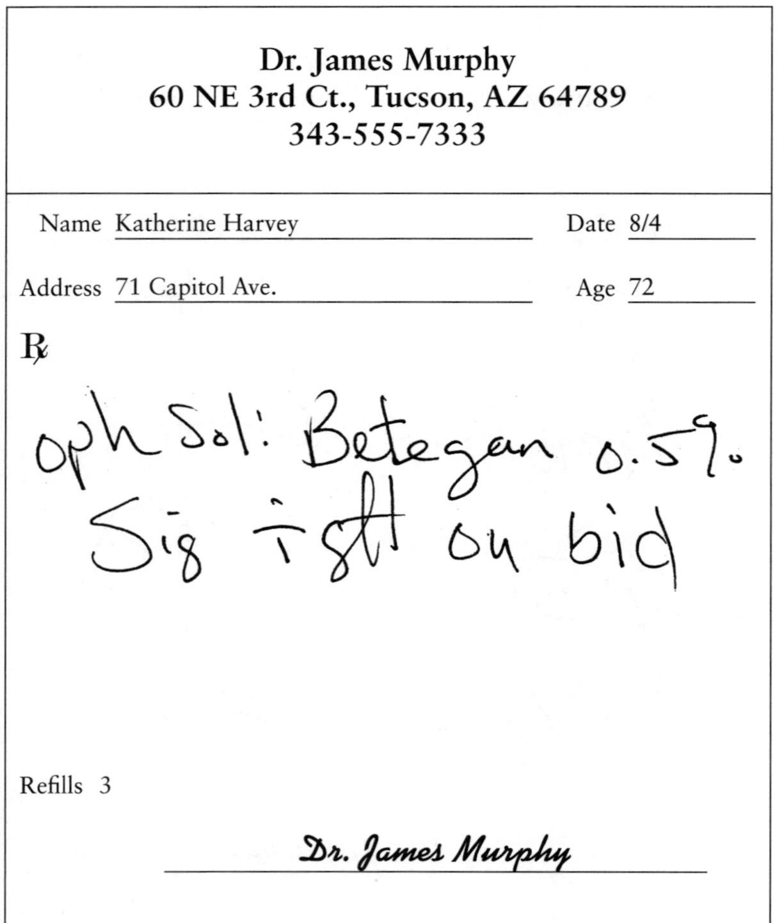

Dr. James Murphy
60 NE 3rd Ct., Tucson, AZ 64789
343-555-7333

Name Katherine Harvey Date 8/4

Address 71 Capitol Ave. Age 72

℞

oph Sol: Betegan 0.5%
Sig i gtt ou bid

Refills 3

Dr. James Murphy

13.3a

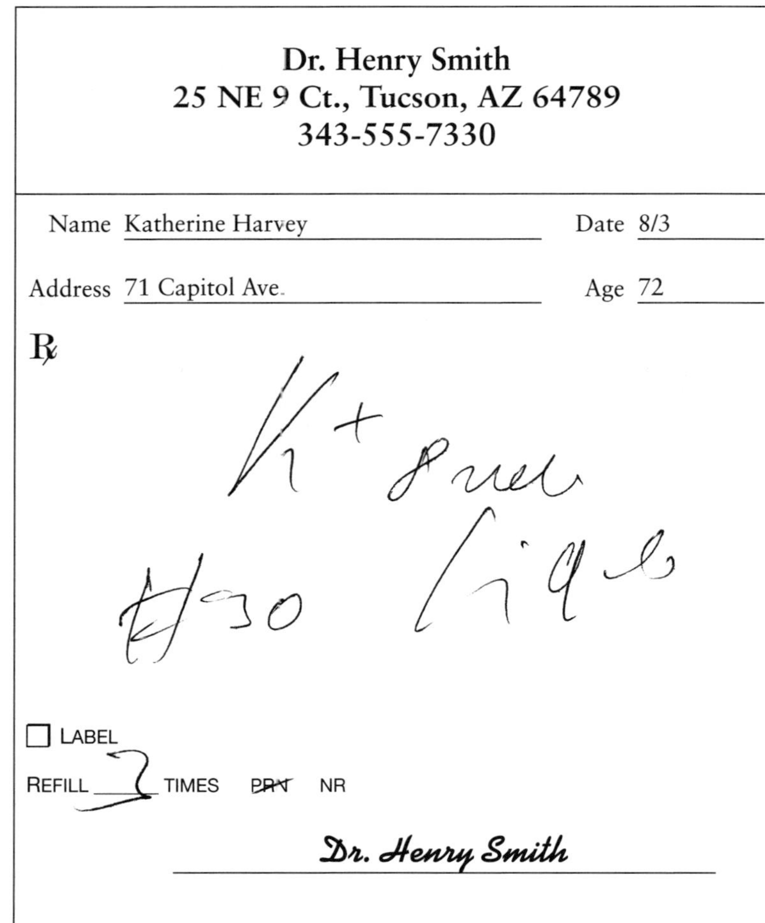

Dr. Henry Smith
25 NE 9 Ct., Tucson, AZ 64789
343-555-7330

Name Katherine Harvey Date 8/3

Address 71 Capitol Ave. Age 72

℞

K+ 8 meq
#30 Sig i qd

☐ LABEL

REFILL 2 TIMES ~~PRN~~ NR

Dr. Henry Smith

13.3b

13.4

PT. NAME: **JEAN EDWARDS** GENDER: **F** ADDRESS: **555 STIRLING RD.** WEIGHT: **188** HEIGHT: **5′ 4″**
AGE: **62** DX: **GLAUCOMA, HTN, CHF, OA PAIN, SINUS PAIN** ALLERGY: **NKA** HX: **ETOH, BARTENDER-WAITRESS**

MEDICATION	SIG.	PRESCRIBER	ORIG. DATE	REFILL DATE	REFILL DATE	REFILL DATE	REFILL DATE
Aldactone 25 mg #28	I qd pc bkfst	Robins	9/6	9/29			
Furosemide 20 mg #30	I qd	Robins	9/6	9/29			
Ultracet 37.5/325 mg #60	I prn pain bid	Robins	4/12	8/15			
Sudafed 30 mg #24	I tid for sinus	OTC	2/2	4/9	8/30	9/28	

Dr. Gloria Crawfords
599 Nova Drive, Fort Lauderdale, FL 44718
463-555-1388

Name Jean Edwards Date 10/2

Address 555 Stirling Rd. Age 62

℞

Oph pilo 4%
Sig gtt i OD qid

REFILL ✓ PRN
_____ TIMES

LABEL ✓ YES
_____ NO

Dr. Gloria Crawfords

13.4a

Dr. Ned Gray
30 Nova Drive, Fort Lauderdale, FL 44718
463-555-8100

Name Jean Edwards Date 10/3

Address 555 Stirling Rd. Age 62

℞

Percocet 5/325
i po PRN pain
Q6H #30

N.R.

Dr. Ned Gray

DEA # BG 1234563

13.4b

13.5

PT. NAME: **JIM LEWIS**	GENDER: **M**	ADDRESS: **224 SE 6TH ST.**	WEIGHT: **140**	BMI: **21**
AGE: **78**	DX: **GLAUCOMA, BPH, HTN, CONSTIPATION**	ALLERGY: **NKA**	HX: **NURSING HOME RESIDENT**	

MEDICATION	SIG.	PRESCRIBER	ORIG. DATE	REFILL DATE	REFILL DATE	REFILL DATE	REFILL DATE
Restoril 15 mg #30	I hs prn sleep	Weiss	6/7				
Diovan HCT 80/12.5 mg #30	I qd	Weiss	4/2	5/I	6/I		
Surfak 240 mg #C	I hs for BM	Weiss	4/2				
Cardura I mg #60	I hs	Weiss	5/30				

Dr. Lydia Krypol
55 Center Ave., Des Moines, IA 55055
705-444-2233

Name Jim Lewis Date 6/12

Address 224 SE 6th St. Age 78

℞

Oph Sol: Cosopt
Sig T gtt ou bid

Refills 4

Dr. Lydia Krypol

13.5a

Dr. Lydia Krypol
55 Center Ave., Des Moines, IA 55055
705-444-2233

Name Jim Lewis Date 6/12

Address 224 SE 6th St. Age 78

℞

Oph Sol:
Xalatan .005%
Sig T gtt ou qhs

Refills 4

Dr. Lydia Krypol

13.5b

13.6

PT. NAME: **BETTY SMITH** GENDER: **F** ADDRESS: **2 TANNER ST.** WEIGHT: **138** BMI: **27**
AGE: **62** DX: **HTN, ANGINA, GLAUCOMA** ALLERGY: **PCN** HX: **CNA FOR ELDERLY PEOPLE**

MEDICATION	SIG.	PRESCRIBER	ORIG. DATE	REFILL DATE	REFILL DATE	REFILL DATE	REFILL DATE
BuSpar 10 mg #30	1 qd	Popovich	9/29	10/30			
Procardia XL 30 mg #30	1 qd	Pray	7/10	8/9	9/10	10/20	
Pilocarpine 1% Opht. gtt 15 mL	1 gtt ou qid	Newtons	4/12	6/15	8/12	10/11	

Dr. Gail Newtons
133 Heine St. NW, West Lafayette, IN 33999
505-777-4443

Name Betty Smith Date 11/7

Address 2 Tanner St. Age 62

℞
Xalatan .005% oph sol
sig 1gtt QHS OU
2.5ml

NOT VALID FOR CONTROLLED SUBSTANCES

Refills prn

Dr. Gail Newtons

13.6a

Dr. Don Perry
400 Blue Drive, West Lafayette, IN 33999
505-777-2100

Name Betty Smith Date 11/7

Address 2 Tanner St. Age 62

℞
Norvasc 5m #60
i PO
/

Refills 1x

Dr. Don Perry

13.6b

13.7 PT. NAME: **JOAN GREEN** AGE: **68** GENDER: **F** DX: **GLAUCOMA, HTN, TYPE 2 DM, ANXIETY, VERTIGO, OA** ADDRESS: **654 SEAGULL CT.** ALLERGY: **NKA** WEIGHT: **136** BMI: **22**

MEDICATION	SIG.	PRESCRIBER	ORIG. DATE	REFILL DATE	REFILL DATE	REFILL DATE	REFILL DATE
Chlorthalidone 25 mg #90	I qd	Robins	7/31	11/27			
Glyburide 5 mg #60	I daily	Robins	6/5	7/31	9/29	11/27	
Naproxen 500 mg #30	I bid	Robins	4/13				
Meclizine 25 mg #30	I tid × 3d, I bid × 3d, I qd	Robins	6/5	6/14	8/30		

Dr. Calvin Robins
7823 Tea Rose Trail, Miami, FL 44718
463-555-8000

Name Joan Green Date 12/1

Address 654 Seagull Ct. Age 68

℞

Timoptic 1/2 %
#i Bottle
Sig: i gtt ou BID

Refills 4

Dr. Calvin Robins

13.7a

Dr. Tom Fay
200 Blake St., Miami, FL 44718
463-555-2199

Name Joan Green Date 12/1

Address 654 Seagull Ct. Age 68

℞

Xanax 1 mg
#30
S. tab i a Dentist

☐ LABEL

REFILL 1X TIMES PRN NR

Dr. Tom Fay

DEA # BF 1234563

13.7b

13.8 PT. NAME: **MARK BLACK** AGE: **73** GENDER: **M** DX: **CHOLESTEROL, GERD, GLAUCOMA, UTI** ADDRESS: **854 S LILLY BLVD.** ALLERGY: **NKA (NKDA)** WEIGHT: **142** HX: **SMOKER FOR MORE THAN 50 YEARS** BMI: **30**

MEDICATION	SIG.	PRESCRIBER	ORIG. DATE	REFILL DATE	REFILL DATE	REFILL DATE	REFILL DATE
Pravachol 20 mg #30	I qd	Green	6/12	7/12	8/9	9/25	
Timoptic 0.5% 15 mL	I gtt ou bid	Manning	7/3	8/9			
Prilosec 20 mg #60	I bid	Green	4/4	5/25	7/10	9/1	10/2
Tylenol PM #C	I hs	OTC	1/10	4/8	8/30		

Dr. Nicole Popovich
38 University Drive, West Lafayette, IN 66444
813-555-7554

Name Mark Black Date 10/3

Address 854 S Lilly Blvd. Age 73

℞

Betoptic S
i gtt ou BID
mitte 1 vial

Refills 2

Dr. Nicole Popovich

13.8a

Dr. Ray Frankel
20 Manning St., West Lafayette, IN 66444
813-555-0021

Name Mark Black Date 10/4

Address 854 S Lilly Blvd. Age 73

℞

NKDA

Bactrim DS po BID
20.

☐ Do Not Refill
☒ Refill 1 Times

Dr. Ray Frankel

13.8b

13.9

PT. NAME: **ALAN JOHNSON**	GENDER: **M**	ADDRESS: **53 IRIS BLVD.**	WEIGHT: **159**	HEIGHT: **5′ 8″**
AGE: **72**	DX: **CHOLESTEROL, HTN, TYPE 2 DM, CHF, GLAUCOMA**	ALLERGY: **PCN**	HX: **SMOKER (50 PACK-YEARS)**	

MEDICATION	SIG.	PRESCRIBER	ORIG. DATE	REFILL DATE	REFILL DATE	REFILL DATE	REFILL DATE
Lomotil #30	1–2 tid prn	Smith	4/8				
Vasotec 10 mg #60	1 am & 1 pm	Smith	6/26	7/31			
DiaBeta 2.5 mg #120	2 bid	Davis	5/21	6/25			
Westcort Ointment 60 g	apply to face bid	Jackson	7/22				
Lanoxin 0.25 mg #60	1 qd ud	Smith	4/9	5/22	6/26	7/6	

Dr. Doug Griffin
7611 147th Terrace, Monterey, CA 38411
705-555-6644

Name Alan Johnson Date 8/9

Address 53 Iris Blvd. Age 72

℞

☒ Alphagan-P % Eye Drops ____ ml
Sig: 1 Drop to OU eye(s) BID

☐ ____ Pills/Capsules # ____
Sig: ____ by Mouth ____

☐ ____ Eye Ointment ____ tube(s)
Sig: Use ____ eye(s) ____

Label

Refill 6 x

Dr. Doug Griffin

13.9a

Dr. Doug Griffin
7611 147th Terrace, Monterey, CA 38411
705-555-6644

Name Alan Johnson Date 8/9

Address 53 Iris Blvd. Age 72

℞

oph Sol: Levobunolol 0.5%
Sig i gtt OU bid

NON REP.
REFILL 1 2 3 (4)

Dr. Doug Griffin

13.9b

13.10

PT. NAME: **DENISE LEWIS** GENDER: **F** ADDRESS: **684 HURRICANE ALLEY** WEIGHT: **229** BMI: **33**
AGE: **74** DX: **HTN, GLAUCOMA, HYPOTHYROID, ANGINA, VERTIGO, COLD SYMPTOMS** ALLERGY: **NKA** HX: **OBESE SINCE CHILDHOOD**

MEDICATION	SIG.	PRESCRIBER	ORIG. DATE	REFILL DATE	REFILL DATE	REFILL DATE	REFILL DATE
Synthroid 0.05 mg #30	1 qd	Davis	5/2	5/23	6/22	7/31	
Nitro Patch 0.1 mg/hr #30	apply qd as directed	Davis	6/22	7/20	8/22		
BuSpar 5 mg #30	1 bid	Davis	8/29				
Nyquil Liquid 6 oz	2 tbs for cold	OTC	8/1				
Dramamine Original Formula #12	1 prn dizziness	OTC	7/30				

Dr. Alfred Sauls
151212 S High Rd., Chicago, IL 23875
954-555-1300

Name Denise Lewis Date 8/30

Address 684 Hurricane Alley Age 74

℞

alphagan P 0.15
15 ml bottle
i gtt ou bid

Refill 3 Times

Dr. Alfred Sauls

13.10a

Dr. Alfred Sauls
151212 S High Rd., Chicago, IL 23875
954-555-1300

Name Denise Lewis Date 8/30

Address 684 Hurricane Alley Age 74

℞

Cosopt
i gtt ou bid
30 d supply

Refill 3 Times

Dr. Alfred Sauls

13.10b

13.11

PT. NAME: **GLADYS BAKER** GENDER: **F** ADDRESS: **184 GREEN ST.** WEIGHT: **120** BMI: **24**
AGE: **77** DX: **HTN, NARROW-ANGLE GLAUCOMA, ANGINA, TIA, CONSTIPATION** ALLERGY: **NKA** HX: **ETOH**

MEDICATION	SIG.	PRESCRIBER	ORIG. DATE	REFILL DATE	REFILL DATE	REFILL DATE	REFILL DATE
Pilocarpine 1% Oph. Sol. 15 mL	I gtt od tid	Howard	4/3	5/10			
HCTZ 25 mg #C	I qod	Weiss	2/3				
Procardia XL 30 mg #90	I q am	Weiss	2/3	5/10			
Nitroglycerin SL 0.4 mg #C	I sl chest pain	Weiss	2/3				
Atropine Sulf. 1% Oph. Sol. 5 mL	I gtt od tid	Howard	5/1				
Colace 100 mg #60	I bid prn	OTC	5/9	6/2	7/4	8/3	

Dr. Mervin Howard
9 Sheridan St., Austin, TX 90902
874-555-9888

Name Gladys Baker Date 8/5

Address 184 Green St. Age 77

℞

Trusopt Ophthal Soln: 2%

Disp: 10 mL

Sig: i gtt OD TID

Refills ad lib rep

Dr. Mervin Howard

13.11a

Dr. Jay Weiss
33 Grant St., Austin, TX 90902
874-555-3300

Name Gladys Baker Date 8/5

Address 184 Green St. Age 77

℞

① Aggrenox 200/25
i po qd
30

② Toprol XL 50 mg
i po qd
30

Refills 3x ea

Dr. Jay Weiss

13.11b

13.12 PT. NAME: **ANDREW PHILLIPS** AGE: **82** GENDER: **M** DX: **GLAUCOMA, CHF, ANEMIA (ELEVATED MCV)** ADDRESS: **774 FANTASTIC ST.** ALLERGY: **PCN** WEIGHT: **140** BMI: **22**

MEDICATION	SIG.	PRESCRIBER	ORIG. DATE	REFILL DATE	REFILL DATE	REFILL DATE	REFILL DATE
Lanoxin 0.125 mg #30	1 qd	Weiss	4/6				
Aldactone 25 mg #30	1 qd	Weiss	4/6				
Lasix 20 mg #30	1 qd	Weiss	4/6				
Folic acid 1 mg #60	1 qd	Weiss	4/6				

Dr. Calvin Robins
7823 Tea Rose Trail, Miami, FL 44718
463-555-8000

Name Andrew Phillips Date 4/30

Address 774 Fantastic St. Age 82

℞

Azopt ophth Sol
10mL
sig ī gtt OU BID

Refills prn

Dr. Calvin Robins

13.12a

Dr. Calvin Robins
7823 Tea Rose Trail, Miami, FL 44718
463-555-8000

Name Andrew Phillips Date 4/30

Address 774 Fantastic St. Age 82

℞

OptiPranolol™ 0.3%
Sig: ī gtt BID OD OS (OU)

Refills prn

Dr. Calvin Robins

13.12b

13.13

PT. NAME: **JACK DAVIS** GENDER: **M** ADDRESS: **5132 GIRAFFE DR.** WEIGHT: **146** HEIGHT: **5′ 5″**
AGE: **78** DX: **HTN, ASTHMA, GLAUCOMA, BACTERIAL CONJUNCTIVITIS** ALLERGY: **NKA**

MEDICATION	SIG.	PRESCRIBER	ORIG. DATE	REFILL DATE	REFILL DATE	REFILL DATE	REFILL DATE
Singulair 10 mg #90	1 qd	Clint	4/18				
Dyazide #60	1 qd	Clint	3/12	5/9	7/5		
Verapamil 80 mg #270	1 tid	Clint	3/12	6/6			
Prednisone 5 mg #90	1 q am	Clint	2/15	5/20			
Proventil HFA 6.7 g	Use prn SOB	Clint	4/18	5/20	6/25		

Dr. Erin Thomas
988 North Ridge, New York, NY 88364
813-555-7554

Name Jack Davis Date 7/5

Address 5132 Giraffe Dr. Age 78

℞

Betoptic .5% gtts
Disp: 2-5cc bottles
Sig: use as directed

Refills prn

Dr. Erin Thomas

13.13a

Dr. Erin Thomas
988 North Ridge, New York, NY 88364
813-555-7554

Name Jack Davis Date 7/5

Address 5132 Giraffe Dr. Age 78

℞

Bleph 10 ophth sol
1 gtt tid OU

Refills NR

Dr. Erin Thomas

13.13b

13.14

PT. NAME: **DANIEL JAMES**	GENDER: **M**	ADDRESS: **1558 DEXTER AVE.**	WEIGHT: **184**	HEIGHT: **6′ 2″**	BMI: **32**
AGE: **32**	DX: **IRRITATED EYES, BACTERIAL CONJUNCTIVITIS**	ALLERGY: **DAIRY PRODUCTS, ERYTHROMYCIN, SULFA, PCN**			

MEDICATION	SIG.	PRESCRIBER	ORIG. DATE	REFILL DATE	REFILL DATE	REFILL DATE	REFILL DATE
Centrum Tablets #200	qd	OTC	3/2	6/8			
Visine A.C. Eye drops 15 mL	1 drop tid for eyes	OTC	5/1	6/7	7/22		
Lactaid Fast Act Chewable tabs #32	2 tab with dairy food	OTC	3/6	4/22	5/29	6/18	7/30

Dr. Mathew Xavier
5456 Southern Trail, Santa Fe, NM 54545
766-555-6600

Name Daniel James Date 8/30

Address 1558 Dexter Ave. Age 32

℞

Tobradex

Ophth ointment

Apply as dir daily

Refills 0

Dr. Mathew Xavier

13.14a

Dr. Mathew Xavier
5456 Southern Trail, Santa Fe, NM 54545
766-555-6600

Name Daniel James Date 8/30

Address 1558 Dexter Ave. Age 32

℞

OCUFLOX EYE SOL

1 gtt O.S QID

Refills 0

Dr. Mathew Xavier

13.14b

13.15

PT. NAME: **BEN SMITH** AGE: **64** GENDER: **M** DX: **ANGINA, HTN, GLAUCOMA, OA BACK PAIN, CONJUNCTIVITIS** ADDRESS: **71 CAPITOL AVE.** ALLERGY: **NKA** WEIGHT: **130** HX: **CARPENTER** BMI: **24**

MEDICATION	SIG.	PRESCRIBER	ORIG. DATE	REFILL DATE	REFILL DATE	REFILL DATE	REFILL DATE
ISMO 20 mg #60	1 bid	Thomas	4/10	5/8	6/3		
HCTZ 25 mg #15	1/2 tab qd	Thomas	4/10	5/8	6/9		
Naproxen 375 mg #60	1 q 12 h for joint pain	Thomas	2/12	3/5	4/8	5/10	
Phospholine Iodide 0.125% 5 mL	1 gtt os q 12 h	Zoeller	6/10				

Dr. Marilyn Zoeller
45 Alabama Place, Detroit, MI 64789
343-555-7771

Name Ben Smith Date 7/1

Address 71 Capitol Ave. Age 64

℞

Timoptic XE 0.5%
Bottle 1 10 mL
Gtts i os qam

LABEL
REFILL 3

Dr. Marilyn Zoeller

13.15a

Dr. Marilyn Zoeller
45 Alabama Place, Detroit, MI 64789
343-555-7771

Name Ben Smith Date 7/1

Address 71 Capitol Ave. Age 64

℞

Ciloxan e/t sol
1 gtt o.u. qid
x 6 days

Refills no

Dr. Marilyn Zoeller

13.15b

13.16

PT. NAME: **CHRISTOPHER BLAKE**	GENDER: **M**	ADDRESS: **575 REDWOOD WAY**	WEIGHT: **185**	HEIGHT: **6′**
AGE: **44**	DX: **BACTERIAL CONJUNCTIVITIS, GLAUCOMA, NASAL ALLERGY, FOOT FUNGUS**	ALLERGY: **SULFA**	HX: **SMOKER (15 PACK-YEARS)**	

MEDICATION	SIG.	PRESCRIBER	ORIG. DATE	REFILL DATE	REFILL DATE	REFILL DATE	REFILL DATE
Allegra Allergy 24 hr tabs #30	1 qd	OTC	3/8	4/12			
Mycolog Cream 15 g	Apply to aa qid prn	Johns	1/28				

Dr. Bernardo Olinisky
7000 SW 1st Ave., Santa Fe, NM 54545
766-555-9097

Name Christopher Blake Date 4/15

Address 575 Redwood Way Age 44

℞

Blephamide ointment
Disp 1 tube

Sig: Apply to [crossed-out word] inner surface right lower lid morning & night

Refills 4

Dr. Bernardo Olinisky

13.16a

Dr. Bernardo Olinisky
7000 SW 1st Ave., Santa Fe, NM 54545
766-555-9097

Name Christopher Blake Date 4/15

Address 575 Redwood Way Age 44

℞

☐ Betagan 0.50%	☐ Flarex	☐ Tobrex
☐ Betagan 0.25%	☐ F.M.L.	☐ TobraDex
☐ Betoptic S 0.25%	☐ F.M.L. Forte	☐ Ciloxan
☐ Timoptic 0.50%	☐ Pred Forte	☐ Gentacidin
☐ Timoptic 0.25%	☐ Econopred 1%	☐ Polytrim
☐ Optipranolol	☐ FML S	☐ Achromycin
☐ Propine 0.1%	☐ Vasocidin	☐ Polysporin
☐ Isopto Carpine ____%	☐ Vasosulf	☐ Vasocon A
☒ Pilocar 1 %	☐ Isopto Cetamide	☐ Naphcon A
☐ Neptazane ____mg	☐ Cetapred	☐ Zovirax 200 mg
☐ Diamox ____mg	☐ Viroptic 1%	
☐ Phospholine Iodide ____%	☐ ________	

DISP: Eye Drops: 5 ml (10 ml) 15 ml 30 ml

SIG: Gtts 1 in: (O.D.); ____ O.S.; ____ O.U.

QD BID (TID) QID QHS

RF ________ Times

Dr. Bernardo Olinisky

13.16b

13.17 PT. NAME: **JOHN BRYAN** AGE: **69** GENDER: **M** DX: **GLAUCOMA, GERD, PARKINSON'S DISEASE, HTN, ANGINA, SEBORRHEIC DERMATITIS** ADDRESS: **34 JACKSON ST.** ALLERGY: **NKA** WEIGHT: **152** BMI: **22**

MEDICATION	SIG.	PRESCRIBER	ORIG. DATE	REFILL DATE	REFILL DATE	REFILL DATE	REFILL DATE
Carbidopa/Levodopa 25/100 #30	1 bid	Chaplin	2/5	2/26	3/30		
Nexium 40 mg #30	1 q am	Kelly	1/28	2/25	3/27		
Torsemide 10 mg #30	1 q am	Chaplin	1/12	2/10	3/11		
NTG 0.4 mg SL #C	1 sl ud	Chaplin	1/12				
Maalox Suspension 12 oz	prn	OTC	1/3	1/29	2/18	3/26	
Omeprazole 20 mg #14	1 bid	OTC	2/5	3/12			
Senokot-S tabs #60	1 prn constipation	OTC	1/5	3/12			
Nizoral A-D 4 oz	Apply 3 × a week	OTC	1/5	3/12			

Dr. Gary Reiss
3 NE 12 Ave, Cherry Hill, NJ 80555
220-555-9871

Name John Bryan Date 4/14

Address 34 Jackson St. Age 69

℞

Travatan Z
i gtt ou qhs
mitte 1 vial

☐ MEDICALLY NECESSARY
LABEL CONTENTS
REFILL 1 - 2 - 3 - NR - PRN (circled: PRN)

Dr. Gary Reiss

13.17a

Dr. Gary Reiss
3 NE 12 Ave, Cherry Hill, NJ 80555
220-555-9871

Name John Bryan Date 4/14

Address 34 Jackson St. Age 69

℞

TRUSOPT
i gtt OS BID
mitte 1 vial

☐ Label

Refill ______ times PRN (circled) NR

Dr. Gary Reiss

13.17b

13.18

PT. NAME: **KELLY LANE** GENDER: **F** ADDRESS: **99 SW 5 ST.** WEIGHT: **154** HEIGHT: **5′ 2″**
AGE: **59** DX: **DEPRESSION, GLAUCOMA, INSOMNIA, SEVERE BACK PAIN** ALLERGY: **NKA** HX: **SMOKES, DRINKS, GAMBLES**

MEDICATION	SIG.	PRESCRIBER	ORIG. DATE	REFILL DATE	REFILL DATE	REFILL DATE	REFILL DATE	REFILL DATE	REFILL DATE
Wellbutrin XL 150 mg #30	1 q am × 3d, then 2 q am	Sachs	9/30						
Wellbutrin XL 300 mg #30	1 q am	Sachs	10/10	11/7	12/9				
Citalopram 20 mg #30	1 q am	Sachs	6/22	7/20	8/28	9/27	10/22	11/15	12/8
Percocet 5/325 mg #30	1 q 4–6 h prn pain	Dunn	5/5						
Percocet 10/325 mg #30	1 q 4–6 h prn pain	Dunn	5/30						
Temazepam 15 mg #30	1 hs	Sachs	5/5	6/3	7/7	8/4	9/5	10/18	
Alprazolam 0.5 mg #30	1 tid prn nerves	Sachs	4/5	6/6	6/19				

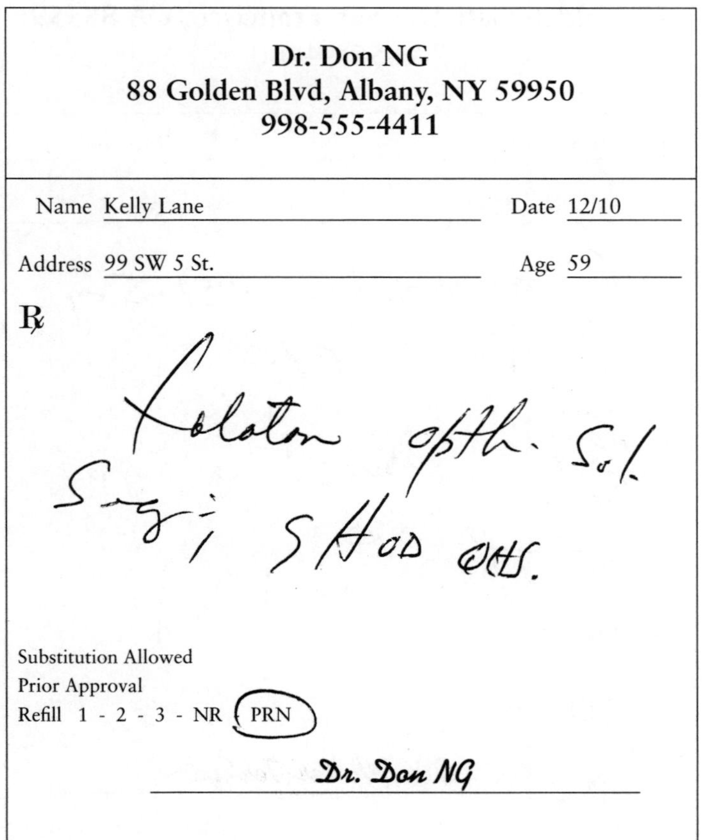
Dr. Don NG
88 Golden Blvd, Albany, NY 59950
998-555-4411

Name Kelly Lane Date 12/10
Address 99 SW 5 St. Age 59

℞
Xalatan opth. Sol.
Sig: i gtt OD qHS.

Substitution Allowed
Prior Approval
Refill 1 - 2 - 3 - NR - (PRN)

Dr. Don NG

13.18a

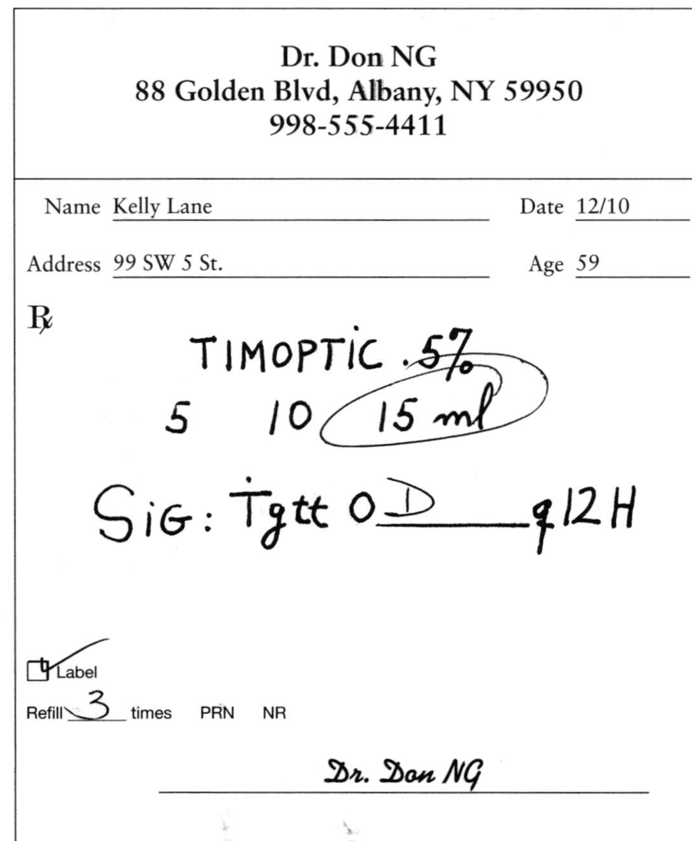
Dr. Don NG
88 Golden Blvd, Albany, NY 59950
998-555-4411

Name Kelly Lane Date 12/10
Address 99 SW 5 St. Age 59

℞
TIMOPTIC .5%
5 10 (15 ml)
Sig: 1gtt OD q12H

☑ Label
Refill 3 times PRN NR

Dr. Don NG

13.18b

13.19

PT. NAME: **SHIRLEY BRAND** | AGE: **65** | GENDER: **F** | DX: **HTN, TYPE 2 DM, HIGH LDL CHOLESTEROL, BACTERIAL EYE INFECTION, HYPOTHYROID** | ADDRESS: **55 MASON ST.** | ALLERGY: **NKA** | WEIGHT: **144** | HX: **GAVE UP SMOKING 5 YEARS AGO, STILL DRINKS** | BMI: **23**

MEDICATION	SIG.	PRESCRIBER	ORIG. DATE	REFILL DATE	REFILL DATE	REFILL DATE	REFILL DATE
Altace 5 mg #30	I q am	Terhyden	1/30	2/27	3/30	4/27	5/28
Glyburide 5 mg #60	I bid	Terhyden	2/27	3/25	4/29	5/30	
Lipitor 10 mg #30	I hs	Terhyden	1/30	2/27	3/30	4/27	5/28
Vitamin D 1000 IU #30	I q am	Terhyden	1/30	2/27	3/30	4/27	5/28

Dr. Lillian Mello
33 Golden Gate Dr., San Francisco, CA 88559
776-555-0505

Name Shirley Brand Date 6/3

Address 55 Mason St. Age 65

℞

Schedule:

Drug Name/Units Qty SIG

Erythromycin ophtalmic ointment apply tid

Allergies

NKDA

Special Instructions:

Refills 0

Dr. Lillian Mello

13.19a

Dr. Walter Terhyden
40 Golden Gate Dr., San Francisco, CA 88559
776-555-4400

Name Shirley Brand Date 6/3

Address 55 Mason St. Age 65

℞ (1) Maxzide 37.5/25mg i qd #30

(2) Synthroid 0.1mg qd #30

☐ No Safety Closure
DEA#
Label
Refill 0 1 2 (3) 4

Dr. Walter Terhyden

13.19b

13.20

PT. NAME: **GABE MILLER** AGE: **63**
GENDER: **M**
DX: **GLAUCOMA, HTN, PUD, DEPRESSION, SINUS CONGESTION**
ADDRESS: **87 COOPER ST.**
ALLERGY: **NKA**
WEIGHT: **177**
HX: **SMOKER (30 PACK-YEARS), DRINKS ETOH**
HEIGHT: **5′ 9″**

MEDICATION	SIG.	PRESCRIBER	ORIG. DATE	REFILL DATE	REFILL DATE	REFILL DATE	REFILL DATE
Pepcid 20 mg #60	1 tab bid	Kimble	8/8	9/4	10/5	11/6	
Lexapro 10 mg #30	1 q am	Kimble	9/4	10/5	11/2		
Furosemide 20 mg #30	1 q am	Kimble	7/7	8/3	9/4	10/15	
Sudafed PE 10 mg Nasal Decongestant tabs #72	1 prn sinus congestion	OTC	6/8	7/1	8/22	9/12	11/3

Dr. Marie Spellman
4946 Marvin Drive, Nutley, NJ 87878
898-555-9811

Name Gabe Miller Date 11/8

Address 87 Cooper St. Age 63

℞

Lumigan
i ou q hs

Substitution Allowed
Prior Approval
Refill 1 - 2 - 3 - NR - (PRN)

Dr. Marie Spellman

13.20a

Dr. Samuel Kimble
1680 Meridian Ave, Nutley, NJ 87878
898-555-1111

Name Gabe Miller Date 11/8

Address 87 Cooper St. Age 63

℞

Corgard 40mg #100
i daily

Refill 5 times

Dr. Samuel Kimble

13.20b

13.21

PT. NAME: **SHARON EVITT** GENDER: **F** ADDRESS: **90 WEST ST.** WEIGHT: **198** HEIGHT: **5′ 11″**
AGE: **68** DX: **GLAUCOMA, TYPE 2 DM, RESPIRATORY INFECTION, NASAL ALLERGY** ALLERGY: **PCN** HX: **RETIRED TEACHER, SMOKER, 20 PACK-YEARS**

MEDICATION	SIG.	PRESCRIBER	ORIG. DATE	REFILL DATE	REFILL DATE	REFILL DATE	REFILL DATE
Cetirizine 10 mg #15	1 qd	Hamilton	2/15	3/1	3/20	4/2	
Metformin 500 mg #60	1 bid	Hamilton	1/20	2/18	3/20	4/19	
Glipizide 5 mg ER #30	1 q am	Hamilton	1/3	2/3	3/2	4/1	5/3
Allegra-D 24 hr tabs #10	1 qd	Hamilton	1/21				
Azithromycin 250 mg pack #6 tabs	Take ud	Hamilton	1/21				

Dr. Howard Pereira
60 South 3000 East, Salt Lake City, UT 84112
440-555-9871

Name Sharon Evitt Date 5/12

Address 90 West St. Age 68

℞

Cosopt #10cc

Sig: i gtt

i ou

BID

Substitution Allowed

Prior Approval

Refill 1 - 2 - (3) - NR - PRN

Dr. Howard Pereira

13.21a

Dr. Howard Pereira
60 South 3000 East, Salt Lake City, UT 84112
440-555-9871

Name Sharon Evitt Date 5/12

Address 90 West St. Age 68

℞

Travatan Z #5cc

Sig: i gtt ou q hs

Substitution Allowed

Prior Approval

Refill 1 - 2 - (3 - NR) - PRN

Dr. Howard Pereira

13.21b

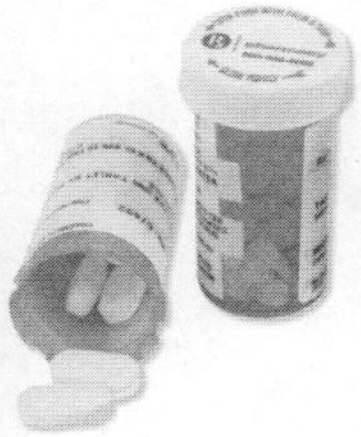

• DIABETES 14

UPON COMPLETION OF THIS CHAPTER,
THE STUDENT WILL BE ABLE TO:

- discuss the importance of taking certain medications at exactly the correct times to make them effective.
- discuss the various types of diabetes and the drug therapy for each.
- compare and contrast each class of agents used in the treatment of diabetes.
- using a person's glycated hemoglobin reading, interpret the 90-day average blood sugar (mg %).
- design a logical plan of action for the person with diabetes to attain consistent "tight" glucose control.
- advise patients on proper syringe selection.
- caution patients regarding food, drug, and vitamin interference with home testing systems.
- counsel patients about the problems inherent in switching insulin brands.
- describe the concept of "sliding scale insulin," using regular or rapid-acting insulin.
- design simple lifestyle changes that would create a better quality of life for the person with diabetes.
- communicate appropriately to the person with diabetes using laymen's terms.
- suggest the "DASH Diet" to lower blood pressure and help glycemic control.

DRUG LIST

Actoplus MET
Amaryl
Avandia/Actos
Byetta/Victoza
Diabinese
Glipizide
Glucophage
Glyburide
Insulin
Januvia/Onglyza/Tradjenta
Metaglip
Prandin/Starlix
Precose/Glyset
Symlin

• DRUG HOT POINTS

Actoplus MET
Combination of ACTOS with metformin

Amaryl
Sulfonylurea agent indicated for use with insulin
Combined use may increase the potential for hypoglycemia
Long acting—once-a-day dose

Avandia/Actos
Activate nuclear receptor (PPAR-γ) resulting in increased insulin sensitivity in target cells; they do not increase insulin secretion
Combined effect with other agents for Type 2 DM
Recommended baseline liver enzyme test, then q 2 months/1 year, then periodically
Cautions: fluid retention, major concerns over CV cautions
Note: Avandia restrictions
Not recommended in patients with symptomatic heart failure

Byetta
Incretin mimetic
Adjunct to diet and exercise to improve glycemic control in adults with Type 2 diabetes mellitus
Subcutaneous injection, BID
Compare with Victoza, QD

Diabinese
Dose: less than 500 mg/day
No alcohol: may cause disulfiram-like syndrome (facial flushing, breathlessness)
May cause SIADH
Longest acting sulfonylurea; unpredictable glycemic control

Glipizide
Glucotrol: regular (IR) & XL (ER)
Second generation—fewer side effects
Take 30 minutes AC
IR absorption is delayed by food
IR maximum daily dose is 40 mg

Glucophage (metformin)
Decreases hepatic glucose production
2550 mg/day: maximum daily dose
Diarrhea—adverse effect (in higher doses)
Renal function, warnings (monitor for lactic acidosis)
Regular and long-acting forms
Glucovance—in combination with glyburide
Metaglip—in combination with Glipizide

Glyburide
Nonantimicrobial sulfonamide structure
DiaBeta, Micronase
Glynase: micronized formulation
Increases beta cell production of insulin & increases target cell insulin sensitivity
May be used together with metformin to produce synergistic effect
Second generation; fewer side effects, more potent than earlier sulfonylureas
All sulfonylureas may produce severe hypoglycemia
Monitor: check symptoms
Remind the patient to eat *prescribed* scheduled meals & snacks

Insulin
Mechanism of action, functions
Compare various types of insulin:
Escherichia coli—Humulin
Baker's yeast—Novolin
Caution: Regular 500 units/mL should be measured with 1 mL TB syringe to avoid incorrect dose
Do not freeze
Order of mixing (if mixing insulin types, measure regular in syringe first)
Do not shake cloudy insulin; roll vial slowly in hands for 5 to 10 slow rolls
Rotate injection sites
Compare insulin "pens" with vials
Refrigerate after opening
Different types of syringes (select size based on prescribed unit amount)
Humalog, NovoLog, Apidra: rapid acting
Lantus and Levemir: long acting
N or NPH (cloudy): intermediate acting
General diabetes counseling (diet, compliance with medicine, low salt, follow meal plan and snacks, see specialists regularly, do A.M. finger stick for fasting blood sugar—record daily results and report to physician or pharmacist, etc.)
Sliding scale insulin—use regular insulin or Humalog/NovoLog
IV insulin: use regular insulin

• DRUG HOT POINTS (continued)

Januvia

Inhibits DPP-IV

Slows inactivation of incretin hormones

Increases insulin synthesis and release from pancreatic beta cells

Lowers glucagon secretion leading to reduced hepatic glucose production

In combination with metformin: Janumet

Compare with Onglyza

Tradjenta: No dose adjustment with renal impairment

Prandin/Starlix

Stimulate insulin release at beta cell by closing K^+ channels, depolarizing the beta cell, which causes Ca^{2+} channels to open, inducing insulin secretion

Starlix has a shorter duration of action, possibly reducing the potential for hypoglycemia

Caution: drug interaction: CYP-450 3A4 inducers (barbiturates, rifampin, carbamazepine) may increase Prandin metabolism, decreasing its effect

CYP-450 inhibitors (itraconazole, fluconazole, erythromycin, clarithromycin, etc.) may inhibit Prandin metabolism, increasing its effect, increasing risk for producing hypoglycemia

Precose

Inhibits alpha-glucosidase & alpha-amylase

Delays digestion of carbohydrates, thereby resulting in a smaller rise in blood glucose following meals; this results in reduced levels of HbA1c in patients with Type 2 DM

Counseling: side effects (gas, pain, diarrhea) caused by undigested carbohydrates in lower GI tract

LFT q 3 m for the first year, periodically thereafter. If elevated transaminases are observed, a reduction in dosage or withdrawal of therapy may be indicated, particularly if the elevations persist

Counseling: take with the first bite of main meals

Watch diet, do mild exercise

Precose prevents the breakdown of table sugar

Glucose, not sucrose or candy, should be available to treat symptoms of low blood sugar

The lowest dose tolerable should be used

Compare with miglitol (Glyset). Similar action and dosing

Symlin

Synthetic amylin analog

Amylin is co-secreted with insulin by pancreatic beta cells in response to food intake

Effects:

- Modulation of gastric emptying
- Prevention of the postprandial rise in plasma glucagon
- Satiety leading to decreased caloric intake and potential weight loss

Adjunctive treatment in Type 1 or Type 2 DM patients who use mealtime insulin therapy and who have failed to achieve desired glucose control despite optimal insulin therapy

Caution: hypoglycemia

• QUESTIONS TO BE ANSWERED IN PREPARATION FOR CHAPTER 14 LAB

- Describe the advantages of the second-generation oral sulfonylurea agents over the first-generation agents.
- What is the mechanism of action of Precose?
- Explain why acarbose commonly causes adverse GI effects.
- Which organisms are used to manufacture recombinant DNA-derived insulin?
- A prescription is presented to you as follows: Diabinese 250 mg QID for an 85-year-old person weighing 120 lb. Would you fill the prescription as written?
- What is the maximum adult daily dose of Glucophage?
- What substance is added to insulin to make NPH insulin longer lasting than regular insulin?
- What is the smallest tablet of metformin in milligrams?
- Which forms of insulin are used for the "sliding scale," or SSI?
- Give an example of a "sliding scale" prescription order.
- If a patient needs 55 units of insulin per dose, which size of insulin syringe should be used: 1, 0.5, or 3/10 cc?
- Explain why Precose should be taken at the "first bite" of food with each meal.
- Define the letters "NPH" when used to refer to insulin.
- What is the maximum recommended adult total daily dose of Micronase in milligrams?
- Name the three mechanisms of action of Glucophage.
- What are the advantages of using Prandin (repaglinide) over the oral sulfonylurea products?
- What is a hidden problem with the use of sorbitol "sugar-free" products?
- Describe the etiology, signs and symptoms, and treatment of diabetic gastroparesis.
- Compare the actions of Symlin and Byetta.
- Describe the mechanism of action of Januvia.
- What would you tell your client about the importance of the prescribed, scheduled afternoon or evening food snack?
- How would you counsel your client about the storage and use of insulin?
- A person who has diabetes requests advice on purchasing a sharp blade to trim the corns and excess calluses on his feet. What would you advise him to do?
- Should Glucotrol IR (immediate release) tablets be taken before, with, or after meals?
- Which sulfonylurea agent is indicated for use with insulin?
- Describe the interaction between the intake of ethanol and chlorpropamide.
- How should a person agitate and disperse the two phases of NPH insulin?
- A person experiences severe itch and rash around the site of injection of NPH insulin. It appears to be an allergic-type reaction. Which insulin would give a longer duration but would be less likely to cause this skin problem?
- Compare the dosing regimens of Lantus and Humalog.
- What are the advantages of combination products such as Glucovance?
- A person with Type 2 diabetes is currently taking glyburide 5 mg BID. He is scheduled to have an afternoon snack at 3 P.M. If he forgets the snack, what adverse effects are likely to occur?
- A person with diabetes requests pseudoephedrine tablets (OTC) for a cold. How would you counsel him or her?
- A person states that he or she takes less oral diabetic medication than the physician prescribed because he or she feels "better" with fewer drugs. How would you counsel him or her?
- What is the brand name of the product that contains pioglitazone and metformin?
- What is an advantage of Victoza over Byetta?
- Describe the cautions for Avandia.

• DIABETES MEDICATION THERAPY MANAGEMENT QUESTIONS AND COMMENTS

- Welcome to our pharmacy. We are here for your first medication therapy management session.
- You have indicated that your doctor wants you to take medication to treat your condition that was identified as diabetes mellitus Type 2. The doctor has written prescriptions for pills and has written orders for you to see an RD. Although the word diabetes is feared by some people, it is an irregularity in a person's metabolism. It really does not fit the description of a disease caused by germs. It is not contagious. It is not anything that you have done wrong. Everyone's body works differently. Yours just needs help in making sugar work the way that it is supposed to work. With monitoring (or checking), medication, lifestyle, and diet, many patients have found that their condition improves. Your day-to-day control of blood sugar should be back to normal as long as you stay on the program. Some pharmacy sessions center on the medications; however, in your case, the way that you adhere to the doctor's overall program will be of most value. Indeed, some of our patients or clients have succeeded over time to reduce the pills or injections to low amounts, and in some cases, to be free of any medications. This will take time, discipline, and collaboration among the members of your team of health care professionals. Here at our pharmacy, we can be an important cornerstone of your total health.
- An important study has shown that patients with diabetes who have worked closely with their pharmacists have had the most success in keeping normal sugar levels and lowering harmful effects of sugar on their bodies. We will begin by discussing the medications that your doctor ordered, how they work, and how to use food and snacks to your advantage along with the medications. Food and snacks are as important as medications. Diabetes medications require exact food planning. The literature that your doctor gave you explains the food choices. Your appointment with the registered dietitian will give you an expert advice to follow. Remember the three elements that will make you successful: food choices, exercises, and medications.
- Monitoring will let you, the doctor, and us know how the program is working. In most cases, adjustments might have to be made to your medications or food choices. We will be available to advise you about blood glucose monitoring. It will give you a daily picture of the progress of your program. Your condition might require adjustments of your medications. As time goes by, we will work with you and your doctor to avoid the damage that would happen to your body without monitoring and treatment.
- Let's get started on our program today, shall we?
- Your doctor has prescribed pills to keep sugar normal in your bloodstream and body. Sometimes one or more medications might be necessary. The main focus is to follow your doctor's medication plan, diet program, and daily exercise program; then, check the sugar in your blood. This is called blood glucose monitoring.
- Because the pills that you will be taking reduce sugar in the blood, your three meals each day along with the prescribed small snacks (sometimes at 3 P.M. and 10 P.M.) must be consistent. The meals and snacks must be taken by-the-clock. An alarm on your watch will act as a reminder. Many of your medications must be skipped if you miss meals. Call us if you need advice. We, as well as your doctor or certified diabetes educator (CDE), are available for unusual problems.
- It is also important to keep a source of sugar with you at all times in case you feel effects of low blood sugar. If that happens, swallowing simple sugars such as orange juice, life savers, or table sugar can help to restore low blood sugar at normal levels. The literature that we are giving you explains the signs and symptoms of low blood sugar. Let's go over to them one by one today.
- Your physician has prescribed an injection of a medication that is a human hormone called *insulin*. There are many forms. This one has been selected for you. I am giving you information on storage and injection technique. You will find that this form of medication, when used appropriately, has few adverse effects compared to what you might have heard many years ago. Remember, insulin will lower

• DIABETES MEDICATION THERAPY MANAGEMENT QUESTIONS AND COMMENTS (*continued*)

blood sugar. It is critical to stay on your prescribed meal and snack plan just as if they were medications. A major take-home point is that high blood sugar can cause harm to the body over time. Low blood sugar can be life threatening in a short period of time.

- Although many people with diabetes use insulin before meals, do not be surprised if your doctor prescribes it with or right after a meal. There are some conditions that require with- or after-food insulin administration. Check with us if you have any questions about this.
- Alcohol is a drink that is truly a drug. In some quantities, it has the potential of dropping your blood sugar to unsafe levels. At all costs, please avoid alcoholic drinks. We recommend that when attending parties or social events, take a glass of sugar-free carbonated drink or lemonade and sip it throughout the event. That will take pressure off you.
- Please avoid so-called dietetic candy and snacks. They actually do contain a form of sugar that would upset your carefully planned food program.
- Every drug has some potential for side effects. The benefit of medication outweighs the risks. If you experience any unusual adverse effect, be sure to contact us or your physician—whoever is available.
- You will notice that with your medication, we include an information paper for you to read. Please read it carefully and keep it close to where you store your medications. The information should be reviewed regularly. If you have questions, please call us to assist you by phone or in person.
- Because you have a low vision, I will put a rubber band around the package, vial, pen, or bottle of regular insulin. Remember that the letter "R" means rubber band and regular. It could also apply to another rapid form. In that case the "R" means rapid. Those are the fast-acting forms.
- The other type that you use is either intermediate or longer acting.
- I notice that you are wearing a device to help your hearing. I will write all these instructions on a separate paper in very big letters.
- Your insulin is in a form of a suspension. It has the letters "NPH" or "N" in the name. Before injecting it, roll it gently 5 to 10 times between the palms of your hands to mix it well.
- Your insulin has been prescribed as a "sliding scale." Please make sure that you use only the form of insulin that the doctor ordered for this, whether short acting or rapid acting; never the intermediate or longer acting forms.
- Because you have been diagnosed with a form of diabetes called "Type 1," let's work together to make sure that your blood glucose monitoring, insulin administration, and meal planning are done appropriately.
- Have you checked your blood pressure? Make sure that your primary physician monitors this carefully. You might be prescribed a blood pressure medication called an "ACE inhibitor" or one called an "ARB." This form of medication is valuable to treat high blood pressure and protect the kidneys, especially for someone with diabetes.
- In our session, it would be appropriate for me to give you a list of physicians who are specialists in the most common problems for patients with diabetes. They include the following: dentists, dermatologists, foot doctors (podiatrists), eye doctors, urologists, and others.
- Please be cautious of claims that might be made by proponents of natural, herbal, complementary, or alternative treatments. Although some natural products might have effects on blood sugar, your condition has been diagnosed by a trained professional physician or other health care professional. Have faith in the treatment and medical plan that he or she has given you. We, here at the pharmacy, are available in person or by phone many hours per week. We welcome your questions.
- Above all, do not become discouraged. Think of how we welcome you to our medication therapy management program and that the word welcome starts with "WE."

14.1

PT. NAME: **JOHN TAYLOR** AGE: **74** GENDER: **M** ADDRESS: **30998 LAKESHORE DR.** WEIGHT: **199** HEIGHT: **5′ 10″** BMI: **29**

DX: **TYPE 2 DM, HTN, HIGH TRIGLYCERIDES, SKIN ALLERGY, RESPIRATORY TRACT INFECTION, LOW LEVELS OF VITAMIN D** ALLERGY: **NKA** HX: **OVERWEIGHT SINCE CHILDHOOD**

MEDICATION	SIG.	PRESCRIBER	ORIG. DATE	REFILL DATE	REFILL DATE	REFILL DATE	REFILL DATE
Claritin 10 mg #30	I qd	Coving	6/6	8/3	9/15		
Augmentin 875 mg #16	I bid	Coving	6/2				
Procardia XL 60 mg #30	I qd	Coving	7/7	8/6	9/8		
Lasix 40 mg #30	I qd	Coving	7/7	8/5	9/8		
Vitamin D 1000 IU Capsules #90	I qd	Coving	7/7				

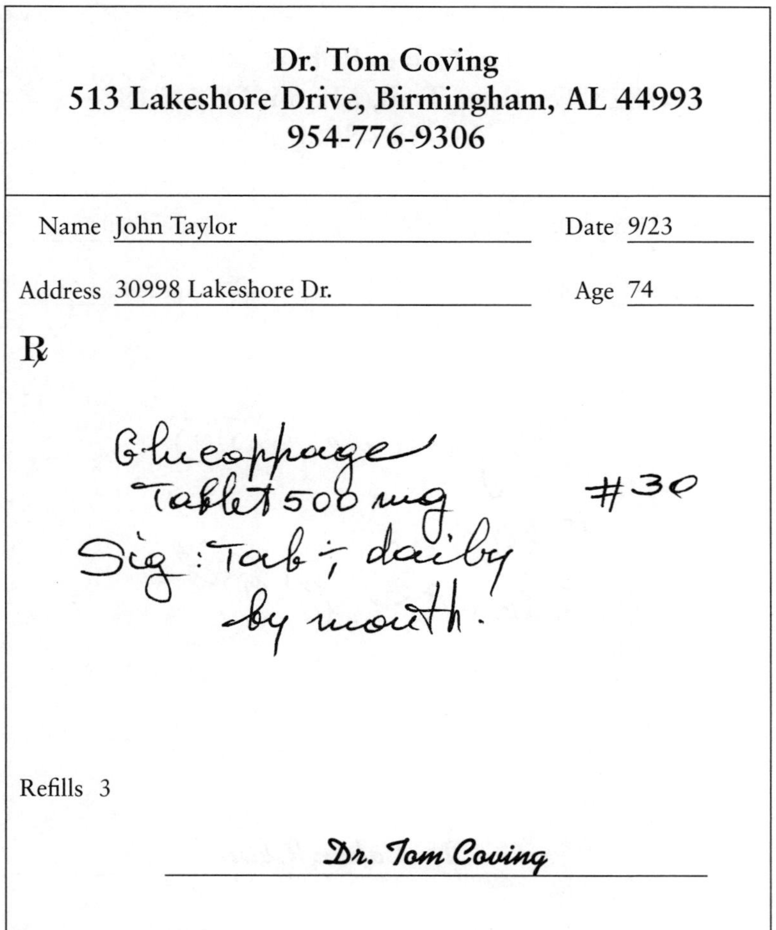

Dr. Tom Coving
513 Lakeshore Drive, Birmingham, AL 44993
954-776-9306

Name John Taylor Date 9/23

Address 30998 Lakeshore Dr. Age 74

℞

Glucophage Tablet 500 mg #30
Sig: Tab i daily by mouth.

Refills 3

Dr. Tom Coving

14.1a

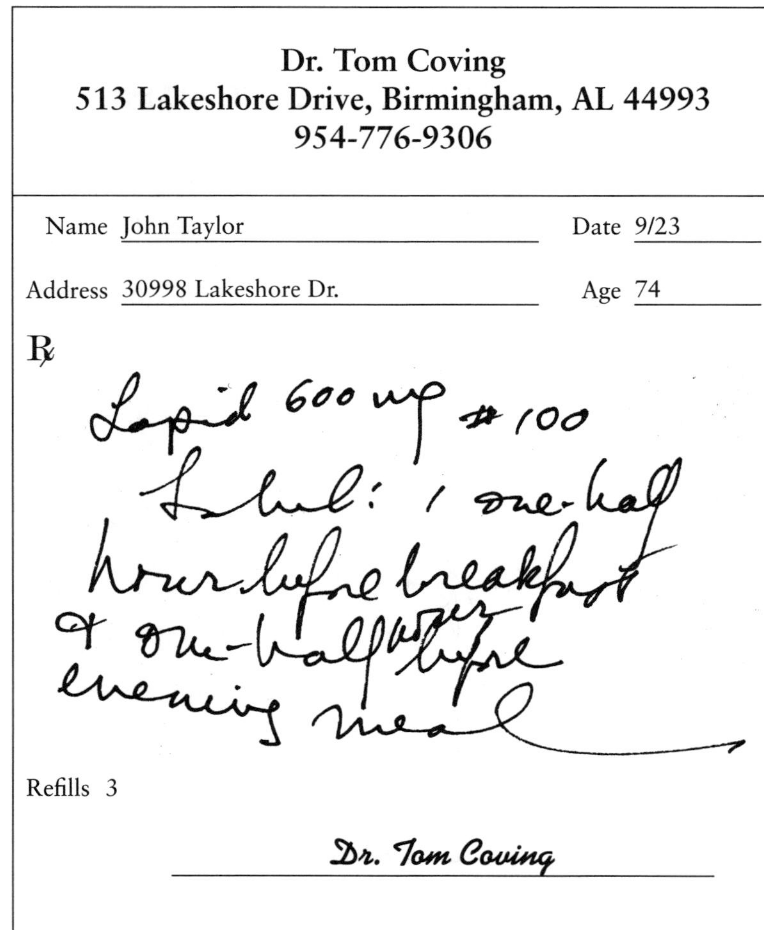

Dr. Tom Coving
513 Lakeshore Drive, Birmingham, AL 44993
954-776-9306

Name John Taylor Date 9/23

Address 30998 Lakeshore Dr. Age 74

℞

Lopid 600 mg #100
Label: 1 one-half hour before breakfast & one-half hour before evening meal

Refills 3

Dr. Tom Coving

14.1b

14.2 PT. NAME: **TOMMY DIVITO** AGE: **64** GENDER: **M** DX: **TYPE 2 DM, HTN, BPH, HIGH CHOLESTEROL, ANXIETY** ADDRESS: **564 COLLINS AVE.** ALLERGY: **ASA** WEIGHT: **189** HX: **SMOKER (30 PACK-YEARS)** HEIGHT: **5′ 9″** BMI: **28**

MEDICATION	SIG.	PRESCRIBER	ORIG. DATE	REFILL DATE	REFILL DATE	REFILL DATE	REFILL DATE
Ativan 1 mg #120	1 qid	Robins	3/14	4/17	5/16	6/14	
Glucophage 500 mg #60	1 bid ac bkfst & dinner	Robins	4/20	6/22			
Proscar 5 mg #30	1 qd	Jones	6/19				
Lipitor 20 mg #30	1 qd	Robins	4/17	5/16	6/16		
Demadex 20 mg #30	1 qd	Robins	3/14	4/17	5/16	6/16	

Dr. Calvin Robins
7823 Tea Rose Trail, Miami, FL 44718
463-555-8000

Name Tommy DiVito Date 7/20

Address 564 Collins Ave. Age 64

℞

Metformin 500g #120

Sig: i bid

Refills 3

Dr. Calvin Robins

14.2a

Dr. Calvin Robins
7823 Tea Rose Trail, Miami, FL 44718
463-555-8000

Name Tommy DiVito Date 7/20

Address 564 Collins Ave. Age 64

℞

glyburide 2.5mg

#30

take one po qd

Refills 3

Dr. Calvin Robins

14.2b

14.3

PT. NAME: **JENNIFER BROWN**	GENDER: **F**	ADDRESS: **321 WEST RD.**	WEIGHT: **195**	HEIGHT: **5′ 6″**	BMI: **31**
AGE: **71**	DX: **HTN, CHF, TYPE 2 DM, HERPES ZOSTER ("SHINGLES")**	ALLERGY: **PCN**	HX: **OVEREATERS ANONYMOUS MEMBER**		

MEDICATION	SIG.	PRESCRIBER	ORIG. DATE	REFILL DATE	REFILL DATE	REFILL DATE	REFILL DATE
Diltiazem 60 mg #90	I q 8 h	Sauls	3/9	4/6	5/11		
Digoxin 0.125 mg #30	I qd	Sauls	2/5	3/15	4/20	5/20	
Norvasc 5 mg #30	I qd	Sauls	3/9	4/20	5/20		
Zovirax Ointment 5% 15 g	Apply to left CW qid	Sauls	4/30	5/4	5/18	5/23	6/1
Tylenol No. 2 #24	I q 6 h prn	Sauls	4/30	5/2	5/6	5/23	6/1
Ecotrin Regular Strength tabs 325 mg #125	I qd	Sauls	2/5	5/30			

Dr. Alfred Sauls
151212 S High Rd., Chicago, IL 23875
954-555-1300

Name Jennifer Brown Date 6/5

Address 321 West Rd. Age 71

℞

Humulin 70/30 # 6 VIALS
i 55 units q AM
U100 Insulin Syringes # 100
i as directed

Refills 4

Dr. Alfred Sauls

14.3a

Dr. Alfred Sauls
151212 S High Rd., Chicago, IL 23875
954-555-1300

Name Jennifer Brown Date 6/5

Address 321 West Rd. Age 71

℞

Glucotrol 5 mg
i BID
1/2 h AC food)
100

Refills 4

Dr. Alfred Sauls

14.3b

14.4

PT. NAME: **DON BLACK** AGE: **68** GENDER: **M** DX: **A-FIB, TYPE 2 DM, CONSTIPATION, DIARRHEA, TENSION HEADACHES** ADDRESS: **566 EAST CT.** ALLERGY: **PCN** WEIGHT: **248** HX: **SEDENTARY LIFESTYLE, BUYS "DIETETIC CANDY"** HEIGHT: **6′ 1″** BMI: **33**

MEDICATION	SIG.	PRESCRIBER	ORIG. DATE	REFILL DATE	REFILL DATE	REFILL DATE	REFILL DATE
Coumadin 2.5 mg #60	1 q am	Griffin	3/22	4/27	7/6		
Lomotil 2.5 mg #100	1–2 qid prn diarrhea	Griffin	4/10	6/3	8/7		
Lanoxin 0.125 mg #90	1 q am	Griffin	3/22	6/30			
Metamucil Original Course Milled 72 doses	1 tsp in water q am	OTC	4/5				

Dr. Doug Griffin
7611 147th Terrace, Monterey, CA 38411
705-555-6644

Name Don Black Date 8/10
Address 566 East Ct. Age 68

℞

Micronase 10mg
10 ʒ po q Am
5mg
2 QAm

Refills prn

Dr. Doug Griffin

14.4a

Dr. Doug Griffin
7611 147th Terrace, Monterey, CA 38411
705-555-6644

Name Don Black Date 8/10
Address 566 East Ct. Age 68

℞

Fioricet 2 q 4h

#100

Refill 3 times

Dr. Doug Griffin

14.4b

14.5	PT. NAME: **RITA MOORLAND**	GENDER: **F**	ADDRESS: **23 SOUTH ST.**	WEIGHT: **155**	HEIGHT: **5′**	BMI: **30**
	AGE: **72**	DX: **CHF, TYPE 2 DM, GERD, DIABETIC GASTROPARESIS, CARDIAC VALVE REPLACEMENT, SPASTIC COLON, LOW VIT. D LEVELS**		ALLERGY: **ASA**	DX: **OBESE MOST OF HER LIFE; "SOCIAL" ETOH DRINKER**	

MEDICATION	SIG.	PRESCRIBER	ORIG. DATE	REFILL DATE	REFILL DATE	REFILL DATE	REFILL DATE
Prilosec 20 mg #30	I qd	Isaacs	10/26	11/29			
Levsin SL 0.125 mg #20	I sl bid prn	Isaacs	10/3	10/16	11/20	12/3	
Coumadin 4 mg #30	I q am report weekly INR	Isaacs	10/3	10/26	11/20		
Lanoxin 0.25 mg #30	I qd	Isaacs	10/3	10/26	11/20		
Furosemide 20 mg #40	I bid	Isaacs	10/3	10/26	11/10		
Vitamin D 1000 IU caps #60	I qd with bkfst	Isaacs	10/3	12/2			

Dr. Howard Isaacs
1115 Turnaround Lane, Detroit, MI 64789
343-555-7000

Name Rita Moorland Date 12/5

Address 23 South St. Age 72

℞

Glucophage 500 T #60

T po BID

Refills 1

Dr. Howard Isaacs

14.5a

Dr. Howard Isaacs
1115 Turnaround Lane, Detroit, MI 64789
343-555-7000

Name Rita Moorland Date 12/5

Address 23 South St. Age 72

℞

Reglan 10 T #30

ī TID AC

☐ Label

Refill ______ times PRN NR

Dr. Howard Isaacs

14.5b

14.6 PT. NAME: **ART HARRIS** AGE: **64** GENDER: **M** DX: **HTN, BPH, TYPE 2 DM, INSOMNIA, POSTNASAL DRIP, OTITIS EXTERNA** ADDRESS: **458 NW 185TH TERRACE** ALLERGY: **IODINE, ASA, CODEINE** WEIGHT: **180** HX: **SMOKER, OVEREATER** HEIGHT: **5′ 6″** BMI: **29**

MEDICATION	SIG.	PRESCRIBER	ORIG. DATE	REFILL DATE	REFILL DATE	REFILL DATE	REFILL DATE
Restoril 15 mg #30	I hs prn sleep	Robins	5/11	8/16			
Lasix 20 mg #90	I qd	Robins	3/14	7/5	8/29		
KCl 750 mg (10 mEq) #90	I qd	Robins	3/9				
Tenormin 25 mg #90	I qd	Robins	3/6	7/5			
Sudafed 30 mg #24	I tid for cold symptoms	OTC	4/6	8/7	9/12		
Hytrin 2 mg #90	I cap hs	Robins	2/7	5/16	8/20		

Dr. Calvin Robins
7823 Tea Rose Trail, Miami, FL 44718
463-555-8000

Name Art Harris Date 9/15

Address 458 NW 185th Terrace Age 64

℞

1) HCTZ 25mg #30
ʒ ī qD

2) Glipizide 10mg #60
ʒ ī BID

Refills 2

Dr. Calvin Robins

14.6a

Dr. Rishi Das
2800 NE 163rd St.
North Miami Beach, FL 44718
463-555-2345

Name Art Harris Date 9/15

Address 458 NW 185th Terrace Age 64

℞

Cortisporin OTIC Soln
#1
2 Drops in Ears
tid x 5 DAYS

Dr. Rishi Das

14.6b

14.7 PT. NAME: **MARTIN EDWARDS** AGE: **63** GENDER: **M** DX: **TYPE 2 DM, OA, HTN, GERD** ADDRESS: **654 EAGLE RUN** ALLERGY: **MSG IN CHINESE FOOD** WEIGHT: **189** HX: **ETOH** HEIGHT: **5′ 11″** BMI: **26**

MEDICATION	SIG.	PRESCRIBER	ORIG. DATE	REFILL DATE	REFILL DATE	REFILL DATE	REFILL DATE
Percocet 5/325 mg #50	1 bid prn pain	Thomas	1/12				
Calan SR 240 mg #50	1/2 tab qd	Thomas	1/12	4/18	7/28		
Triamcinolone Cream 0.1% 80 g	Apply ud	Gaines	2/15	4/28			
Prevacid 30 mg #30	1 qd	Thomas	6/14				

Dr. Erin Thomas
988 North Ridge, New York, NY 88364
813-555-7554

Name Martin Edwards Date 7/29

Address 654 Eagle Run Age 63

℞

Aciphex
20 mg
qd
#30

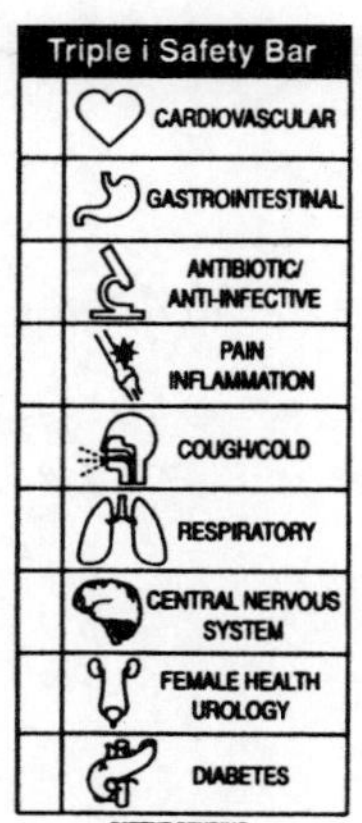

Refills 1

Dr. Erin Thomas

14.7a

Dr. Janet Halloway
4414 W Bridge Rd., New York, NY 88364
813-555-8200

Name Martin Edwards Date 7/30

Address 654 Eagle Run Age 63

℞

Glucovance 5/500
(60)

sig tab i bid

Refills 1

Dr. Janet Halloway

14.7b

14.8

PT. NAME: **JIM LOTHAR** | AGE: **71** | GENDER: **M** | DX: **GOUT, HTN, ANEMIA, TYPE 2 DM, UTI, "SHINGLES"** | ADDRESS: **7541 NORTH AVE.** | ALLERGY: **SULFA, DAIRY PRODUCTS** | WEIGHT: **182** | HX: **NERVOUS PERSONALITY** | HEIGHT: **5′ 4″** | BMI: **31**

MEDICATION	SIG.	PRESCRIBER	ORIG. DATE	REFILL DATE	REFILL DATE	REFILL DATE	REFILL DATE
Colchicine 0.6 mg #90	1 qd	Isaacs	2/10				
Doxycycline 100 mg #14	1 q 12 h × 7 d	Isaacs	3/20				

Dr. Howard Isaacs
1115 Turnaround Lane, Detroit, MI 64789
343-555-7000

Name Jim Lothar Date 4/10

Address 7541 North Ave. Age 71

℞

Glucophage 500mg
T qd #90

Folic Acid 1mg #90

Inderal 40mg T Bid #90

Allopurinol 300mg
T qd #90

Refills 0

Dr. Howard Isaacs

14.8a

Dr. Paul Magelan
1110 Turnaround Lane, Detroit, MI 64789
343-555-7001

Name Jim Lothar Date 4/10

Address 7541 North Ave. Age 71

℞

#35

Zovirax 200mg
i Po 5x daily for 7 days

Refills N.R.

Dr. P. Magelan

14.8b

14.9

PT. NAME: **LYNN SMITH** AGE: **70** GENDER: **F** DX: **HTN, ANGINA, GERD, TYPE 2 DM** ADDRESS: **61 GREEN ST.** ALLERGY: **CATS** WEIGHT: **185** HX: **SMOKER MOST OF HER LIFE** HEIGHT: **5′7″** BMI: **29**

MEDICATION	SIG.	PRESCRIBER	ORIG. DATE	REFILL DATE	REFILL DATE	REFILL DATE	REFILL DATE
Imdur 30 mg #90	I hs	Weiss	5/1	8/10			
K-Dur 20 mEq #30	I q am	Weiss	5/1	5/27			
Altace 1.25 mg cap #30	I qd	Weiss	6/28	7/27	8/25	9/21	
Pepcid 20 mg #30	I hs	Weiss	4/4				
Glucophage 500 mg #120	I bid	Weiss	5/17	8/21	10/8		

Dr. Barry Weiss
901 Sheridan St., Austin, TX 90902
874-555-9000

Name Lynn Smith Date 10/20
Address 61 Green St. Age 70

℞

Tenormin 25 #100
~~BID~~ ASDir
D.A.W.

Refills 2

Dr. Barry Weiss

14.9a

Dr. Barry Weiss
901 Sheridan St., Austin, TX 90902
874-555-9000

Name Lynn Smith Date 10/20
Address 61 Green St. Age 70

℞

Prandin 4 mg
i PO AC TID
#280

Refills 2

Dr. Barry Weiss

14.9b

14.10

PT. NAME: **JANET GOODMAN** AGE: **58** GENDER: **F** DX: **TYPE 2 DM, DEPRESSION, INFECTION, CHRONIC RHINITIS** ADDRESS: **500 HICKORY LANE** ALLERGY: **NKA** WEIGHT: **189** HX: **POSTAL EMPLOYEE** HEIGHT: **5′ 3″** BMI: **33**

MEDICATION	SIG.	PRESCRIBER	ORIG. DATE	REFILL DATE	REFILL DATE	REFILL DATE	REFILL DATE
Allegra 60 mg #10	I bid prn	Gilman	8/3				
Augmentin 875 mg #8	I bid	Gilman	6/22				
Sudafed 30 mg #24	I prn	Gilman	1/15	2/10	3/12	4/15	7/25
Prozac 20 mg #30	I qd	Updyke	8/15				

Dr. Arnold Gilman
33 Spruce St., St. Louis, MO 99545
766-555-8000

Name Janet Goodman Date 8/20

Address 500 Hickory Lane Age 58

℞

Glycotro 10 mg
#60
Take i p.o. BID

☐ Label

Refill 1 times PRN NR

Dr. Arnold Gilman

14.10a

Dr. Arnold Gilman
33 Spruce St., St. Louis, MO 99545
766-555-8000

Name Janet Goodman Date 8/20

Address 500 Hickory Lane Age 58

℞

Metforanin 500 mg
#30
Take i p.o. QD

☐ Label

Refill 1 times PRN NR

Dr. Arnold Gilman

14.10b

14.11

PT. NAME: **GRETCHEN BLACK** AGE: **69** GENDER: **F** DX: **TYPE 2 DM, HTN, OA** ADDRESS: **5633 FLAMINGO CT.** ALLERGY: **AMINOGLYCOSIDES, PCN** WEIGHT: **163** HX: **ETOH, SMOKER** HEIGHT: **5′ 1″** BMI: **31**

MEDICATION	SIG.	PRESCRIBER	ORIG. DATE	REFILL DATE	REFILL DATE	REFILL DATE	REFILL DATE
Celebrex 200 mg #30	1 qd	Griffin	10/4	11/9	12/8		
Monopril 40 mg #30	1 qd	Griffin	10/4	12/15			
Lasix 20 mg #30	1 qd	Griffin	10/4	11/9			

Dr. Donna Johns
7000 SW 1st Ave., Santa Fe, NM 54545
766-555-9097

Name Gretchen Black Date 12/20

Address 5633 Flamingo Ct. Age 69

℞ Novolin N

#1 X 10ml

Sig: 12 units q am
11 units q pm

☑ Label

Refill three times PRN NR

Dr. Donna Johns

14.11a

Dr. Donna Johns
7000 SW 1st Ave., Santa Fe, NM 54545
766-555-9097

Name Gretchen Black Date 12/20

Address 5633 Flamingo Ct. Age 69

℞ Novolin R

#1 X 10ml.

Sig: 12 units q am
11 units q pm.

☑ Label

Refill three times PRN NR

Dr. Donna Johns

14.11b

14.12

PT. NAME: **ALAN JOHNSON** AGE: **62** GENDER: **M** DX: **TYPE 2 DM, HTN, HIGH LDL CHOLESTEROL, DYSPEPSIA** ADDRESS: **854 MAROON ST.** ALLERGY: **NKA** WEIGHT: **198** HX: **OBESITY** HEIGHT: **5′ 2″** BMI: **36**

MEDICATION	SIG.	PRESCRIBER	ORIG. DATE	REFILL DATE	REFILL DATE	REFILL DATE	REFILL DATE
HCTZ 25 mg #90	1 q am	Celestin	2/4	5/16			
Carafate 1 g #120	1 qid ac with water	Celestin	1/3	2/20	4/10		
Lipitor 10 mg #90	1 q am for cholesterol	Celestin	1/20	5/22			

Dr. Daniel Keller
5007 Turtle Drive, Miami, FL 98887
247-555-9876

Name Alan Johnson Date 5/30

Address 854 Maroon St. Age 62

℞

① Glucophage 500mg #60
1 BID

② Actos 30mg
#30
1 T. QD

Refills 0

Dr. Daniel Keller

14.12a

Dr. Karl Celestin
2121 NE 164th St. N, Miami, FL 98887
247-555-6543

Name Alan Johnson Date 5/28

Address 854 Maroon St. Age 62

℞

Zocor 20mg
#30
1 PO

Refills X 3

Dr. Karl Celestin

14.12b

14.13 PT. NAME: **FRED LICHTENSTEIN** AGE: **72** GENDER: **M** ADDRESS: **1920 ELECTRON DR.** DX: **HTN, HIGH LDL CHOLESTEROL, MIGRAINES, CONSTIPATION, DEPRESSED, TYPE 2 DM** WEIGHT: **132** ALLERGY: **NKA** HEIGHT: **5′ 4″** HX: **ETOH** BMI: **23**

MEDICATION	SIG.	PRESCRIBER	ORIG. DATE	REFILL DATE	REFILL DATE	REFILL DATE	REFILL DATE
Questran Light packets #60	I pack tid	James	2/7	4/6			
Paxil 20 mg #30	I qd	James	1/17	2/16			
Lipitor 20 mg #30	I qd	James	3/20	5/3	6/1		
DiaBeta 5 mg #50	I q am	James	4/10				
Lasix 40 mg #30	I qd	James	2/20	3/19	4/20	5/19	
Docusate Sodium 100 mg caps #100	I bid with water	OTC	4/9				

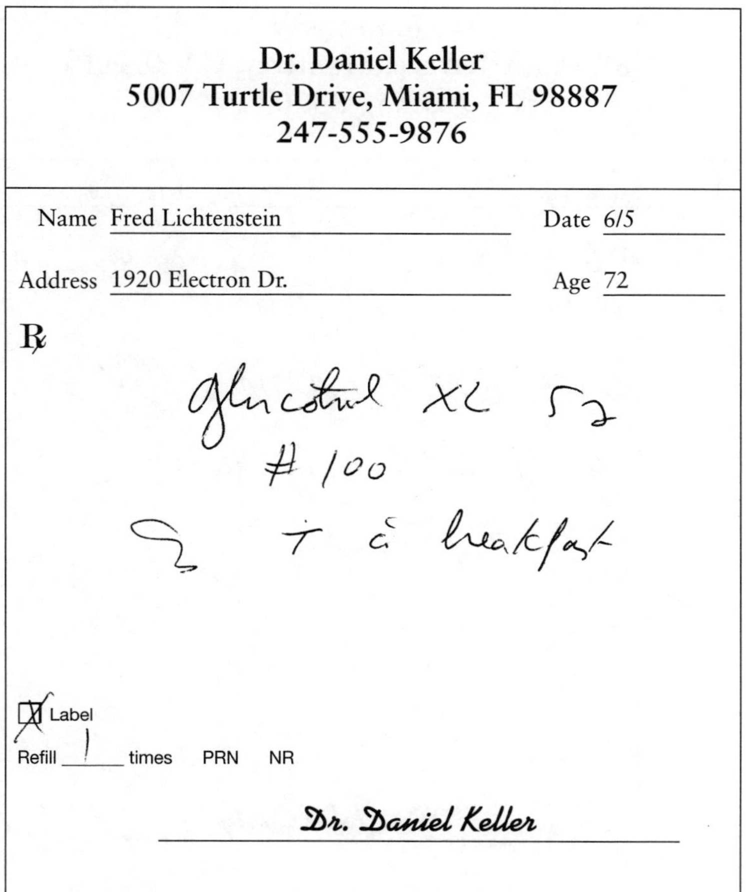
Dr. Daniel Keller
5007 Turtle Drive, Miami, FL 98887
247-555-9876

Name Fred Lichtenstein Date 6/5
Address 1920 Electron Dr. Age 72

℞
Glucotrol XL 5mg
#100
q i c̄ breakfast

☒ Label
Refill 1 times PRN NR

Dr. Daniel Keller

14.13a

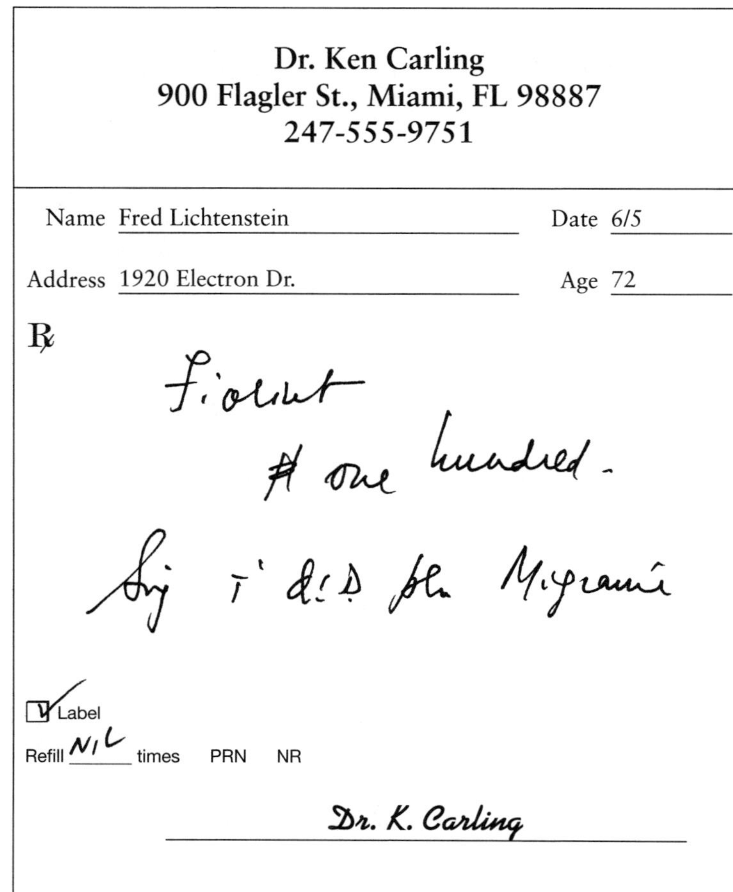
Dr. Ken Carling
900 Flagler St., Miami, FL 98887
247-555-9751

Name Fred Lichtenstein Date 6/5
Address 1920 Electron Dr. Age 72

℞
Fioricet
one hundred.
Sig i q.i.d. prn Migraine

☑ Label
Refill N/C times PRN NR

Dr. K. Carling

14.13b

14.14

PT. NAME: **LAURA BAKER** | AGE: **68** | GENDER: **F** | ADDRESS: **445 LINCOLN AVE.** | DX: **TYPE 2 DM, TOENAIL FUNGUS, HEARTBURN, VAGINAL YEAST (CANDIDIASIS)** | WEIGHT: **199** | ALLERGY: **NKA** | HEIGHT: **5′ 3″** | HX: **ATTENDS OVEREATERS ANONYMOUS** | BMI: **35**

MEDICATION	SIG.	PRESCRIBER	ORIG. DATE	REFILL DATE	REFILL DATE	REFILL DATE	REFILL DATE
Terazol 7 vaginal cream 0.4% 45 g	Insert PV at hs × 7 d	Griffin	5/12	6/15	7/19		
Maalox Regular Susp. 12 oz	10 mL prn	Griffin	3/12	4/15	5/29	6/30	
Lamisil AT Cream 12 g	Apply to feet bid	OTC	4/12	5/30			

Dr. Doug Griffin
7611 147th Terrace, Monterey, CA 38411
705-555-6644

Name Laura Baker Date 7/20
Address 445 Lincoln Ave. Age 68

℞

glucotrol XL 10
#100
i qD

Refill XY times

Dr. Doug Griffin

14.14a

Dr. John Carty
9988 145th Terrace, Monterey, CA 38411
705-555-3470

Name Laura Baker Date 7/20
Address 445 Lincoln Ave. Age 68

℞

Sporonox 100mg #168
Sig: i BID x 12wks

Refills NR

Dr. John Carty

14.14b

14.15 PT. NAME: **LISA FORTUNA** AGE: **78** GENDER: **F** ADDRESS: **1 MAIN ST.** DX: **HTN, TYPE 2 DM, CHF, GLAUCOMA, ALZHEIMER'S DISEASE, "SHINGLES"** WEIGHT: **209** ALLERGY: **SULFA** HEIGHT: **5′ 7″** HX: **SMOKER, ETOH** BMI: **33**

MEDICATION	SIG.	PRESCRIBER	ORIG. DATE	REFILL DATE	REFILL DATE	REFILL DATE	REFILL DATE
Lasix 20 mg #90	I q am	Isaacs	4/12	8/15			
Toprol XL 50 mg #60	I qd	Isaacs	4/24	5/17	6/19	7/22	
Aricept 5 mg #30	I am	Isaacs	3/17				
Aricept 10 mg #30	I am	Isaacs	4/17	5/8	6/21	7/14	
Xalatan 0.005% 2.5 mL	I gtt ou hs	Rand	4/30				

Dr. Daniel Keller
5007 Turtle Drive, Miami, FL 98887
247-555-9876

Name Lisa Fortuna Date 8/15

Address 1 Main St. Age 78

℞

Glucotrol
1/2 of 5mg tablet daily
50

REFILL 5 TIMES

Dr. Daniel Keller

14.15a

Dr. Daniel Keller
5007 Turtle Drive, Miami, FL 98887
247-555-9876

Name Lisa Fortuna Date 8/15

Address 1 Main St. Age 78

℞

Zostrix HP—generic
apply QID
arm

Zovirax #20
i tid 400mg

Refill 4 times

Dr. Daniel Keller

14.15b

14.16

PT. NAME: **DENNIS DAVIS**	GENDER: **M**	ADDRESS: **4589 BLUEJAY LANE**	WEIGHT: **162**	HEIGHT: **5′ 4″**	BMI: **28**
AGE: **70**	DX: **RECURRENT UTI, TYPE 2 DM, HTN, GERD**	ALLERGY: **PCN**	HX: **HYPOGLYCEMIC EPISODES**		

MEDICATION	SIG.	PRESCRIBER	ORIG. DATE	REFILL DATE	REFILL DATE	REFILL DATE	REFILL DATE
Bactrim DS #90	I qd	Farris	4/12	7/9	10/10		
Ativan 1 mg #30	I bid, q am + 6 pm	Farris	5/15	6/12			
Prevacid 30 mg #30	I qd	Farris	2/12	4/15	6/12	8/20	
Reglan 10 mg #120	I tid 1/2 h ac	Farris	2/14	4/6	6/12		
Lotrisone cream 45 g	Apply bid ud	Farris	2/14	3/12	4/30	6/15	
Lisinopril 10 mg #30	I qd	Farris	5/6	6/5	7/7	8/10	10/15

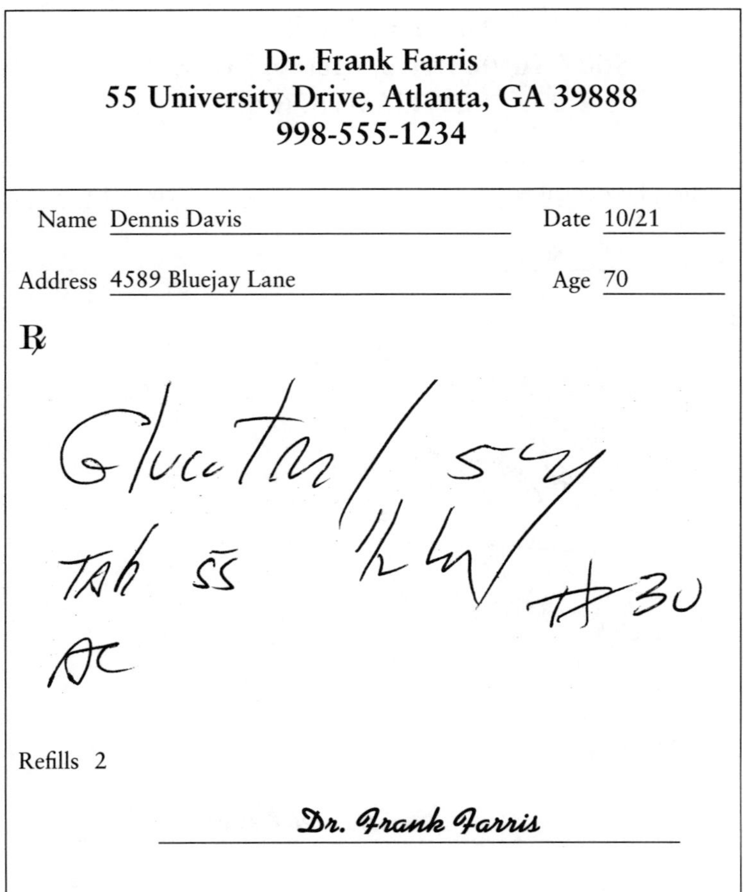
Dr. Frank Farris
55 University Drive, Atlanta, GA 39888
998-555-1234

Name Dennis Davis Date 10/21

Address 4589 Bluejay Lane Age 70

℞

Glucotrol 5 mg
Tab ss ½ hr AC #30

Refills 2

Dr. Frank Farris

14.16a

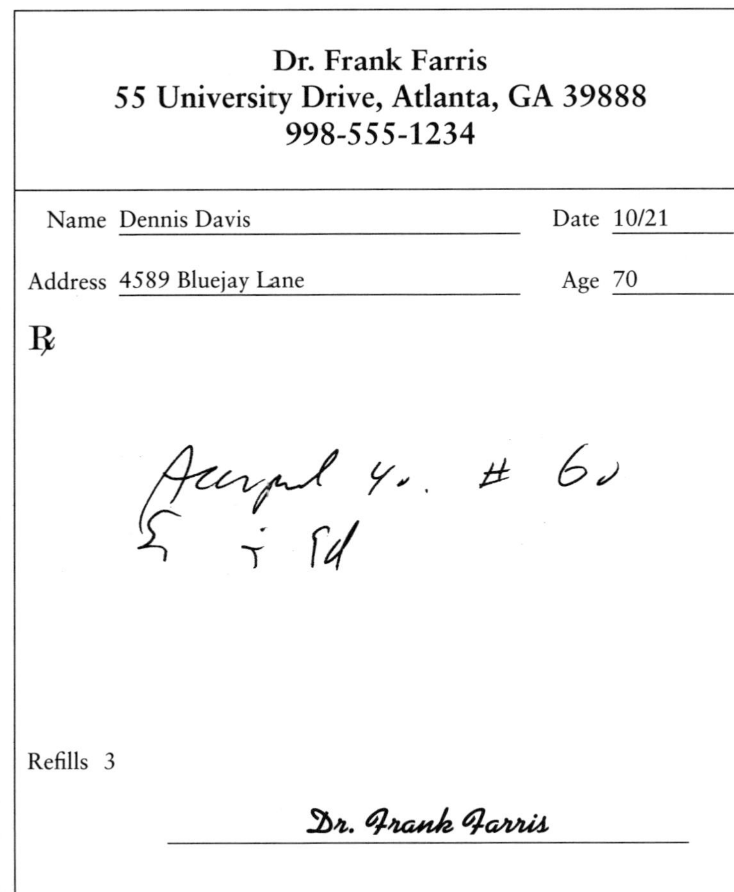
Dr. Frank Farris
55 University Drive, Atlanta, GA 39888
998-555-1234

Name Dennis Davis Date 10/21

Address 4589 Bluejay Lane Age 70

℞

Accupril 40 #60
Sig i qd

Refills 3

Dr. Frank Farris

14.16b

14.17

PT. NAME: **ANTHONY JOHNSON**
AGE: **69**
GENDER: **M**
DX: **HTN, TYPE 2 DM, GOUT, ANEMIA, URINARY HESITANCY**
ADDRESS: **774 STATE ST.**
ALLERGY: **NKA**
WEIGHT: **165**
HEIGHT: **5′ 8″**
BMI: **25**
HX: **ETOH, SMOKER (40 PACK-YEARS)**

MEDICATION	SIG.	PRESCRIBER	ORIG. DATE	REFILL DATE	REFILL DATE	REFILL DATE	REFILL DATE
Zyloprim 300 mg #90	1 q am	Thomas	2/4	5/14			
Lasix 20 mg #90	1 qd	Thomas	2/4	5/14			
Folic acid 1 mg #C	2 qd	Thomas	2/4	4/20			
Saw Palmetto caps 450 mg #C	2 bid	OTC	1/20	3/22	5/11		

Dr. Erin Thomas
988 North Ridge, New York, NY 88364
813-555-7554

Name Anthony Johnson Date 5/20

Address 774 State St. Age 69

℞

Premarin 1.25 mg
Disp #31
Sig: i qd

Refills 1

Dr. Erin Thomas

14.17a

Dr. Erin Thomas
988 North Ridge, New York, NY 88364
813-555-7554

Name Anthony Johnson Date 5/20

Address 774 State St. Age 69

℞

Glipizide ī
200
ī po TID

☐ LABEL

REFILL _____ TIMES (PRN) NR

Dr. Erin Thomas

14.17b

14.18

PT. NAME: **MONROSE GIFFORD**	GENDER: **M**	ADDRESS: **23 NW 4TH CT.**	WEIGHT: **NOT ON FILE**
AGE: **67**	DX: **HTN, TYPE 2 DM, PARKINSON'S, DIABETIC GASTROPARESIS, ANXIETY, INSOMNIA, GERD**	ALLERGY: **SHELLFISH, CHOCOLATE**	HX: **OBESITY, UNCONTROLLED HYPERGLYCEMIA**

MEDICATION	SIG.	PRESCRIBER	ORIG. DATE	REFILL DATE	REFILL DATE	REFILL DATE	REFILL DATE
Sinemet 25/100 #90	1 tab tid	Vargas	7/14	8/3			
Protonix 40 mg #30	1 tab qd	Salerno	6/5	7/3	8/2		
Ativan 1 mg #10	1 bid prn	Salerno	6/5	7/3	8/2		
Restoril 30 mg #30	1 cap hs	Salerno	6/5	7/3	8/2		
Insulin syringes 1/2 cc #C	ud	Salerno	8/16				
Zestril 5 mg #90	1 qd	Salerno	2/1	5/8	8/9		

Dr. Eleanor Salerno
2799 Victory Place, East Brunswick, NJ 33838
400-555-3344

Name Monrose Gifford Date 8/16

Address 23 NW 4th Ct. Age 67

℞

☐ENTER ☐DO NOT ENTER...NAME AFTER ℞ ON LABEL. | MG./CC | QUAN. | TIMES REFILL

℞1 Humulin NPH | 1 bottle | refill 2 (circled)
SIG. 25U each morning
℞2 20U each evening
SIG.
℞3 Regular Humulin Insulin | 1 bottle | refill 2 (circled)
SIG. SSI – use per scale given

Dr. E. Salerno

14.18a

Dr. Eleanor Salerno
2799 Victory Place, East Brunswick, NJ 33838
400-555-3344

Name Monrose Gifford Date 8/16

Address 23 NW 4th Ct. Age 67

℞

Reglan 10 mg # 100
sig. i tab. T.I.D. ac

Pepcid 40 mg # 30
sig. i tab. Q.D

☐ Label

Refill ______ times (PRN circled) NR

Dr. E. Salerno

14.18b

14.19

PT. NAME: **TANIA LEOPOLD** GENDER: **F** ADDRESS: **91 PINE ST.** WEIGHT: **169** HEIGHT: **5′ 1″** BMI: **32**

AGE: **61** DX: **TYPE 2 DM, HTN, ANXIETY, DEPRESSION, PAINFUL DIABETIC NEUROPATHY, CONSTIPATED** ALLERGY: **PCN, ASA** HX: **SMOKES 1 PACK/WEEK**

MEDICATION	SIG.	PRESCRIBER	ORIG. DATE	REFILL DATE	REFILL DATE	REFILL DATE	REFILL DATE
HCTZ 25 mg #30	1 q am	Riley	6/19	7/20	8/23	9/15	10/20
Amitriptyline 10 mg #60	1 hs	Riley	8/1	10/4			
Percocet 5/325 mg #30	1 q 4–6 h prn	Riley	9/3				
Neurontin 100 mg #60	1 hs × 7 d, then 1 tid	Brock	11/8				
Hydroxyzine HCl 25 mg #50	1 bid	Riley	7/15	8/30			
Metformin 500 mg #60	1 bid	Riley	8/17	9/19	10/20		
Fleet Enema Saline 113 mL #6	prn BM	OTC	8/6	9/6	10/22		

Dr. Sean Riley
1750 NE 190 St., Arlington, VA 23445
239-555-0033

Name Tania Leopold Date 11/18

Address 91 Pine St. Age 61

℞

metaglib
5/500
#60
1 with B ✓
1 " Dinner

Refills 2X

Dr. Sean Riley

14.19a

Dr. Hal Brock
80 Fort Meyer Drive, Arlington, VA 23445
239-555-1023

Name Tania Leopold Date 11/18

Address 91 Pine St. Age 61

℞

Neurontin
300.
t.i.d
#100

Refills 5X

Dr. Hal Brock

14.19b

14.20

PT. NAME: **HARVEY WILSON** | AGE: **58** | GENDER: **M** | DX: **TYPE 2 DM, HTN, ASTHMA, COPD, UTI, URTICARIA** | ADDRESS: **48 OAK ST.** | ALLERGY: **NKA** | WEIGHT: **249** | HEIGHT: **6′ 4″** | BMI: **30** | HX: **OBESE MOST OF HIS LIFE; SMOKING HX: 10 PACK-YEARS; QUIT 5 YEARS AGO**

MEDICATION	SIG.	PRESCRIBER	ORIG. DATE	REFILL DATE	REFILL DATE	REFILL DATE	REFILL DATE
Lantus insulin SoloSTAR pen 5 X 3 mL	Use SC ud	Reiner	1/6	2/18	3/30		
Glyburide 5 mg #60	1 bid	Reiner	1/6	2/7	3/3		
Temazepam 15 mg #30	1 hs	Reiner	2/8	3/6	4/1		
Albuterol inhaler 8.5 g	Use prn, ud	Reiner	1/20	3/26			
Lisinopril 5 mg #30	1 qd	Reiner	1/6	2/4	3/6	4/1	
Levaquin 500 mg #7	1 qd	Reiner	1/20				

Dr. Jim Reiner
38 Dalton St, Raleigh, NC 84723
333-555-9990

Name Harvey Wilson Date 4/3

Address 48 Oak St. Age 58

℞

Glucovance 2.5/500
Sig: i q 8 AM
#30

Refills 2X

Dr. Jim Reiner

14.20a

Dr. Alice Sawyer
400 West Drive, Raleigh, NC 84723
333-555-1116

Name Harvey Wilson Date 4/3

Address 48 Oak St. Age 58

℞

Triamcinolone cream 0.1% 80 g
Sig: apply BID

PLEASE LABEL

☐ NO REFILL

☐ REFILL 3 TIMES

Dr. Alice Sawyer

14.20b

14.21

PT. NAME: **GLORIA HAMILTON** GENDER: **F** ADDRESS: **41 GRAPEFRUIT DR.** WEIGHT: **160** HEIGHT: **5′** BMI: **31**

AGE: **53** DX: **TYPE 2 DM, HTN, HYPERLIPIDEMIA, DIABETIC NEUROPATHY** ALLERGY: **PCN** HX: **OBESE, SEDENTARY LIFESTYLE, WIDOWED**

MEDICATION	SIG.	PRESCRIBER	ORIG. DATE	REFILL DATE	REFILL DATE	REFILL DATE	REFILL DATE
Quinapril 20 mg #60	1 bid	Duvalle	6/5	7/3	8/1	9/2	
Lipitor 10 mg #30	1 qd for cholesterol	Duvalle	9/1				
Glucophage 500 mg #60	1 bid	Duvalle	3/2	4/1	5/2	6/3	
Glucophage 500 mg #60	2 bid	Duvalle	7/2	7/14	8/1	8/15	9/1
Metoprolol tartrate 25 mg #60	1 bid	Duvalle	1/15	2/20			
HCTZ 25 mg #30	1 qod	Duvalle	1/15	3/10	5/9	7/10	9/11
Neurontin 100 mg #30	1 tid	Dunston	9/5				

Dr. Ray Duvalle
300 Orange Dr., Dunedin, FL 88811
223-555-0266

Name Gloria Hamilton Date 9/15

Address 41 Grapefruit Dr. Age 53

℞

glucophage 850 mg
#100

Sig: i BID

☑ LABEL

REFILL 3 TIMES PRN NR

Dr. Ray Duvalle

14.21a

Dr. George Dunston
28 Gray St., Dunedin, FL 88811
223-555-1101

Name Gloria Hamilton Date 9/15

Address 41 Grapefruit Dr. Age 53

℞

Effexor XR
75 mgs po
ii QAM #50
Neurontin
~~800 mgs~~
400 mgs po ii TID
#100

Refills NR

Dr. George Dunston

14.21b

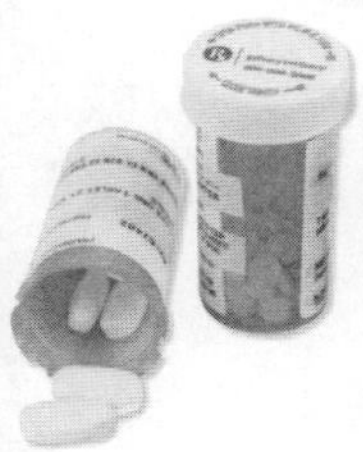

• MISCELLANEOUS PRODUCTS 15

UPON COMPLETION OF THIS CHAPTER, THE STUDENT WILL BE ABLE TO:

- ensure that full patient warnings have been given concerning side effects of antihistamines.
- discuss appropriate weight loss methods with overweight clients.
- illustrate the correct method of instilling ear and eye products, as well as correctly applying topical creams and ointments.
- counsel patients about the increased risk of cardiovascular problems associated with combining oral contraceptives and smoking.
- discuss alternative methods of birth control and their relative effectiveness.
- counsel patients on the potential risks and benefits of miscellaneous products.
- recall all the material needed for appropriate, cautious filling of prescriptions and continue to study into the future to be able to give correct counseling to the patient.
- take charge of his or her profession by staying active, interacting with all people, and never forgetting the awesome power and responsibility that goes with OUR PROFESSION!

DRUG LIST

Allegra
Bactroban
Benadryl
Chlorhexidine
Claritin/Clarinex
Cortisporin Otic
Hycodan
Hydroxyzine
Imitrex and other triptans
Lotrisone
Midrin
Mycolog
Oral contraceptives
Periactin
Phenergan
Silvadene
Sudafed
Tessalon
Treximet
Tussionex
Tussi-Organidin
Tussi-Organidin DM
Xenical, Alli
Xyzal
Zyrtec

• DRUG HOT POINTS

Allegra
Nonsedating H_1 receptor blocker
Rx and OTC

Bactroban
Topical; active against Staph & Strep
Binds to bacterial enzymes, inhibits tRNA, bacterial protein, RNA synthesis
Ointment, cream, intranasal

Benadryl
Different uses: allergy, sleep, sleep aid (OTC), parkinsonism, drug-induced EPS, motion sickness, antitussive
Topically: local anesthetic
Counsel on anticholinergic side effects
Warning: alcohol and driving, Beers list

Chlorhexidine
Topical antimicrobial, oral rinse, hand wash, surgical scrub
Adsorbed onto bacterial cell wall; this results in cell wall leakage & cell death
Caution: mouthwash may discolor teeth
Oral rinse: use after brushing and flossing

Claritin—Regular and D
Long-acting nonsedating antihistamine: Rx and OTC
No significant anticholinergic activity
One (10 mg) daily on empty stomach
Regular tablets and RediTabs (rapidly disintegrating tablets)
Differences in Claritin D (12 and 24 hours)
Compare with Clarinex regular and D

Cortisporin Otic Solution and Suspension
Hydrocortisone, neomycin, polymyxin B
Antimicrobial/anti-inflammatory
Suspension: shake well
Do not use in eye; caution with eye and ear Rxs
Make sure drops are retained in ear

Hycodan
Antitussive; contains hydrocodone with homatropine to discourage deliberate abuse
Take with lots of water for best antitussive effect
Schedule III caution: monitor for abuse

Hydroxyzine
Sedating, anticholinergic, used for anxiety & to potentiate narcotics
Atarax: (HCl), Vistaril PO: (Pamoate)

Imitrex
Serotonin (5-HT_1) agonist; constricts vessels in brain and decreases inflammatory neuropeptides
Tablets, nasal spray, & injection; note maximums
Compare with Zomig, Maxalt, Amerge, Axert, Relpax, Frova
Combination with Naproxen: Treximet

Lotrisone
Antifungal with corticosteroid
Apply sparingly by the "dot method"
Compare with Mycolog

Midrin
Analgesic, sedative, vasoconstrictor
May be discontinued

Oral Contraceptives
Take q 24 h (same time daily)—use other methods of birth control during first week
Antibiotic interaction
Counsel against smoking, missed dose strategy
Vitamin deficiency; take supplements

Periactin
A piperidine H_1 & serotonin antagonist
Antihistamine: counsel on drowsiness
Uses: appetite stimulant, urticaria, anorgasmia due to SSRIs (may reverse effects)
Used as a "street drug" for sexual purposes

Phenergan
Antihistamine with phenothiazine structure
Anticholinergic effects
Use: for motion sickness, antiemetic, for itch
Included in cough syrups as mild antitussive
Boxed warning: avoid in patients younger than 2 years of age

Silvadene
Antimicrobial cream; silver damages cell wall
Warning: sulfa-allergic patients

Sudafed
Sympathomimetic, alpha-adrenergic agonist
Orally taken nasal decongestant
Caution: BPH, DM, HTN, potential for abuse
Limits and documentation for OTC sales

• DRUG HOT POINTS (*continued*)

Tessalon
Local anesthetic, may inhibit cough centrally
Do not chew or dissolve contents in mouth: could cause anesthesia of mouth & choking

Tussionex
Extended-release suspension of hydrocodone & chlorpheniramine (q 12 h dosing)
Indicated for relief of cough & upper respiratory symptoms
Schedule III narcotic; caution for overuse
Must be shaken well
Compare with Tussi-Organidin (and DM)

Xenical
Inhibits GI lipase; obesity management
Blocks absorption of dietary fat
Take only with meals containing 30% fat
Caution: take fat-soluble vitamins at bedtime
Caution: gas and fecal incontinence
OTC: Alli

Zyrtec—Regular and D
The active metabolite of hydroxyzine
Greater affinity for H_1 receptor
Rapid onset, long duration of action
Indicated for urticaria, allergic rhinitis, etc.
Compare with Xyzal

• QUESTIONS TO BE ANSWERED IN PREPARATION FOR CHAPTER 15 LAB

- Describe some common uses for Benadryl.
- Benadryl causes drowsiness. Explain the mechanism.
- Compare the structural formulas of acetylcholine, diphenhydramine, and loratadine. Using the formulas, can you predict which antihistamine has more anticholinergic side effects?
- Describe the differences between Cortisporin otic solution and suspension.
- Explain the mechanism whereby Tussionex, a suspension, is dosed twice a day.
- Why is an anticholinergic agent included in the formula of Hycodan liquid?
- Explain the reason for counseling patients to take Hycodan liquid with lots of water.
- Claritin is available in combination with a decongestant. What are the two strengths? What is the advantage of combining the two agents? How would you fill a prescription written "Claritin D"?
- Describe the various dosage forms of Claritin.
- Name some common uses for cyproheptadine.
- Why should a person who is using Periactin avoid driving?
- Explain the reason why promethazine commonly causes drowsiness.
- Describe the various dosage forms of Phenergan.
- What is the boxed warning for promethazine?
- Your client is taking Sinemet, Symmetrel, Mirapex, and Comtan. Why would it not be appropriate for him to take Phenergan?
- Compare and contrast the different dosages and formulations of Atarax and Vistaril.
- How is Zyrtec related to Atarax?
- What is the brand name of the active isomer of cetirizine?
- To which illegal substance is Sudafed converted?
- Describe the mechanism of action of pseudoephedrine in the treatment of rhinorrhea.
- Explain the reason for insomnia that may occur with the use of Sudafed.
- Illustrate, by sketching a picture of the autonomic receptors in the urinary bladder, trigone, sphincter, and urethra, the effect that Sudafed would have on the flow of urine in an elderly man or woman.
- Describe the mechanism of action of orlistat.
- What is the name of the OTC product that is the same medication as Xenical?
- Give examples of some cautions that must be observed with the use of Xenical.
- What is the reason for the recommendation that a person who is taking Xenical should take vitamin tablets at bedtime?
- In pharmacologic terms, explain how taking an oral antibiotic may decrease the effectiveness of an oral contraceptive, leading to an unwanted pregnancy.
- Give the proposed mechanism of action of Tessalon.
- Name some patient counseling points for the person who is using Peridex.
- Explain the mechanism of action of Bactroban as an antimicrobial agent.
- What are the various commercial forms of Bactroban?
- What are the two therapeutic actions of Lotrisone?
- Give some counseling points for the topical administration of Lotrisone.
- Compare and contrast Imitrex with the other "triptan" medications.
- Describe some contraindications to the use of the "triptan" agents.
- Which "triptan" has the longest duration of action?
- Explain the reason for combining an NSAID (naproxen) with sumatriptan in Treximet.

• MISCELLANEOUS PRODUCTS MEDICATION THERAPY MANAGEMENT QUESTIONS AND COMMENTS

- Your prescription is written for an antihistamine. Let's have a discussion to talk about the appropriate method of taking it and cautions about its action. First, avoid alcohol while taking this product. The major caution is that in combination with medications, or alone, alcohol will cause decreased ability to function either with muscle coordination, movement, or mental processes. This includes driving, cooking, and moving about in general.
- Your narcotic cough syrup is a potent medication. It should not be refilled more than required, based on the dose that was recommended by your doctor. I notice that you are refilling it more frequently than it should be refilled. Would you mind having a conference with us to discuss this? If there are reasons why you must take more than the usual, we can contact the doctor to justify the dose. Then this can be documented and we can make a rational decision about refilling your cough syrup.
- Your prescription rinse product, chlorhexidine, has an important caution. Your doctor has written to follow the instructions on the prescription; however, in order to use it correctly, before using the prescription mouthwash, you should brush your teeth thoroughly, floss well, rinse well with water, and then use the prescription. Do not rinse after using the prescription. This should limit the dark tooth discoloration that sometimes occurs with this product. Also, remember to use it only for the amount of time that the dentist prescribed. Would you like to have a private discussion about oral hygiene products and how to use them?
- Your doctor has prescribed a drug called a "triptan." It is useful in treating migraine headaches. Would you like to have a meeting with us to discuss the things called "triggers"? We can go through our OTC department to mention certain painkillers that might be causing your migraines. Then we can supply you with literature about foods and other substances to avoid.
- We are dispensing your oral contraceptive prescription. If this is the first time for you, it would be useful to have a short meeting about this medication. There are issues that we should reinforce concerning side effects that need to be reported if they occur, as they sometimes do. We can also discuss what to do if a dose is missed. In addition, it would be a good idea for us to call the prescriber to ask if a folic acid vitamin supplement would be good for you to take. It is wise for women of child-bearing age to make sure to take daily folic acid tablets.
- Your prescription is for a cream that is applied to the skin. It contains an anti-inflammatory drug plus another drug to treat fungus or yeast infection. We should discuss the appropriate manner of applying it. This cream should be used only as prescribed by the doctor. It should not be used indefinitely because it could harm the skin over a long period of time. Some physicians recommend the application as the "dot" method, where a small amount, the size of a pea, is applied and then lightly spread over the affected area. Let's have a short meeting to demonstrate with a small amount of cold cream as an example.
- Your doctor has prescribed orlistat. This medication limits the absorption of fats from your food. However, there is an important caution to be aware about. Let's go over the enclosed literature to make sure that you use this medication properly and avoid any problems.
- Your prescription medication Tessalon, or benzonatate capsules, should be swallowed, not chewed or crushed. It contains a local anesthetic. This would not be good if it were released on your tongue or the back of the throat.

  Would you like to meet for a brief private visit now to discuss your cough and the appropriate manner of using your medications? A small amount of water or soothing cough drops taken during the day would also be helpful. At this time, we also should review your total medication profile from all the sources from which you receive medications.
- Now that we have had our medication therapy management meeting, do you feel more empowered to play an active role in your well-being?
- This is not the end of our partnership. We will always be available and welcome your questions.

15.1

PT. NAME: **ALAN HUPP** | AGE: **28** | GENDER: **M** | DX: **ALLERGIES TO HOUSEHOLD DUST, COUGH** | ADDRESS: **54 NORTH AVE.** | ALLERGY: **ASA, PCN** | WEIGHT: **186** | HX: **SMOKER, ETOH** | BMI: **29**

MEDICATION	SIG.	PRESCRIBER	ORIG. DATE	REFILL DATE	REFILL DATE	REFILL DATE	REFILL DATE
Vitamin C 1000 mg #CC	1 tid	OTC	6/18	8/2			
Chlor-Trimeton 12 mg #24	1 bid	OTC	6/18	8/12			
Echinacea 500 mg #C	1 bid	OTC	5/22	7/14			
Nyquil Cold and Flu liquid 10 oz	15 mL (1 tbs) prn hs	OTC	6/4	7/9			

Dr. Daniel Keller
5007 Turtle Drive, Miami, FL 98887
247-555-9876

Name Alan Hupp Date 8/25

Address 54 North Ave. Age 28

℞

Tussionex ℥ IV

Sig ʒ i q12h

Refills 3

Dr. Daniel Keller

DEA# AK1234563

15.1a

Dr. Daniel Keller
5007 Turtle Drive, Miami, FL 98887
247-555-9876

Name Alan Hupp Date 8/25

Address 54 North Ave. Age 28

℞

CLARITIN 10 mg tabs

#15

i p.o. daily on empty stomach

Refill x2

Dr. Daniel Keller

15.1b

15.2

PT. NAME: **KRISTY GREEN** AGE: **35** GENDER: **F** DX: **MORBID OBESITY, TYPE 2 DM, SKIN FUNGUS, GERD, DIARRHEA, ALLERGIES** ADDRESS: **3 EAST CT.** ALLERGY: **NKA** WEIGHT: **350+** HX: **INHERITED A FORTUNE; HAS UNHAPPY, PROMISCUOUS LIFE** HEIGHT: **5′ 10″** BMI: **50**

MEDICATION	SIG.	PRESCRIBER	ORIG. DATE	REFILL DATE	REFILL DATE	REFILL DATE	REFILL DATE
DiaBeta 5 mg #60	1 bid	Griffin	1/5	3/1	4/20		
Lotrisone Cream 45 g	Apply bid	Griffin	3/10	3/22	4/12	4/28	5/8
Lomotil 2.5 mg #60	1 qid prn diarrhea	Griffin	2/19	3/12	4/10	5/9	
Prilosec 20 mg #30	1 qd	Griffin	3/25	4/24			

Dr. Doug Griffin
7611 147th Terrace, Monterey, CA 38411
705-555-6644

Name Kristy Green Date 5/10

Address 3 East Ct. Age 35

℞

Lantus Insulin 54 units HS subQ
2 VIALS +syringes
18 unit q AHS . 64

Refills 0

Dr. Doug Griffin

15.2a

Dr. Doug Griffin
7611 147th Terrace, Monterey, CA 38411
705-555-6644

Name Kristy Green Date 5/10

Address 3 East Ct. Age 35

℞

Benadryl 50 mg #30
i q hs

Refills 0

Dr. Doug Griffin

15.2b

15.3

PT. NAME: **DONNA JONES**	GENDER: **F**	ADDRESS: **7 SOUTH ST.**	WEIGHT: **148**	HEIGHT: **5′ 10″**
AGE: **62**	DX: **MIGRAINES, OA WRIST PAIN, HTN, CHRONIC OTITIS EXTERNA WITH PRURITUS**	ALLERGY: **PCN**	HX: **SOCIAL DRINKER**	

MEDICATION	SIG.	PRESCRIBER	ORIG. DATE	REFILL DATE	REFILL DATE	REFILL DATE	REFILL DATE
Furosemide 20 mg #30	1 qd	Isaacs	5/30				
Cozaar 50 mg #30	1 qd	Isaacs	5/30				
Mobic 7.5 mg #30	1 qd	Isaacs	6/15				
Ecotrin Regular Strength tablets 325 mg #125	1 tid prn	OTC	3/6	5/7	6/14		

Dr. Daniel Keller
5007 Turtle Drive, Miami, FL 98887
247-555-9876

Name Donna Jones Date 6/21

Address 7 South St. Age 62

℞

Midrin
sig: i prn headache
max 5/day
#100
max 12/week

Refills 5

Dr. Daniel Keller

15.3a

Dr. Josephine Norwood
61 Turtle Drive, Miami, FL 98887
247-555-9833

Name Donna Jones Date 6/21

Address 7 South St. Age 62

℞

Cortisporin otic soln
10cc
Sig: iii gtts in
each ear tid PRN itch
ATARAX 25 mg #30
Sig: i q 4-6h PRN
itching

☒ Label

Refill 1 times PRN NR

Dr. Josephine Norwood

15.3b

15.4

PT. NAME: **TERRY SMITH** | AGE: **70** | GENDER: **F** | DX: **HTN, CONSTIPATION, DEPRESSION, UTI, LOW VITAMIN D LEVEL** | ADDRESS: **894 WEST RD.** | ALLERGY: **NKA** | WEIGHT: **142** | HX: **CASHIER IN PHARMACY** | HEIGHT: **5′ 3″**

MEDICATION	SIG.	PRESCRIBER	ORIG. DATE	REFILL DATE	REFILL DATE	REFILL DATE	REFILL DATE
Norvasc 5 mg #30	I q am	Johns	5/30	6/29	7/31	8/23	
Levaquin 500 mg #7	I qd	Johns	7/12				
Paxil 10 mg #90	I tid	Johns	5/4	6/4	6/25	7/13	8/20
St. John's wort 300 mg #60	I bid prn	OTC	2/4	8/1			
Vitamin D 1000 IU capsules #60	I qd	Johns	5/30	7/31	8/20		

Dr. Donna Johns
7000 SW 1st Ave., Santa Fe, NM 54545
766-555-9097

Name Terry Smith Date 8/25
Address 894 West Rd. Age 70

℞
Lotrisone Cream
Sig ī apply BID
affected Areas
15 gm tube

Refills 1

Dr. Donna Johns

15.4a

Dr. Mathew Xavier
5456 Southern Trail, Santa Fe, NM 54545
766-555-6600

Name Terry Smith Date 8/25
Address 894 West Rd. Age 70

℞
Lactulose
15cc po bid
#500cc

Refills 1

Dr. Mathew Xavier

15.4b

15.5 PT. NAME: **ASHLEY MUDD** AGE: **58** GENDER: **F** DX: **GERD, CONJUNCTIVITIS, ANXIETY, INFECTION, COUGH** ADDRESS: **2 JOSEPHINE RD.** ALLERGY: **ASA** WEIGHT: **128** HX: **HAS USED ALKA-SELTZER FOR UPSET STOMACH FOR YEARS** HEIGHT: **5′ 3″**

MEDICATION	SIG.	PRESCRIBER	ORIG. DATE	REFILL DATE	REFILL DATE	REFILL DATE	REFILL DATE
Ativan 0.5 mg #30	I bid prn	Keller	4/4	5/1			
Keflex 500 mg #40	I qid × 10 d	Keller	5/8				
Peridex 0.12% liq. 473 mL	Rinse ud	Barkus, DDS	2/14	5/12			
Pepcid 20 mg #60	I bid	Keller	3/12	4/13	5/18		

Dr. Antonio Madpak
44 SW 5th Ave., Metairie, LA 50023
604-555-2345

Name Ashley Mudd Date 5/29

Address 2 Josephine Rd. Age 58

℞

Tussi organidin DM (syrup)

Sig: i 1/2 tsp tid #6 oz

Refills x 1

Dr. Antonio Madpak

DEA# AM1234563

15.5a

Dr. Augusta Aruna
4466 W Napoleon Ave., Metairie, LA 50023
604-555-9987

Name Ashley Mudd Date 5/29

Address 2 Josephine Rd. Age 58

℞

Cortisporin Ophthalmic soln
#1 bottle

Sig: ii drops in eyes QID

☑ Label

Refill 1 times PRN NR

Dr. Augusta Aruna

15.5b

15.6

PT. NAME: **DONALD WILSON** GENDER: **M** ADDRESS: **62 RATTLER DR.** WEIGHT: **248** HEIGHT: **6′ 4″** BMI: **30**

AGE: **42** DX: **COPD, OA, SKIN INFECTION, MIGRAINES** ALLERGY: **SNAKE VENOM** HX: **RETIRED FOOTBALL COACH, STILL SMOKES 1 PACK/DAY**

MEDICATION	SIG.	PRESCRIBER	ORIG. DATE	REFILL DATE	REFILL DATE	REFILL DATE	REFILL DATE
Z-Pak	Take ud	Honeywell	1/15				
Celexa 20 mg #30	1 daily	Inge	2/1	2/29			
Tylenol No. 3 #25	1 q 6–8 h prn pain	Inge	2/1	3/20			
Theophylline SR 300 mg #C	1 bid	Inge	1/15	4/3			

Dr. Leon Inge
201 Dyson Ave., Tallahassee, FL 99555
408-222-3345

Name Donald Wilson Date 4/5

Address 62 Rattler Dr. Age 42

℞ Bactroban ointment.

Sig: TID to affected area.

Refill 1 times

Dr. Leon Inge

15.6a

Dr. Leon Inge
201 Dyson Ave., Tallahassee, FL 99555
408-222-3345

Name Donald Wilson Date 4/5

Address 62 Rattler Dr. Age 42

℞ Zomig 2.5

i po QD PRN

#twenty-

Refill 2 times

Dr. Leon Inge

15.6b

15.7

PT. NAME: **PAT LARSON** | GENDER: **M** | ADDRESS: **564 E 11TH AVE.** | WEIGHT: **128** | HEIGHT: **5′ 1″**

AGE: **39** | DX: **CHRONIC COUGH, JOCK ITCH, ANXIETY, LOW BACK PAIN** | ALLERGY: **PCN, ASA, EGGS, SHELLFISH** | HX: **SMOKER FOR 24 YEARS**

MEDICATION	SIG.	PRESCRIBER	ORIG. DATE	REFILL DATE	REFILL DATE	REFILL DATE	REFILL DATE
Lorazepam 0.5 mg #60	1 bid prn	Giles	10/12	11/9			
BuSpar 15 mg #60	1/2 tab bid	Giles	11/1				
Tylenol No. 3 #7	1 q 6 h prn pain	Giles	8/12				

Dr. Joseph Giles
2400 E 10th Ave., Denver, CO 44999
998-555-1234

Name Pat Larson Date 11/15

Address 564 E 11th Ave. Age 39

℞

Mycolog Crm
30 g

S [illegible] b.i.d.

Refills PRN

Dr. Joseph Giles

15.7a

Dr. Joseph Giles
2400 E 10th Ave., Denver, CO 44999
998-555-1234

Name Pat Larson Date 11/15

Address 564 E 11th Ave. Age 39

℞

Tussi Organidin DM
Expect.
℥ VI

S [illegible] q 4-6 h prn
cough

Refills: ii

Dr. Joseph Giles

15.7b

15.8

PT. NAME: **JENNIFER ANDERSON** GENDER: **F** ADDRESS: **321 WEST RD.** WEIGHT: **132** HEIGHT: **5′ 6″**

AGE: **42** DX: **GERD, OTITIS EXTERNA, UTI, COUGH, INSOMNIA, BRONCHITIS** ALLERGY: **SULFA** HX: **ETOH; HOBBY: SCUBA DIVING**

MEDICATION	SIG.	PRESCRIBER	ORIG. DATE	REFILL DATE	REFILL DATE	REFILL DATE	REFILL DATE
Aciphex 20 mg #30	1 q am	Yountz	3/18	4/14	5/16		
Restoril 30 mg #30	1 hs prn	Yountz	2/29	3/26	4/27	5/30	
Levaquin 500 mg #7	1 qd	Yountz	6/1				

Dr. Andrew Yountz
888 NW 27th Ave., Miami, FL 98885
247-555-6613

Name Jennifer Anderson Date 6/2

Address 321 West Rd. Age 42

℞

Tessalon Perles
100 mg
Sig: i po tid
#27

Refills: 0

Dr. Andrew Yountz

15.8a

Dr. Andrew Yountz
888 NW 27th Ave., Miami, FL 98885
247-555-6613

Name Jennifer Anderson Date 6/2

Address 321 West Rd. Age 42

℞

Cortisporin otic (clean)
i unit
2 gtts in AS + AD bid

Refill x 2

Dr. Andrew Yountz

15.8b

15.9

PT. NAME: **CAROL SMITH** | GENDER: **F** | ADDRESS: **14 HALL ST.** | WEIGHT: **150** | HEIGHT: **5′ 8″**

AGE: **70** | DX: **HYPOTHYROID, GLAUCOMA, HTN, ANGINA, LEG CRAMPS, COUGH** | ALLERGY: **NKA**

MEDICATION	SIG.	PRESCRIBER	ORIG. DATE	REFILL DATE	REFILL DATE	REFILL DATE	REFILL DATE
Nitro Patch 0.1 mg/hr #30	Apply 1 daily	Yountz	6/22	7/20	8/22		
Procardia XL 30 mg #90	1 daily	Yountz	6/22				
Synthroid 50 mcg #90	1 qd	Yountz	5/2	8/10			
Tylenol PM #C	1 hs	OTC	4/1	7/9			
Timoptic 0.5% 15 mL	1 gtt ou bid	Troutman	3/5	5/9	7/20		

Dr. Andrew Yountz
888 NW 27th Ave., Miami, FL 98885
247-555-6613

Name Carol Smith Date 8/30

Address 14 Hall St. Age 70

℞

Quinine sulfate 324 mg
#100
1 i po hs at direct

Refills 2

Dr. Andrew Yountz

15.9a

Dr. Andrew Yountz
888 NW 27th Ave., Miami, FL 98885
247-555-6613

Name Carol Smith Date 8/30

Address 14 Hall St. Age 70

℞

Phenergan with codeine

6 oz

1 tsp q4h prn cough

Label

Refill 1 times

Dr. Andrew Yountz

15.9b

15.10

PT. NAME: **TERRY KELLER** GENDER: **F** ADDRESS: **6 NW 3RD ST.** WEIGHT: **142** HEIGHT: **5′ 10″**
AGE: **39** DX: **LUMBAR PAIN, URTICARIA, INSOMNIA, PERIODONTAL SURGERY** ALLERGY: **SHELLFISH, ASA** HX: **SMOKER SINCE TEEN YEARS**

MEDICATION	SIG.	PRESCRIBER	ORIG. DATE	REFILL DATE	REFILL DATE	REFILL DATE	REFILL DATE
Advil Liqui-Gel #120	1 q 4 h prn pain	Karig	9/5	10/3	11/1		
Percocet 5/325 mg #12	1–2 q 4–6 h prn pain	McComb, DDS	10/15				
Amoxicillin 500 mg #28	1 tid	McComb DDS	10/15				
Allegra 60 mg #30	1 bid	Karig	8/3				
Ambien 5 mg #50	1 hs prn	Karig	7/5	8/8	9/12	10/20	11/23

Dr. Andrew Karig
100 Calhoun St., Charleston, SC 49999
909-555-5554

Name Terry Keller Date 12/20

Address 6 NW 3rd St. Age 39

℞

Peri Actin 4mg
#30
i AC TID
+ HS

Refills 2

Dr. Andrew Karig

15.10a

Jane McComb, DDS
2 Calhoun St., Charleston, SC 49999
909-555-1234

Name Terry Keller Date 12/20

Address 6 NW 3rd St. Age 39

℞

Peridex rinse

as dir

Refills 2

Jane McComb, DDS

15.10b

15.11

PT. NAME: **ANN RILEY** GENDER: **F** ADDRESS: **564 CAPITOL AVE.** WEIGHT: **128** HEIGHT: **5′ 6″**

AGE: **78** DX: **SEIZURES, HYPOTHYROID, SKIN TEARS, VERTIGO, SKIN STAPH INFECTION** ALLERGY: **NOT ON FILE** HX: **RESIDENT IN ALF**

MEDICATION	SIG.	PRESCRIBER	ORIG. DATE	REFILL DATE	REFILL DATE	REFILL DATE	REFILL DATE
Synthroid 0.125 mg #90	1 qd	Johnson	1/23	4/24	7/20		
Dilantin 100 mg #90	3 hs	Johnson	3/27	4/24	5/28	6/30	7/22
Keflex 250 mg #28	1 qid	Johnson	2/27				

Dr. Kevin Johnson
6258 Garrett St., New York, NY 88364
813-555-7554

Name Ann Riley Date 7/24

Address 564 Capitol Ave. Age 78

℞

Silvadene cream
1lb jar
Sig: bid

☑ Label

Refill ______ times (PRN) NR

Dr. Kevin Johnson

15.11a

Dr. Kevin Johnson
6258 Garrett St., New York, NY 88364
813-555-7554

Name Ann Riley Date 7/24

Address 564 Capitol Ave. Age 78

℞

Phenergan 250mg
#50
Sig: i tab q 4-6h prn

☐ LABEL

REFILL ______ TIMES

Dr. Kevin Johnson

15.11b

15.12

PT. NAME: **JENNA WILLIAMS**	GENDER: **F**	ADDRESS: **321 WEST RD.**	WEIGHT: **110**	BMI: **19**
AGE: **59**	DX: **POOR APPETITE, NERVES, SKIN IRRITATIONS**	ALLERGY: **NKA**	HX: **POOR PATIENT; LIVES ALONE**	

MEDICATION	SIG.	PRESCRIBER	ORIG. DATE	REFILL DATE	REFILL DATE	REFILL DATE	REFILL DATE
Benadryl 25 mg #24	1 hs	OTC	6/3	8/9	10/20		
Vitamin B-1 Tablets 100 mg #C	1 bid	OTC	5/20	7/13	8/22	10/4	11/10
Geritol Tonic Liquid 12 oz	1 tsp bid	OTC	5/20	6/14	7/20	8/22	10/30

Dr. Marilyn Zoeller
45 Alabama Place, Detroit, MI 64789
343-555-7771

Name Jenna Williams Date 11/21

Address 321 West Rd. Age 59

℞

Lotrisone Cream
45gm
Sig: Apply BID

REFILL NR 1 2 3 4 (PRN)

Dr. Marilyn Zoeller

15.12a

Dr. Marilyn Zoeller
45 Alabama Place, Detroit, MI 64789
343-555-7771

Name Jenna Williams Date 11/21

Address 321 West Rd. Age 59

℞

Ciproheptadine 125mg/5ml
1 teasp. Bid
disp 1 pint

Refills NR

Dr. Marilyn Zoeller

15.12b

15.13

PT. NAME: **BARBARA ERICKSON**	GENDER: **F**	ADDRESS: **566 EAST CT.**	WEIGHT: **153**	HEIGHT: **5′ 7″**
AGE: **39**	DX: **MIGRAINES, VAGINAL YEAST INFECTION, UTI**	ALLERGY: **PCN**	HX: **FAST LIFESTYLE**	

MEDICATION	SIG.	PRESCRIBER	ORIG. DATE	REFILL DATE	REFILL DATE	REFILL DATE	REFILL DATE
Excedrin Migraine tablets #100	2 at onset of headache	OTC	3/2	5/2	7/13		
Bactrim DS #20	1 bid	Yountz	3/28				
Cipro 500 mg #14	1 bid × 7 days	Yountz	7/4	8/14			
Diflucan 150 mg #1	Take as 1 dose	Smith	7/31				

Dr. Andrew Yountz
888 NW 27th Ave., Miami, FL 98885
247-555-6613

Name Barbara Erickson Date 8/16

Address 566 East Ct. Age 39

℞

Imitrex 25

#9

1 q6h
prn migraine

Refills 6

Dr. Andrew Yountz

15.13a

Dr. Deborah Smith
9746 Physician's Way, Miami, FL 98885
247-555-6912

Name Barbara Erickson Date 8/16

Address 566 East Ct. Age 39

℞

Ortho Novum 777
Refill x 6
Sig: as directed

REFILL 1 - 2 - 3 - NR - PRN

Dr. Deborah Smith

15.13b

15.14

PT. NAME: **HARRIET WILSON** GENDER: **F** ADDRESS: **23 SOUTH ST.** WEIGHT: **118** HEIGHT: **5′ 2″**
AGE: **72** DX: **IBS, DIZZINESS, COUGH, CONSTIPATION, RHINORRHEA** ALLERGY: **NKA** HX: **SMOKER, 60 PACK-YEARS**

MEDICATION	SIG.	PRESCRIBER	ORIG. DATE	REFILL DATE	REFILL DATE	REFILL DATE	REFILL DATE
Antivert 25 mg #90	I tid for dizziness	Thomas	5/13	6/20			
Levsin 0.125 mg #30	I sl q 6 h prn	Thomas	2/12	3/5	4/30	6/30	7/29
Sudafed 30 mg #24	I prn runny nose	Thomas	1/12	3/12			
Fleet Enema Saline 113 mL #3	I prn bowel movement	OTC	4/20	5/13	6/19	7/25	8/20

Dr. Erin Thomas
988 North Ridge, New York, NY 88364
813-555-7554

Name Harriet Wilson Date 8/23

Address 23 South St. Age 72

℞

Hycodan Liquid
5 cc po Q6h prn
4 oz

Refills 0

Dr. Erin Thomas

15.14a

Dr. Erin Thomas
988 North Ridge, New York, NY 88364
813-555-7554

Name Harriet Wilson Date 8/23

Address 23 South St. Age 72

℞

Scopolamine Patches

#5

Sig: i patch to mastoid process
q 72°

☐ LABEL

REFILL 2 TIMES PRN NR

Dr. Erin Thomas

15.14b

15.15

PT. NAME: **KENNETH KLINE**	GENDER: **M**	ADDRESS: **654 EAGLE RUN**	WEIGHT: **148**	HEIGHT: **5′ 8″**
AGE: **24**	DX: **EARS FILLED WITH FLUID, PRURITUS**	ALLERGY: **NKA**	HX: **SURFER**	

MEDICATION	SIG.	PRESCRIBER	ORIG. DATE	REFILL DATE	REFILL DATE	REFILL DATE	REFILL DATE
Sudafed 30 mg #24	1 tid for sinus	OTC	9/24	10/8	11/18		
Zinc Oxide Ointment 20% 1 oz	Sun protection	OTC	10/10	11/8	11/20		
Diphenhydramine 25 mg capsules #24	2 prn skin itch	OTC	10/1	10/30			

Dr. Lynn Jacobson
4850 NW 10th St., Austin, TX 90902
874-555-8200

Name Kenneth Kline Date 12/1

Address 654 Eagle Run Age 24

℞

① Claritin 1 qd #30

② nasal decongest

Refills 0

Dr. Lynn Jacobson

15.15a

Dr. John Neber
100 NW 10th St., Austin, TX 90902
874-555-9988

Name Kenneth Kline Date 11/21

Address 654 Eagle Run Age 24

℞

Atarax 10mg

#50

Sig: 1 q8h prn itch

(Label)

Refill 1 times

Dr. John Neber

15.15b

15.16

PT. NAME: **KRISTINA O'BRIEN** GENDER: **F** ADDRESS: **7541 NORTH AVE.** WEIGHT: **150** HEIGHT: **5′ 9″**

AGE: **47** DX: **GERD, IBS, N/V** ALLERGY: **CHOCOLATE, DAIRY PRODUCTS** HX: **ETOH**

MEDICATION	SIG.	PRESCRIBER	ORIG. DATE	REFILL DATE	REFILL DATE	REFILL DATE	REFILL DATE
Librax #50	1 tid ac prn	Flaharty	4/12	5/30	6/18	7/20	
Tagamet 800 mg #30	1/2 tab qd	Flaharty	4/2	5/2	6/1	7/1	
Xanax 0.25 mg #30	1/2 tab hs prn	Flaharty	4/2	6/1	8/2		
Pepto-Bismol liquid 12 oz	30 mL prn N/V	OTC	5/10	7/7			

Dr. Janice Flaharty
654 Western Ridge, Austin, TX 90902
954-555-9090

Name Kristina O'Brien Date 8/5

Address 7541 North Ave. Age 47

℞

Phenergan supp
25mg i q 8h prn
vomiting #six

Refills 0

Dr. Janice Flaharty

15.16a

Dr. Lynn Jacobson
4850 NW 10th St., Austin, TX 90902
874-555-8200

Name Kristina O'Brien Date 8/5

Address 7541 North Ave. Age 47

℞

Bentyl 20mg. #20
1 q 6h prn abd. distress

Refills 0

Dr. Lynn Jacobson

15.16b

15.17

PT. NAME: **JOHN TORRES** AGE: **27** GENDER: **M** DX: **ALLERGIES, CONGESTION, COUGH** ADDRESS: **61 GREEN ST.** ALLERGY: **NKA** WEIGHT: **185** HX: **SALESMAN; YEARS OF COLDS** HEIGHT: **6′ 1″**

MEDICATION	SIG.	PRESCRIBER	ORIG. DATE	REFILL DATE	REFILL DATE	REFILL DATE	REFILL DATE
Zyrtec 10 mg #30	1 qd prn	Isaacs	4/12	5/15			
Sudafed 30 mg tablets #24	1 prn	Isaacs	3/15	4/20	5/20		
Benzedrex Inhaler #1	Use prn runny nose	OTC	2/5	3/7	4/6	5/9	
Afrin Nasal Spray 1/2 oz (15 mL)	1 puff bid	OTC	2/5	3/5	4/22	5/28	

Dr. Marilyn Zoeller
45 Alabama Place, Detroit, MI 64789
343-555-7771

Name John Torres Date 5/29

Address 61 Green St. Age 27

℞

Tussionex ℥iii

[illegible]

Refills 2

Dr. Marilyn Zoeller

15.17a

Dr. Marilyn Zoeller
45 Alabama Place, Detroit, MI 64789
343-555-7771

Name John Torres Date 5/29

Address 61 Green St. Age 27

℞

[illegible] D

#20

T [illegible]

Refills 2

Dr. Marilyn Zoeller

15.17b

15.18

PT. NAME: **MARK SWANSON** AGE: **49** GENDER: **M** DX: **MIGRAINE HA, ACNE ROSACEA** ADDRESS: **500 SE 2 ST.** ALLERGY: **NKA** WEIGHT: **142** HX: **YEARS OF MIGRAINE HEADACHES** HEIGHT: **5′ 7″**

MEDICATION	SIG.	PRESCRIBER	ORIG. DATE	REFILL DATE	REFILL DATE	REFILL DATE	REFILL DATE
Excedrin Migraine tablets #C	1–2 prn headache	Zoeller	1/14	2/20			
Tylenol PM caplets #C	1–2 prn	OTC	1/14	2/28			

Dr. Marilyn Zoeller
45 Alabama Place, Detroit, MI 64789
343-555-7771

Name Mark Swanson Date 3/8

Address 500 SE 2 St. Age 49

℞

MAXALT MLT 10mg
DISP: #3
SIG: i PO PRN

Refills 1

Dr. Marilyn Zoeller

15.18a

Dr. Erin Thomas
988 North Ridge, Detroit, MI 64789
343-555-7554

Name Mark Swanson Date 3/8

Address 500 SE 2 St. Age 49

℞

Metro Gel
#1
Sig Apply BID x 5 D

Refill ∅ times

Dr. Erin Thomas

15.18b

15.19

PT. NAME: **JOHN NELSON** GENDER: **M** ADDRESS: **5633 FLAMINGO CT.** WEIGHT: **116** HEIGHT: **5′ 4″**
AGE: **67** DX: **SEIZURES, HTN, CA, THROAT PAIN, N/V** ALLERGY: **NKA** HX: **TERMINALLY ILL HOSPICE PATIENT, THROAT CA**

MEDICATION	SIG.	PRESCRIBER	ORIG. DATE	REFILL DATE	REFILL DATE	REFILL DATE	REFILL DATE
Adalat CC 30 mg #30	1 qd	Bauman	8/17				
ASA 325 mg #C	1 qd	Bauman	8/17				
Atenolol 100 mg #30	1 q am	Bauman	8/17				
Dilantin 100 mg #30	3 hs	Bauman	8/17				
Morphine Sulfate solution 20 mg/mL #30 mL	60 mg sl prn q 2 h	Bauman	8/17				

Dr. Debra Bauman
455 Park Place, St. Louis, MO 48484
358-555-7789

Name John Nelson Date 8/25

Address 5633 Flamingo Ct. Age 67

℞

Hycodan syrup, 1 quart
5cc po q4h

Refills 0

Dr. Debra Bauman

15.19a

Dr. Debra Bauman
455 Park Place, St. Louis, MO 48484
358-555-7789

Name John Nelson Date 8/25

Address 5633 Flamingo Ct. Age 67

℞

Vistaril 25mg
Disp #20
Sig i po QID
prn nausea

Refills 0

Dr. Debra Bauman

15.19b

15.20 PT. NAME: **DEBRA KLAPP** GENDER: **F** ADDRESS: **854 GATOR ST.** WEIGHT: **183** BMI: **21**
AGE: **58** DX: **ULCERATIVE COLITIS, HAY FEVER, ACNE VULGARIS, ALLERGIC RHINITIS** ALLERGY: **NKA** HX: **SMOKES 1 PACK/DAY, HEAVY COFFEE DRINKER**

MEDICATION	SIG.	PRESCRIBER	ORIG. DATE	REFILL DATE	REFILL DATE	REFILL DATE	REFILL DATE
Asacol 400 mg #180	2 tid	Foote	1/13	1/31			
Flagyl 250 mg #90	1 tid	Foote	1/13				

Dr. Chris Doering
400 University Drive, Gainesville, FL 88364
833-555-7666

Name Debra Klapp Date 3/10
Address 854 Gator St. Age 58

℞

Claritin Reditabs
T QD
#30

Refill 0 - 1 - 2 - 3 - 4 - 5 P.R.N.

Dr. Chris Doering

15.20a

Dr. Chris Doering
400 University Drive, Gainesville, FL 88364
833-555-7666

Name Debra Klapp Date 3/10
Address 854 Gator St. Age 58

℞

Retin A .05% cream gels
n x 5 gm

Refills 3

Dr. Chris Doering

15.20b

15.21

PT. NAME: **JOHN FRANKLIN** AGE: **57** GENDER: **M** DX: **HTN, TYPE 2 DM, IBS, ANXIETY, FLATULENCE** ADDRESS: **56 BROAD ST.** ALLERGY: **NKA** WEIGHT: **296** HEIGHT: **6′ 2″** BMI: **38** HX: **OVEREATER ALL OF HIS LIFE; SEDENTARY LIFESTYLE**

MEDICATION	SIG.	PRESCRIBER	ORIG. DATE	REFILL DATE	REFILL DATE	REFILL DATE	REFILL DATE
Glucotrol 5 mg #90	I tab po tid pc	Ham	3/2	4/1	5/20	6/28	
Xanax 0.25 mg #60	I po bid prn	Ham	3/2	5/20			
Precose 50 mg #90	I po with meals	Ham	3/2	4/2	5/5	7/11	
Beano #C	I prn abdominal discomfort	OTC	3/6	4/7	5/8		
Mylanta Gas Tablets #24	I prn gas	OTC	3/6	4/7	5/8	6/30	
Altace 2.5 mg #30	I po q am	Ham	3/2	4/2	5/1	6/1	7/1

Dr. David Ham
300 N 34th St., Philadelphia, PA 88859
247-555-6613

Name John Franklin Date 7/12

Address 56 Broad St. Age 57

℞

XENICAL 120mg
Disp # 90
Sig: i TID AC

☐ LABEL

REFILL (6) SIX TIMES PRN NR

Dr. David Ham

15.21a

Dr. David Ham
300 N 34th St., Philadelphia, PA 88859
247-555-6613

Name John Franklin Date 7/12

Address 56 Broad St. Age 57

℞

ACCUPRIL 10mg
Disp # 30
Sig: i DAILY

☐ LABEL

REFILL (12) TWELVE TIMES PRN NR

Dr. David Ham

15.21b

15.22

PT. NAME: **JANE AYERS** AGE: **52**
GENDER: **F**
DX: **ASTHMA, HTN, LOW BACK PAIN, GUM INFECTION, ANXIETY**
ADDRESS: **2900 KITTRELL AVE.**
ALLERGY: **NKA**
WEIGHT: **146**
HX: **SMOKER, 52.5 PACK-YEARS**
HEIGHT: **5′ 6″**

MEDICATION	SIG.	PRESCRIBER	ORIG. DATE	REFILL DATE	REFILL DATE	REFILL DATE	REFILL DATE
Allegra 60 mg #30	1 qd	Ford	8/3				
Xanax 0.25 mg #33	1 tab q 8 h prn	Ford	8/3				
Prednisone 5 mg #120	2 bid	Ford	8/3				
HCTZ 25 mg #30	1 tab qd	Ford	8/22				
Theophylline SR 300 mg #60	1 bid	Ford	6/29	7/28	8/27		
ProAir HFA MDI 3 × 8.5 g	Use prn SOB	Ford	5/9	6/1	7/1	8/3	9/1

Tamara Jenkins, DMD
555 Hampton Ave., Hampton, VA 33344
399-555-4343

Name Jane Ayers Date 9/9

Address 2900 Kittrell Ave. Age 52

℞

Peridex
16 sixteen oz
Dip proxabrush into peridex and
use on upper left tooth

☐ LABEL

REFILL ____ TIMES

Tamara Jenkins, DMD

15.22a

Dr. Kathy Ford
28 Red Road, Hampton, VA 33344
399-555-1237

Name Jane Ayers Date 9/9

Address 2900 Kittrell Ave. Age 52

℞

① Vicodin ī qHS
PRN #30 (thirty)

② Celebrex 100 mg
BID #60

N.R.

Dr. Kathy Ford

15.22b

15.23

PT. NAME: **MARGIE RODRIGUEZ** GENDER: **F** ADDRESS: **501 PENN ST.** WEIGHT: **140** HEIGHT: **5′ 7″**

AGE: **67** DX: **SKIN TEARS, MIGRAINES, UTI, SEASONAL ALLERGIC RHINITIS, LEG WOUND, POSTMENOPAUSAL SYMPTOMS** ALLERGY: **POLLEN, CATS, DOGS** HX: **RETIRED PHARMACIST**

MEDICATION	SIG.	PRESCRIBER	ORIG. DATE	REFILL DATE	REFILL DATE	REFILL DATE	REFILL DATE
Imitrex 25 mg #9	1 tab daily	Spadaro	1/21	2/18	3/10	5/2	6/1
Diazepam 5 mg #10	1 prn	Spadaro	1/7	2/5	3/9	6/15	
Premarin Vaginal Cream 42.5 g	Apply PV biw	Spadaro	2/28				
Noroxin 400 mg #10	1 tab bid	Spadaro	3/10				
Prempro 0.45/1.5 mg #28	1 qd ud	Spadaro	3/9	4/8	5/7	6/9	6/29

Dr. Don Spadaro
3410 S Markham, Little Rock, AR 55775
334-555-7654

Name Margie Rodriguez Date 7/2

Address 501 Penn St. Age 67

℞

Silvadene Cream
apply to medial leg
wound only BID
45 gram

LABEL ______
REFILL 0
DEA NO. ______

Dr. Don Spadaro

15.23a

Dr. Don Spadaro
3410 S Markham, Little Rock, AR 55775
334-555-7654

Name Margie Rodriguez Date 7/2

Address 501 Penn St. Age 67

℞

Allegra D
#30
1 tab BID no generic

☐ Label
Refill 6 times PRN NR

Dr. Don Spadaro

15.23b

15.24

PT. NAME: **ADAM H. CAT (FELINE)** GENDER: **M** ADDRESS: **9 NOVA DR.** WEIGHT: **NOT ON FILE**
AGE: **15** DX: **HYPERTHYROID, CARDIAC ARRHYTHMIA, CONJUNCTIVITIS, FUNGAL SKIN RASH** ALLERGY: **DOGS** HX: **ALLEY CAT/PET**

MEDICATION	SIG.	PRESCRIBER	ORIG. DATE	REFILL DATE	REFILL DATE	REFILL DATE	REFILL DATE
Tapazole 10 mg #C	Give 1/2 tab daily	Hardigan	8/9				
Lotrisone Cream 15 g	Apply to affected areas qd	Hardigan	8/9				

Will Hardigan, DVM
3200 S University Dr., Davie, FL 98885
247-555-6613

Name Adam H. Cat (Feline) Date 9/9
Address 9 Nova Dr. Age 15

℞

Atenolol suspension 12.5mg/ml 2oz
sig: 1/2 ml p.o. q. 24hrs

MAY BE REFILLED
0 – 1 – (2) – 3 – 4 – PRN

REG. NO. ______

Will Hardigan, DVM

15.24a

Will Hardigan, DVM
3200 S University Dr., Davie, FL 98885
247-555-6613

Name Adam H. Cat (Feline) Date 9/9
Address 9 Nova Dr. Age 15

℞

TOBRADEX
SIG ii GTTS TID
x 5 DAYS.
#5cc

Label

Refill ______ times

Will Hardigan, DVM

15.24b

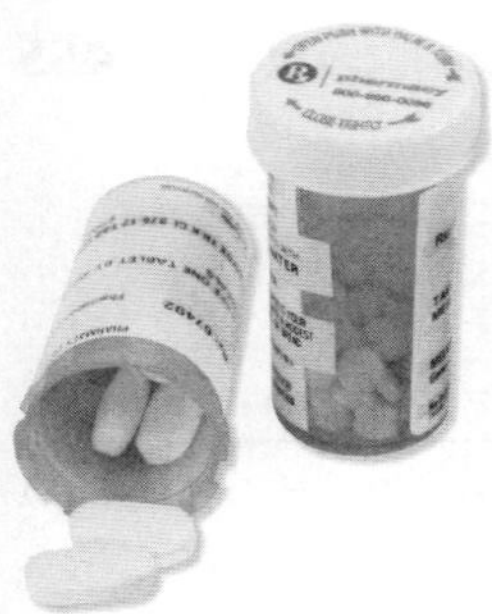

Appendix A • Supplemental Prescriptions

Appendix A

Dr. Richard Penno
488 North Ridge, New York, NY 88364
813-555-7554

Name Harriet Kronkheit Date 3/10

Address 854 Maroon St. Age 48

℞

Humulin 70/30
#2 vial

Insulin syringe 50U/cc
#100

☐ Label

Refill PRN times

Dr. Richard Penno

A.1

Dr. Dennis Wortheng
11 North Ridge, New York, NY 88364
813-555-8554

Name Harris Haverstraw Date 3/10

Address 84 Green St. Age 58

℞

Glucotrol 10 mg #30
Give 1 tablet
1x day

Refills 3

Dr. Dennis Wortheng

A.2

Appendix A

Dr. Dave Kingman
10 North Ridge, New York, NY 88364
813-555-7099

Name Al Smith Date 3/10

Address 668-65 St St. Age 77

℞

[illegible]
[illegible] #30
[illegible]

REFILL TIMES

LABEL ☐

DEA NUMBER

Dr. Dave Kingman

A.3

Dr. Robert Banting
9998 North Ridge, New York, NY 88364
813-555-7111

Name Alf Landon Date 3/10

Address 99 President St. Age 88

℞

[illegible] [illegible]
#28
[illegible]
Every month

☑ LABEL

REFILL 11 TIMES

Dr. Robert Banting

A.4

Appendix A

Dr. Martin Schwartz
98 North Ridge, New York, NY 88364
813-455-7554

Name Mary Green Date 3/10

Address 81 SW 6th St. Age 70

℞

Coumadin 5 mg

#30

Sig: i p.o. daily

☑ Label

Refill ______ times (PRN) NR

Dr. Martin Schwartz

A.5

Dr. Marie Schwartz
988 North Ridge, New York, NY 88364
813-455-7554

Name Joe Hatton Date 3/10

Address 877 NW 3rd St. Age 78

℞

Synthroid 0.1

i qd #100

Refill 3 times

Dr. Marie Schwartz

A.6

Appendix A

Dr. Dave Johnson
988 North Ridge, New York, NY 88364
813-555-7000

Name Ronald Dickstein   Date 3/10

Address 85 Collins Ave.   Age 49

℞

Zantac 150mg
Sig: 150mg po BID
#60

Refills 3

Dr. Dave Johnson

A.7

Dr. Dan Avilla
1 North Ridge, New York, NY 88364
813-555-7098

Name Harold Gluck   Date 3/10

Address 22 NW 44th St.   Age 66

℞

Remeron 30mg i qhs #15

Xanax 2mg i tid #60

Elavil 100mg i qhs #15

Advil 200mg [illegible] #100

Zoloft 50mg i qd #15

Ambien 10mg ii qhs #30

Dr. Dan Avilla

A.8

Appendix A

Dr. Rod Presnelli
8 North Ridge, New York, NY 88364
813-555-7004

Name John Taylor Date 3/10

Address 54 Tallahassee St. Age 98

℞

BACTRIM SS tabs

#60

i p.o. BID

Refill one times

Dr. Rod Presnelli

A.9

Dr. Jameson Powers
77 North Ridge, New York, NY 88364
813-555-0000

Name Andrew Robeson Date 3/10

Address 854 Maroon St. Age 38

℞

Dyazide

#30

Sig: i daily 4-5 days of each month

LABEL AS SUCH

Refill: 0 - (2) - 3 - 12 - P.R.N.

Dr. Jameson Powers

A.10

Appendix A

Dr. Nellie Bly
11 North Ridge, New York, NY 88364
813-555-4444

Name Gladys Gooding Date 3/10

Address 22 Bedford Ave. Age 89

℞ Metoprolol 50 mg
#90
1/2 BID
3 mo supply

☑ Label

Refill 2 times

Dr. Nellie Bly

A.11

Dr. Milton Stock
90 North Ridge, New York, NY 88364
813-555-1238

Name Bruce Edwards Date 3/10

Address 80 DeKalb Ave. Age 58

℞ Ventolin Spray
use as directed

☐ Label

Refill ______ times (PRN) NR

Dr. Milton Stock

A.12

Appendix A

Dr. Karen Daniel
93 North Ridge, New York, NY 88364
813-555-0909

Name Julio Rodriguez Date 3/10

Address 89 W 4th St. Age 68

℞ Thyroid gr ii

#100

Sig: i daily

☑ LABEL

REFILL 0 TIMES

Dr. Karen Daniel

A.13

Dr. Leanne Lai
91 North Ridge, New York, NY 88364
813-555-7989

Name Joe Spillane Date 3/10

Address 84 University St. Age 55

℞ Ativan 1 mg

#30

i at hs

☒ LABEL

REFILL Two TIMES PRN NR

Dr. Leanne Lai

A.14

Appendix A

Dr. Justin Molitano
99 North Ridge, New York, NY 88364
813-555-7144

Name Mary Daddio Date 3/10

Address 1666 Benson Ave. Age 55

℞

Oxybutynin 5 mg

#100

Sig: i TID

☐ Label

Refill PRN times

Dr. Justin Molitano

A.15

Dr. Anthony Lagano
77 North Ridge, New York, NY 88364
813-555-6666

Name Santo Marcucci Date 3/10

Address 1433 Bay 14 St. Age 66

℞

[illegible] i mg

Disp: #90

Sig: i po TID

REFILL 1☐ 2☐ 3☐ 4☐ NR☒
LABEL ☐
MEDICALLY NECESSARY ☐
DEA# ________

Dr. Anthony Lagano

A.16

Appendix A

Dr. Richard Angorno
77 North Ridge, New York, NY 88364
813-555-9999

Name David Brushwood Date 3/10

Address 88 SW 6th St. Age 72

℞

ECDEPASC 5g II 70
i po bid

LABEL CONTENTS

REFILL 1 2 3 NR PRN

Dr. Richard Angorno

A.17

Dr. Ozzie Araujo
66 North Ridge, New York, NY 88364
813-555-7588

Name Wayne Reitz Date 3/10

Address 554 Archer St. Age 77

℞

Dilantin 50mg
#30
i at 3PM c a
100mg cap

Refills 3

Dr. Ozzie Araujo

A.18

Appendix A

Dr. Gary Yee
66 North Ridge, New York, NY 88364
813-555-1111

Name Haywood Sullivan Date 3/10

Address 66 SW 4th St. Age 55

℞

Imdur 60
1 T daily
150

REFILL 1 - 2 - 3 - NR - (PRN)
LABEL WITH NAME OF MEDICATION
DISPENSED

Dr. Gary Yee

A.19

Dr. William Hadley
988 North Ridge, New York, NY 88364
813-555-7000

Name Barnett Borrego Date 3/10

Address 2500 Marble Ave. Age 46

℞

Aciphex 20
hs

60

Label

Refill ______ times

Dr. William Hadley

A.20

Appendix A

Dr. Steven Grossman
99 North Ridge, New York, NY 88364
813-555-7500

Name William Lindsey Date 3/10

Address 85 Surf Ave. Age 55

℞

Lithium CO_3 300mg #150

i PO 5x/day

☐ Label

Refill 6 times

Dr. Steven Grossman

A.21

Dr. Mary Campbell
55 North Ridge, New York, NY 88364
813-555-7777

Name Doris Feinstein Date 3/10

Address 80 Taylor St. Age 77

℞

ALBUTEROL MDI.

2 PUFFS QID

1 CANISTER

Label

Refill ______ times

Dr. Mary Campbell

A.22

Appendix A

Dr. Henry Cohen
66 North Ridge, New York, NY 88364
813-555-1111

Name Stanley Feifer Date 3/10

Address 88 Stillman Ave. Age 28

℞

Ativan 1mg #60

BID

Refill X times

Dr. Henry Cohen

A.23

Dr. Judy Castellanos
99 North Ridge, New York, NY 88364
813-555-2222

Name Robert Bellantone Date 3/10

Address 88 Info Ave. Age 66

℞

Valium 2, # 20

Sig: i q6h prn vertigo

REFILL 1 - 2 - 3 - NR - PRN

LABEL WITH NAME OF MEDICATION

DISPENSED

Dr. Judy Castellanos

A.24

Appendix A

Dr. Roberto Mangiore
99 North Ridge, New York, NY 88364
813-555-6275

Name Denise Balog Date 3/10

Address 854 Utopia St. Age 18

℞

Clarinex 5mg

i T, 1D

#110

Refills 3

Dr. Roberto Mangiore

A.25

Dr. Marco Gillespie
88 North Ridge, New York, NY 88364
813-555-9876

Name Veronica Novy Date 3/10

Address 55 Jamaica St. Age 58

℞

Micronase 5mg

#75

Sig: 2½ tab PO qd

Refills 3

Dr. Marco Gillespie

A.26

Appendix A

Dr. Richard Maddox
910 North Ridge, New York, NY 88364
813-555-1685

Name Timothy Bloom Date 3/10

Address 510 Buies St. Age 88

℞

Lamisil Cr

#I

apply tid

Refills 3

Dr. Richard Maddox

A.27

Dr. Emanuel Dilibert
1695 North Ridge, New York, NY 88364
813-555-1697

Name Robert Garrett Date 3/10

Address 910 NE 61st St. Age 44

℞

Synthroid .2

#100

1 qd

Refills 3

Dr. Emanuel Dilibert

A.28

Appendix A

Dr. Walter Campbell
919 North Ridge, New York, NY 88364
813-555-1123

Name Kim Brouwer Date 3/10

Address 7030 Beard St. Age 33

℞

[illegible]

Librax #50

Sig T cap PO 1/2 hour AC

Refills 3

Dr. Walter Campbell

A.29

Dr. Frederick Eckler
55 North Ridge, New York, NY 88364
813-555-8888

Name Tina Brock Date 3/10

Address 44 NW 5th St. Age 22

℞

Zoloft 50mg

1 qd #30

Refills 3

Dr. Fred Eckler

A.30

Appendix A

Dr. Marvin Roth
988 North Ridge, New York, NY 88364
813-555-7000

Name Harriet Brown Date 3/10

Address 11 Canal St. Age 78

℞

Periactin 4mg
#30

i po q h

Refills 3

Dr. Marvin Roth

A.31

Dr. Agnes Cooper
55 North Ridge, New York, NY 88364
813-555-7777

Name Dennis Williams Date 3/10

Address 33 Paine St. Age 38

℞

prednisone 10mg
XXX (30)
Sig i q.o.D.

NOT VALID FOR CLASS II DRUGS

☒ LABEL

REFILL 2 TIMES PRN NR

Dr. Agnes Cooper

A.32

Appendix A

Dr. Calvin Peterson
44 North Ridge, New York, NY 88364
813-555-6469

Name Agnes Harrington Date 3/10

Address 343 Sudro St. Age 68

℞

Cortisporin Otic Susp
#10cc
Sig: gtts V AD TID

Refills 3

Dr. Calvin Peterson

A.33

Dr. Clarence Schnell
7000 North Ridge, New York, NY 88364
813-555-3636

Name Kathy Gardner Date 3/10

Address 701 NE 1st St. Age 58

℞

Diabeta 5mg
#100

Sig 1/2 qd

Refill 3 times

Dr. Clarence Schnell

A.34

Appendix A

Dr. Ronald Bryant
66 North Ridge, New York, NY 88364
813-555-0404

Name Donald Stansloski Date 3/10

Address 9898 NE 44th Ave. Age 77

℞

ZAMIXYUN 2.5 g

100

1 tb3 MWF

☐ LABEL

REFILL 6 TIMES PRN NR

Dr. Ronald Bryant

A.35

Dr. Paul Smithe
66 North Ridge, New York, NY 88364
813-555-7770

Name Pauline Lucas Date 3/10

Address 555 S Main St. Age 82

℞

Vancomycin 125mg
Disp# 40 (forty)
Sig: i p.o. QID X 10days

☐ LABEL

REFILL 0 TIMES PRN NR

Dr. Paul Smithe

A.36

Appendix A

Dr. James Cassady
44 North Ridge, New York, NY 88364
813-555-2266

Name John Bauer Date 3/10

Address 854 Columbus St. Age 66

℞

Captopril 25
1/2 po BID
#100

Refills 3

Dr. James Cassady

A.37

Dr. Henry Cable
9 North Ridge, New York, NY 88364
813-555-2588

Name Kristin Casper Date 3/10

Address 500 W 12th St. Age 66

℞

Vistaril 50mg
Disp #30#
Sig: i or ii po q HS prn sleep

Refills 3

Dr. Henry Cable

A.38

Appendix A

Dr. Jeff Dalton
67 North Ridge, New York, NY 88364
813-555-7099

Name Carolyn Brackett Date 3/10

Address 866 Ohio St. Age 55

℞

		Amt.	Refill
℞ 1	Vicoprofen	60	∅
Sig:	i PO q12	Sixty	
℞ 2	Celebrex 100 mg	60	∅
Sig:	i PO BID		

Dr. Jeff Dalton

A.39

Dr. Frank Pope
44 North Ridge, New York, NY 88364
813-555-6622

Name John Coyle Date 3/10

Address 55 Benson Ave. Age 77

℞

Synthroid .175

\# 90

i Daily

Refills 3

Dr. Frank Pope

A.40

Appendix A

Dr. David Acosta
67004 North Ridge, New York, NY 88364
813-555-4372

Name Carol Caperel Date 3/10

Address 77 Rhizome St. Age 66

℞

[illegible]

Refills 3

Dr. David Acosta

A.41

Dr. Helen Feuer
820 North Ridge, New York, NY 88364
813-555-7554

Name Harriet Browning Date 3/10

Address 854 Maroon St. Age 48

℞

prilosec 20mg
#30
1 tablet po qd

cardizem CD 180mg
#50
1 tablet po qd

Refills 3

Dr. Helen Feuer

A.42

Appendix A

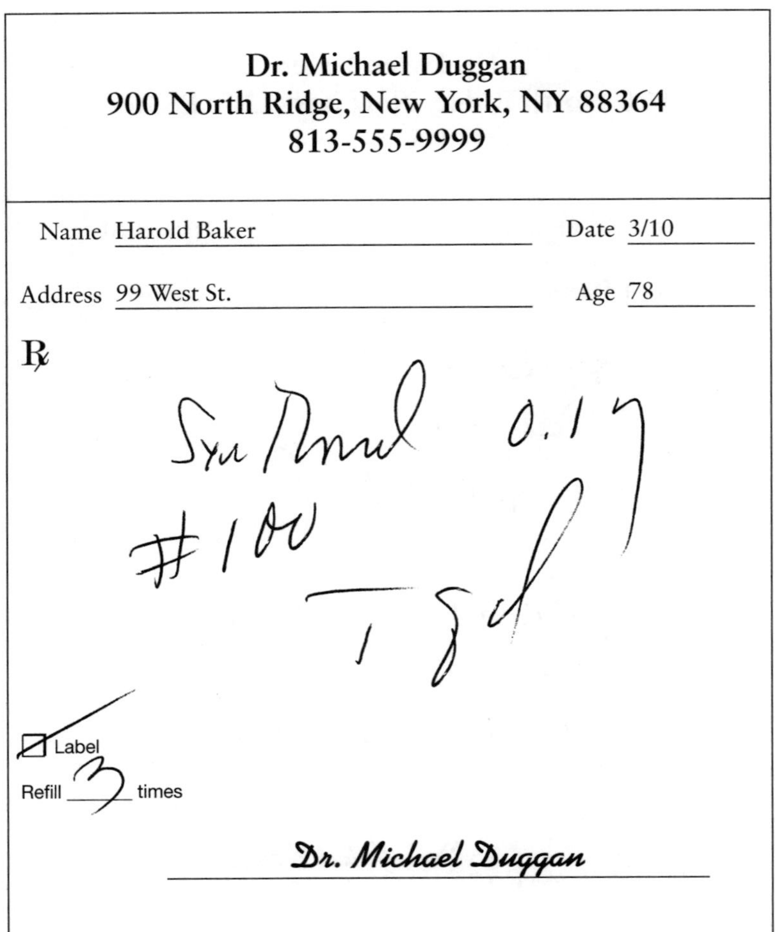

Dr. Michael Duggan
900 North Ridge, New York, NY 88364
813-555-9999

Name Harold Baker Date 3/10

Address 99 West St. Age 78

℞

#100

Label

Refill 3 times

Dr. Michael Duggan

A.43

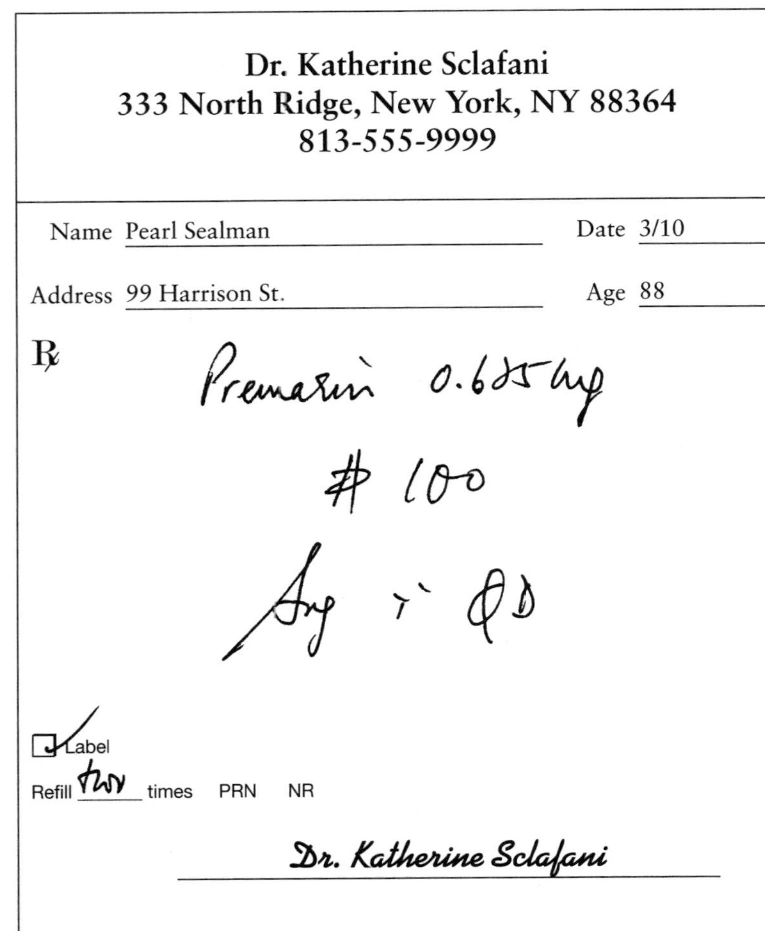

Dr. Katherine Sclafani
333 North Ridge, New York, NY 88364
813-555-9999

Name Pearl Sealman Date 3/10

Address 99 Harrison St. Age 88

℞

Premarin 0.625 mg

#100

Label

Refill two times PRN NR

Dr. Katherine Sclafani

A.44

Appendix A

Dr. Robert Bass
988 North Ridge, New York, NY 88364
813-555-7554

Name Harmon Kiljoy Date 3/10

Address 22 Washington St. Age 88

℞

ZESToretic 10-12.5
#100

Sig 1 tablet p day

☐ Label

Refill ______ times PRN NR

Dr. Robert Bass

A.45

Dr. Erin Grinwal
66 North Ridge, New York, NY 88364
813-555-7001

Name George Smathing Date 3/10

Address 44 West Lake Dr. Age 81

℞

Bactrim DS
6

Sig 1 bid x 3 days

☐ Label

Refill ______ times

Dr. Erin Grinwal

A.46

Appendix A

Dr. George Bouchard
77 North Ridge, New York, NY 88364
813-555-6556

Name Mark Lafebre Date 3/10

Address 22 St. Marie St. Age 78

℞

Tamoxifen 10mg

i PO BID

#100

Refill 5 times

Dr. George Bouchard

A.47

Dr. Harry Schleussler
66 North Ridge, New York, NY 88364
813-555-1230

Name Grace Frank Date 3/10

Address 55 N Park Slope Age 67

℞

LABEL

Midrin #30

i Tab P.O. Q4H PRN

Refills 3

Dr. Harry Schleussler

A.48

Appendix A

Dr. Patrick McCoy
55 North Ridge, New York, NY 88364
813-555-7557

Name Gilbert Frank Date 3/10

Address 4100 Aston Blvd. Age 77

℞

Tobradex eye drops
1 drop TID

Refill [illegible] times

Dr. Patrick McCoy

A.49

Dr. Moses Bromley
1 North Ridge, New York, NY 88364
813-555-9999

Name Harriet Carnover Date 3/10

Address 28 Belle Dr. Age 90

℞

K Dur 10 meq
Disp #14
Sig one daily

Refills 3

Dr. Moses Bromley

A.50

Appendix A

Dr. Ronald Krakow
13 North Ridge, New York, NY 88364
813-555-1313

Name Dove Harnick Date 3/10

Address 45 NE 33rd Ave. Age 44

℞

Leukeran 2 mg #32 tabs

Sig: 8 tabs daily for 4 days

N.R.
P.R.N.
REFILL ____ TIMES

Dr. Ronald Krakow

A.51

Dr. Dave Samples
9888 North Ridge, New York, NY 88364
813-555-7978

Name Herbert Rudolph Date 3/10

Address 9500 NE 2nd Ave. Age 68

℞

Elavil 20mg

#30

S i hs

Refill 3 times

Dr. Dave Samples

A.52

Appendix A

Dr. Gaudy Sotolongo
55 North Ridge, New York, NY 88364
813-555-7557

Name David Brushwood   Date 3/10

Address 88 SW 6th St.   Age 77

℞

Glucophage 500mg
i bid c̄

☐ Label

Refill ______ times (PRN) NR

Dr. Gaudy Sotolongo

A.53

Dr. Rachel Molino
1 North Ridge, New York, NY 88364
813-555-9999

Name William Lindsey   Date 3/10

Address 85 Surf Ave.   Age 90

℞

Glyburide 5mg tab
#100
i daily.

Label yes

Refill 1x 1yr.

Dr. Rachel Molino

A.54

Appendix A

Dr. Branford Wildcrest, Jr.
13 North Ridge, New York, NY 88364
813-555-1313

Name Denise Balog Date 3/10

Address 854 Utopia St. Age 44

℞

Betapace 80 mg i po BID #60
Digoxin 0.25 mg i po QD #30
Coumadin 4 mg i po QD #30
Clonidine 0.2 mg i po TID #90

Dr. Branford Wildcrest, Jr.

A.55

Dr. Glenn Packer
9888 North Ridge, New York, NY 88364
813-555-7978

Name Carolyn Brackett Date 3/10

Address 866 Ohio St. Age 68

℞

Asacol 400 mg
#240
d: iiii po BID

Refills 3

Dr. Glenn Packer

A.56

Appendix A

Dr. Glenn Davis
55 North Ridge, New York, NY 88364
813-555-7557

Name Paul Lucas   Date 3/10

Address 555 S Main St.   Age 77

℞

Buspar 10 mg
Sig: i tab po q AM
Disp #60

☐ LABEL
REFILL Ø TIMES

Dr. Glenn Davis

A.57

Dr. Don Blanchard
1 North Ridge, New York, NY 88364
813-555-9999

Name Pearl Sealman   Date 3/10

Address 99 Harrison St.   Age 90

℞

SYNTHROID 0.1 mg
Sig i PO QD
Disp #30

Label
Refill x3 Times

Dr. Don Blanchard

A.58

Appendix A

Dr. Lawrence Krinsky
13 North Ridge, New York, NY 88364
813-555-1313

Name Harold Baker Date 3/10

Address 99 West St. Age 44

℞

Restoril 15

T po HS PRN

#30

Refills 3

Dr. Lawrence Krinsky

A.59

Dr. Burton Travis
9888 North Ridge, New York, NY 88364
813-555-7978

Name Dennis Williams Date 3/10

Address 33 Paine St. Age 68

℞

Eskalith CR. 450mg

#100

Sig i q AM c 1½ gls.

☒ Label

Refill 3 times PRN NR

Dr. Burton Travis

A.60

Appendix A

Dr. Leon Goldman
99 North Ridge, New York, NY 88364
813-555-9990

Name Ozzie Lam Date 3/10

Address 99 Inside Blvd. Age 88

℞

[illegible] T̄ 20
BID #30

☐ Label

Refill 3 times

Dr. Leon Goldman

A.61

Dr. Jeff Halpern
1 North Ridge, New York, NY 88364
813-555-9999

Name Nelson Randolph Date 3/10

Address 28 Belle Dr. Age 44

℞

Viagra 100mg
#15
Sig i qd prn

Refills 3

Dr. Jeff Halpern

A.62

Appendix A

Dr. Nina Elan
88 North Ridge, New York, NY 88364
813-555-8880

Name Harry Koch Date 3/10

Address 88 Outside Blvd. Age 66

℞

Tegretol 100g
100
ī tid

Refills 3

Dr. Nina Elan

A.63

Dr. Joel Graff
9888 North Ridge, New York, NY 88364
813-555-7978

Name Daniel Lawson Date 3/10

Address 9500 NE 2nd Ave. Age 68

℞

Amoxicillin 500 mg po Tid
for 7 days.

#21

Refills 3

Dr. Joel Graff

A.64

Appendix A

Dr. Glenn Davis
99 North Ridge, New York, NY 88364
813-555-9990

Name Allen Banker　　Date 3/10

Address 99 28th Blvd.　　Age 78

℞

Sinemet CR 50-200
(200 tablets)

Sinemet 25-100
(200 tablets)

Dr. Glenn Davis

A.65

Dr. Moses Bromley
1 North Ridge, New York, NY 88364
813-555-9999

Name Chester Gold　　Date 3/10

Address 281 31st Dr.　　Age 90

℞

Pyridium 200 mg
9

Sig i tid

☐ Label

Refill ______ times

Dr. Moses Bromley

A.66

Appendix A

Dr. Don Blanchard
88 North Ridge, New York, NY 88364
813-555-8880

Name Sherwood Braun   Date 3/10

Address 88 89th Blvd.   Age 66

℞

Vasotec 5 mg
#30
Sig: one daily

Refills 3

Dr. Don Blanchard

A.67

Dr. Dave Samples
9888 North Ridge, New York, NY 88364
813-555-7978

Name Willie Hardigan   Date 3/10

Address 9500 NE 76th Ave.   Age 68

℞

Glucotrol XL 5 mg
#100
one bid

☐ Label

Refill 3 times

Dr. Dave Samples

A.68

Appendix A

Dr. Lawrence Krinsky
28 Lakefront Place, Cincinnati, OH 44499
404-555-7777

Name Vanessa Fleming Date 3/8

Address 55 Koenig Ave. Age 33

℞

Celebrex 200 mg
60

☐ LABEL

REFILL ______ TIMES

Dr. Lawrence Krinsky

A.69

Dr. Lawrence Krinsky
28 Lakefront Place, Cincinnati, OH 44499
404-555-7777

Name Herb Teitler Date 3/8

Address 231 Second Ave. Age 33

℞

Dilantin 100 mg
100
U.D

Dilantin 50 mg
100
U.D

☐ Label

Refill ______ times PRN NR

Dr. Lawrence Krinsky

A.70

Appendix A

Dr. Rosemary Finkello
888 NW 27th Ave., Miami, FL 98885
247-555-6613

Name Margie Fritz Date 5/10

Address 84 Farragut St. Age 72

℞

(1) Lipitor 10mg i po qd #30
(2) Synthroid 0.112mg i po qd #30
(3) Triamterene/HCTZ 75/50mg i po qd #30

Refills 3

Dr. Rosemary Finkello

A.71

Dr. Debra Lawson
888 NW 27th Ave., Miami, FL 98885
247-555-6613

Name Virginia Millhouse Date 12/15

Address 678 Apple St. Age 49

℞

Amoxicillin Cap.
250

Sig: i 3 Times daily
as needed for
cloudy urine for 3 days
Disp. # 30

☐ Label

Refill 1 times

Dr. Debra Lawson

A.72

Appendix A

Dr. Lawrence Braun
28 Lakefront Place, Cincinnati, OH 44499
404-555-7777

Name Harriet Brown Date 3/1

Address 11 Canal St. Age 66

℞

Mellaril 50 mg
Disp # 60
Sig: one in AM + ii HS

REFILL X1 TIMES

Dr. Lawrence Braun

A.73

Dr. Alfred Albano
28 Lakefront Place, Cincinnati, OH 44499
404-555-7777

Name Kim Brouwer Date 3/1

Address 7030 Beard St. Age 75

℞

NTG gr 1/150
Disp #C
Sig T SL prn

Dr. Alfred Albano

A.74

Appendix A

Dr. Jerry Fields
28 Lakefront Place, Cincinnati, OH 44499
404-555-7777

Name Bob Andrews Date 3/8

Address 877 Eleventh St. Age 33

℞

Cap diphenhydramine
50 mg
#100
S - ii @ HS.

☒ LABEL

REFILL 1 TIMES

Dr. Jerry Fields

A.75

Dr. Bob Grayson
28 Lakefront Place, Cincinnati, OH 44499
404-555-7777

Name Vanessa Wright Date 3/8

Address 77 NW 10th St. Age 59

℞

Oph Sol: Trusopt 2%
Sig i gtt OU TID

NON REP.

REFILL 1 2 3 (4)

Dr. Bob Grayson

A.76

Appendix A

Dr. John Allison
33 NW 2nd Pl., Brooklyn, NY 44040
404-555-4444

Name Harry Miller   Date 3/1

Address 44 NW 55 St.   Age 66

℞

Ketek 400 mg #10
Sig 1 tab p.o. BID.

℞ Flonase
Sig 1 puff in each nostril after a hot shower

Dr. John Allison

A.77

Dr. Marie Goldman
77 NE 88th St., Miami, FL 33399
305-555-6543

Name Laura Turner   Date 3/1

Address 44 NW Flamingo Dr.   Age 45

℞

Clinoril 200 mg #60
Sig: i BID p̄ breakfast & dinner

LABEL . ✓ . . . .
REFILL . . ×3 . . . . .
NO REFILL . . . .
SUBSTITUTION ALLOWED . . . .
PRIOR APPROVAL REQUIRED . . . .

Dr. Marie Goldman

A.78

Appendix A

Dr. Marvin Lane
99 NW 125th St., Cincinnati, OH 44499
404-555-3333

Name Baron Capizzi Date 3/8

Address 16799 NW Palm Dr. Age 77

℞

Cosopt Eye Gtts
Disp: OP
Si: 1gtt ou bid

REFILL ___ PRN
___ TIMES
LABEL ___ YES
___ NO

Dr. Marvin Lane

A.79

Dr. Barry Blondel
99 NW 55th Ave., Cincinnati, OH 44499
404-555-4444

Name Debbie Langford Date 3/8

Address 99 University Dr. Age 78

℞

Tobrex Ophthalmic Drops
Sig 1gtt OS q1h on Monday,
q2h Tuesday & Wednesday
No refill

Dr. Barry Blondel

A.80

Appendix A

Dr. Charles Furillo
3600 NE 3rd Ave., Brooklyn, NY 44499
404-555-0987

Name Angie Madpak Date 3/8

Address 55 Green Ave. Age 33

℞

Risperdal 3 mg
Disp # 60
Sig: i BID

LABEL

Refill 3 times

Dr. Charles Furillo

A.81

Dr. Peter Reiser
28 Prospect Place, Vero Beach, FL 44499
404-555-5550

Name Vanessa Harris Date 3/8

Address 7854 28th St. Age 43

℞

TOBRADEX EYE DROPS
1 BOTTLE 15cc

SIG: i gtt BID OD
x 1 WEEK

☑ Label

Refill 3 times PRN NR

Dr. Peter Reiser

A.82

Appendix A

Dr. Jackson Robbins
888 NW 27th Ave., Miami, FL 98885
247-555-6613

Name Branch Rickman Date 3/3

Address 55 28th St. Age 68

℞

NTG Nitrodur .2 mg Patch
sig: apply patch to chest qd
#30

☑ Label

Refill - 0 - 1 - 2 - 3 - (4) - PRN

Dr. Jackson Robbins

A.83

Dr. Melvin Ott
888 NW 27th Ave., Miami, FL 98885
247-555-6613

Name Mary Polo Date 7/7

Address 28 Harlem Dr. Age 50

℞

		MG. or cc.	No.	SIG.	Rep.
1	Toradol	10mg	#15	BID, 8+6	
2					
3					
4					
5		Refill x1			

☐ DRUGS TOTAL (when applicable)
☐ Not Label
☐ Substitution Allowed
☐ Prior Approval

Dr. Melvin Ott

A.84

Appendix A

Patient Name: John XXXXXX

Prescriber Name: Dr. AAA AAAAAA

****

Rx Quantity 30

Refills allowed 4

DAW code

Date Written 7/09/2010

Prior Authorization #

Product: Citalopram tabs 10 mg

NDC #---

Strength 10

Dose Unit

Sig: ONCE A DAY

A.85

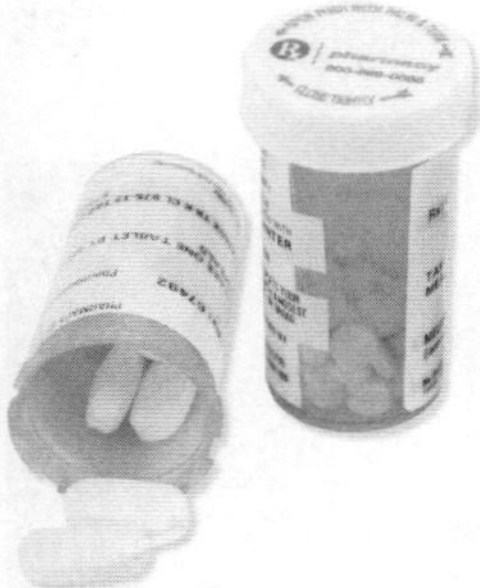

Appendix B • Puzzles and Problems

Appendix B

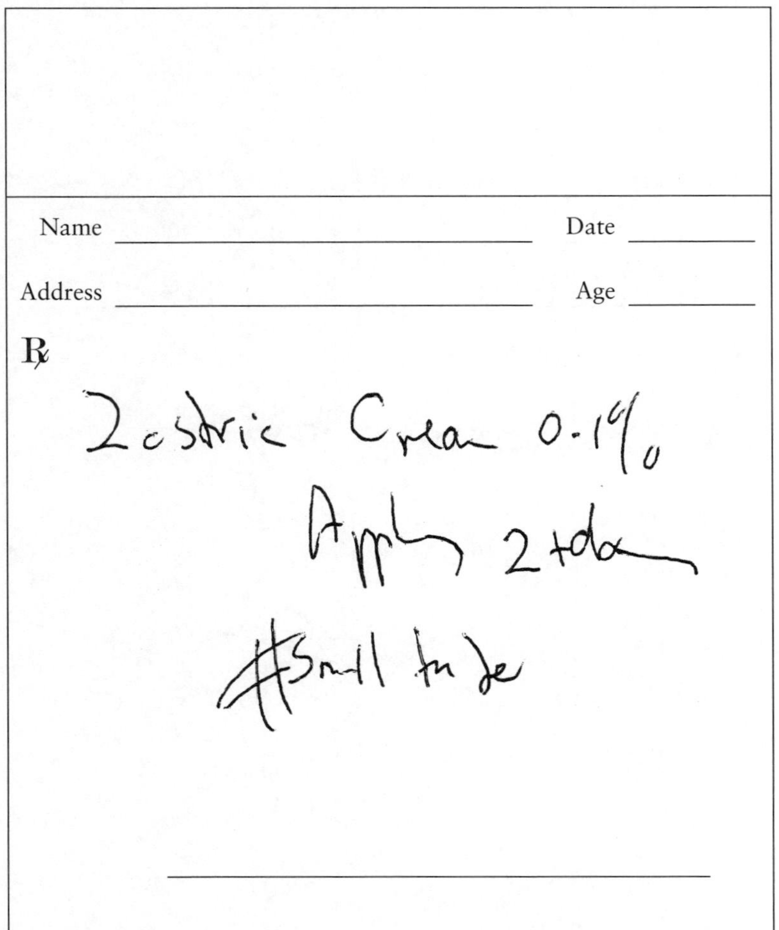

B.1

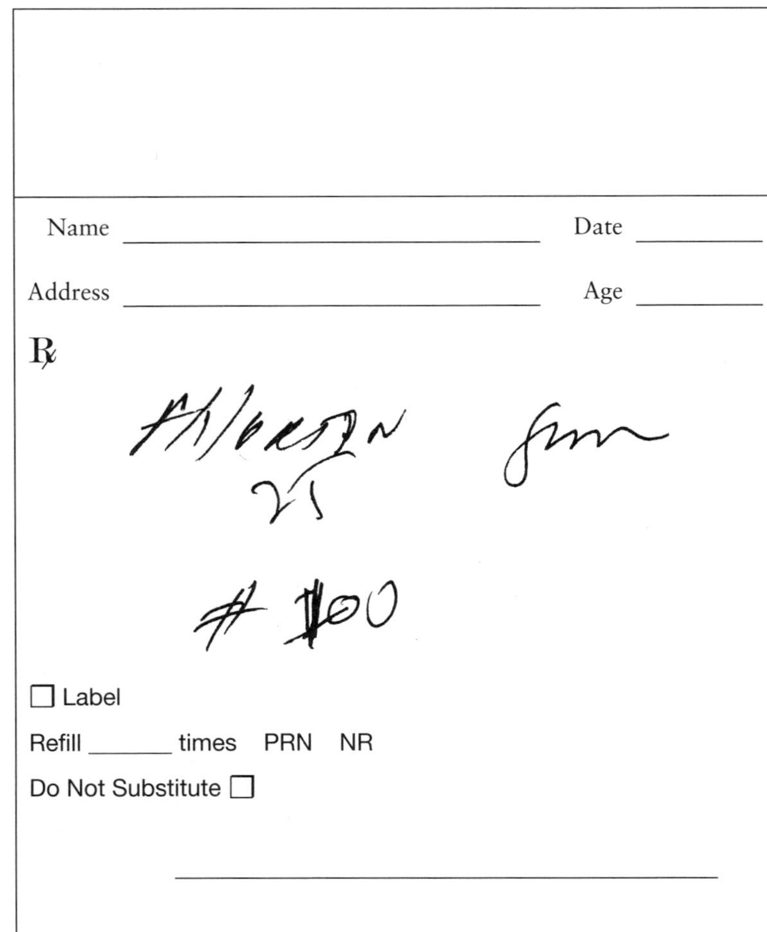

B.2

Appendix B

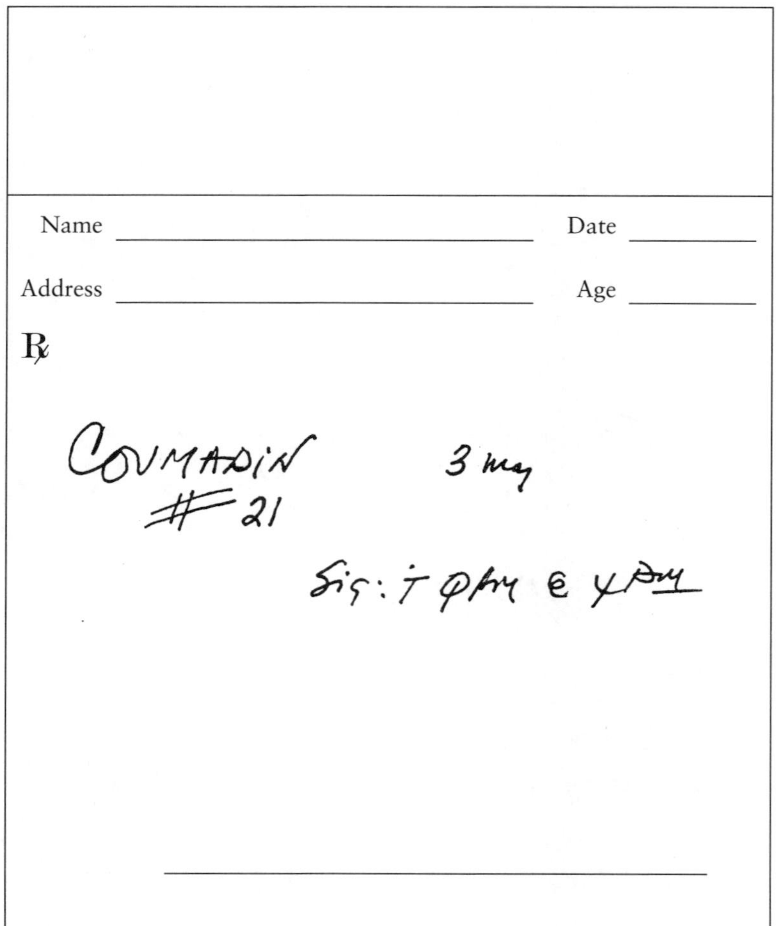

Name ______ Date ______

Address ______ Age ______

℞

COUMADIN 3 mg

21

Sig: ī q PM ē x PM

B.3

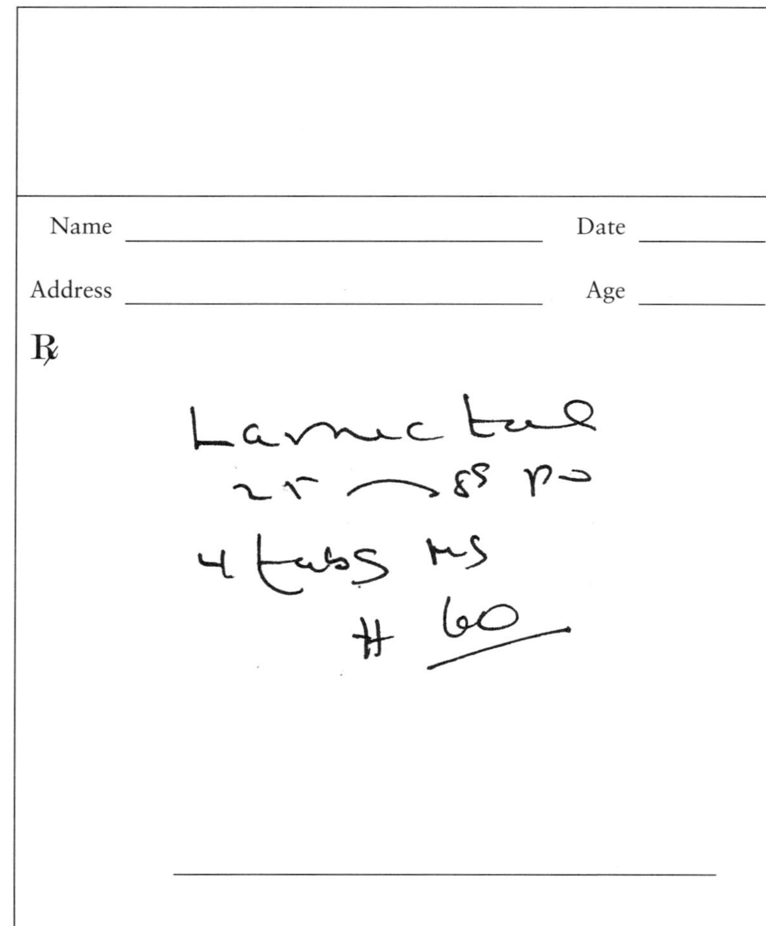

Name ______ Date ______

Address ______ Age ______

℞

Lamictal

4 tabs hs

60

B.4

Appendix B

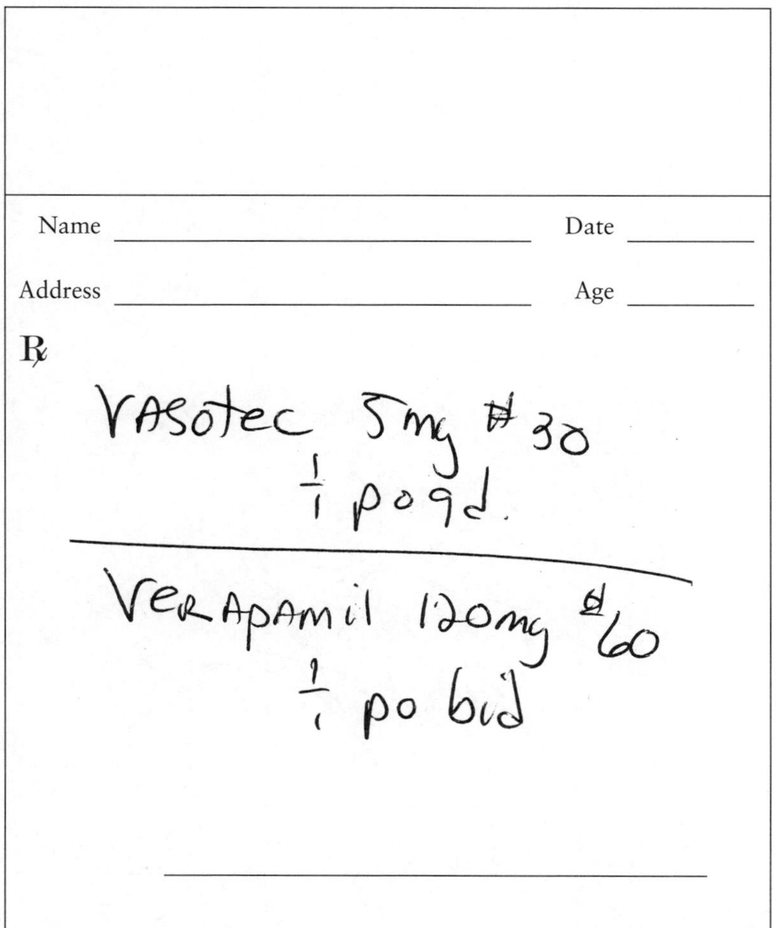

B.5

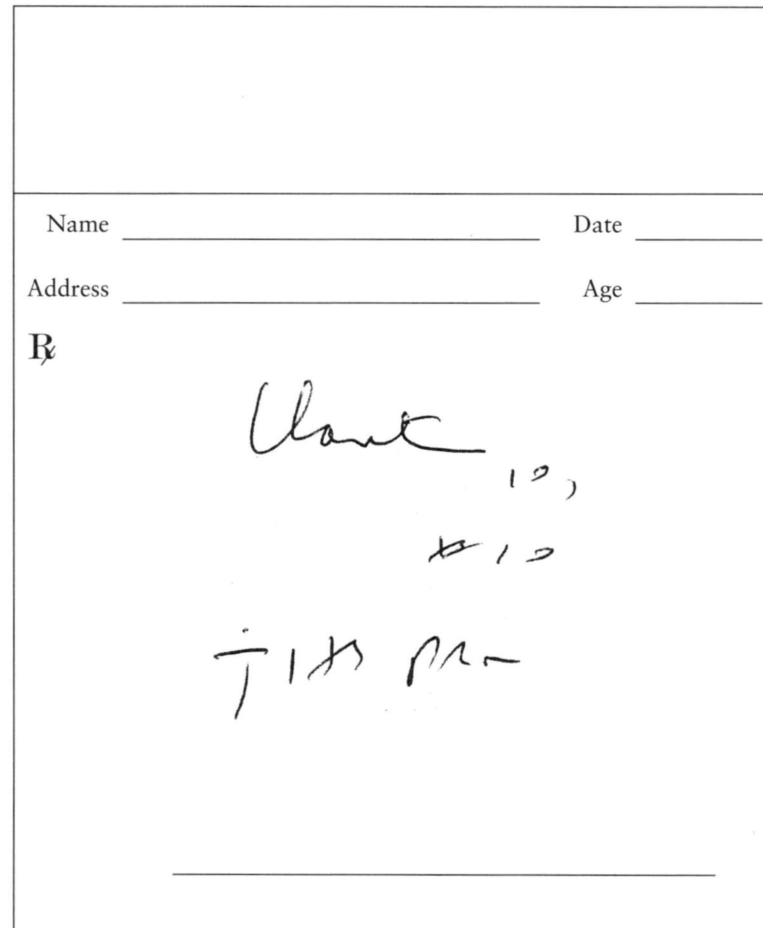

B.6

Appendix B

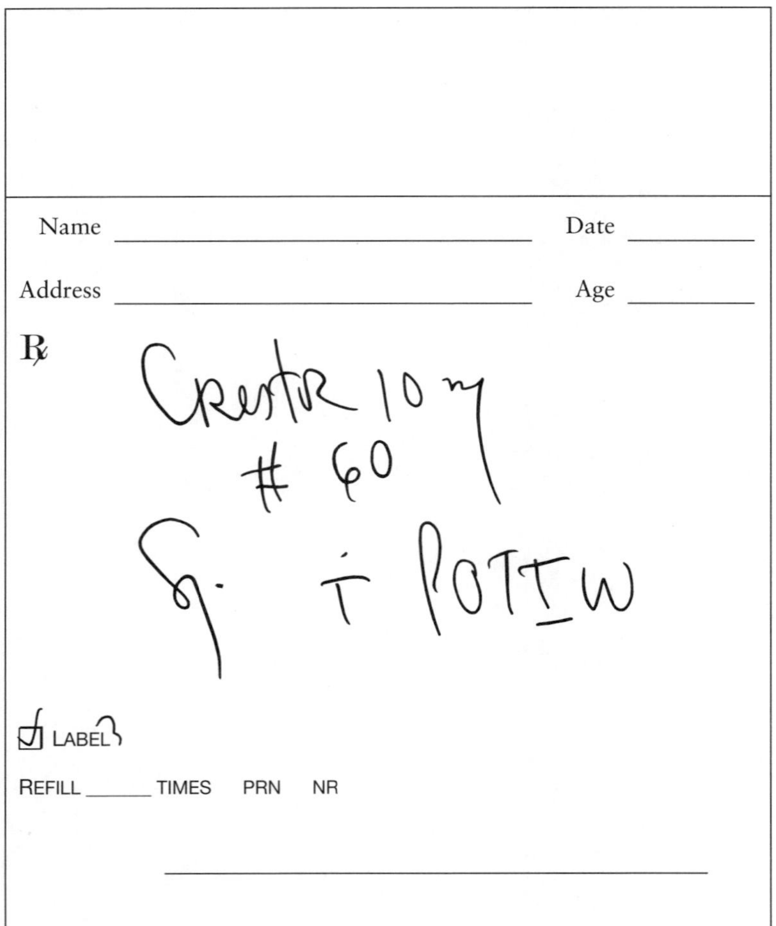

B.7

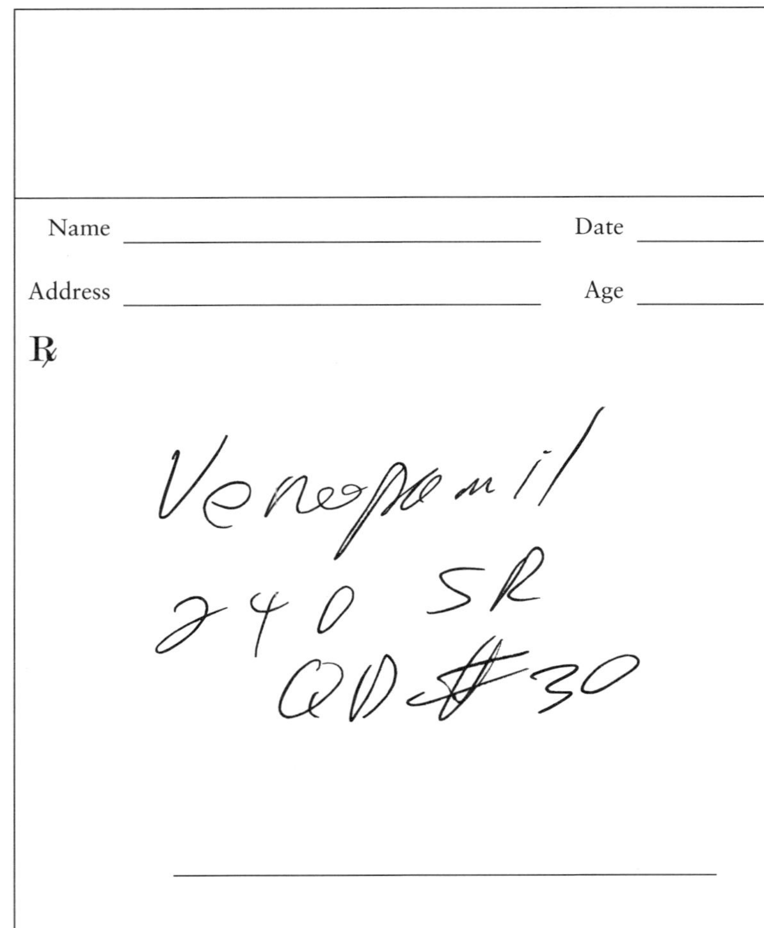

B.8

Appendix B

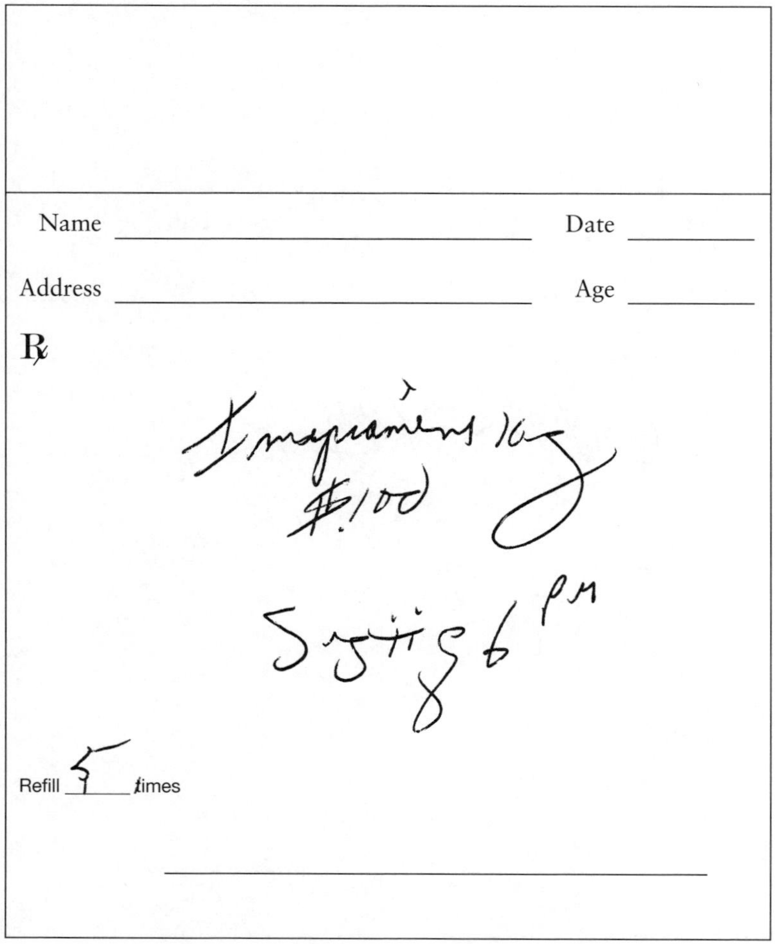
Name ______ Date ______

Address ______ Age ______

℞

#100

Refill 5 times

B.9

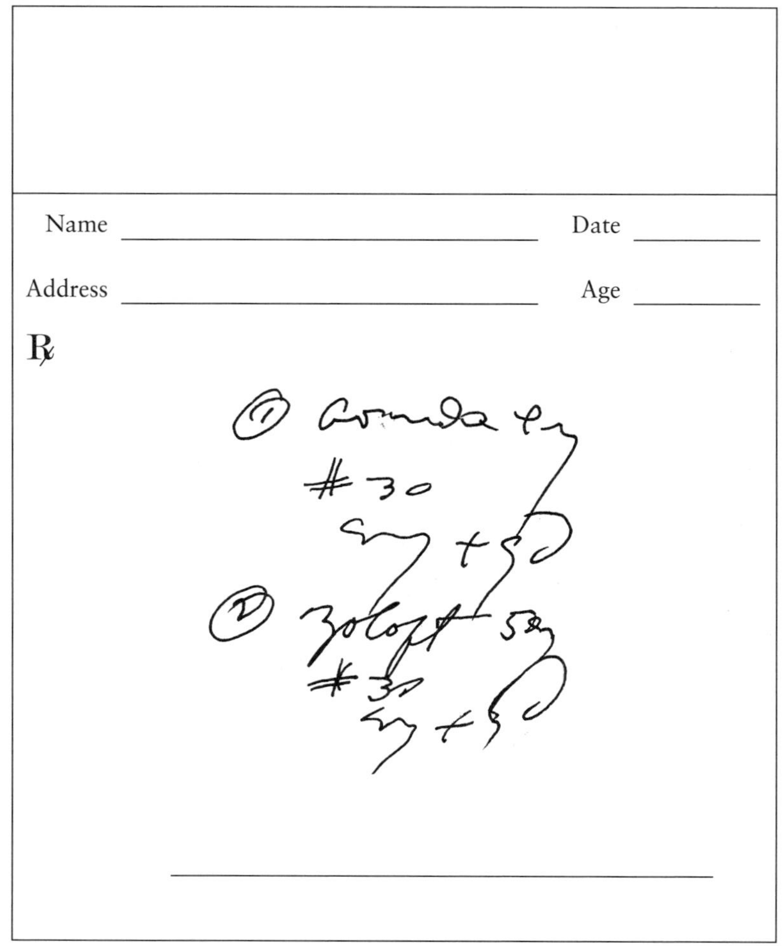
Name ______ Date ______

Address ______ Age ______

℞

#30

#30

B.10

Appendix B

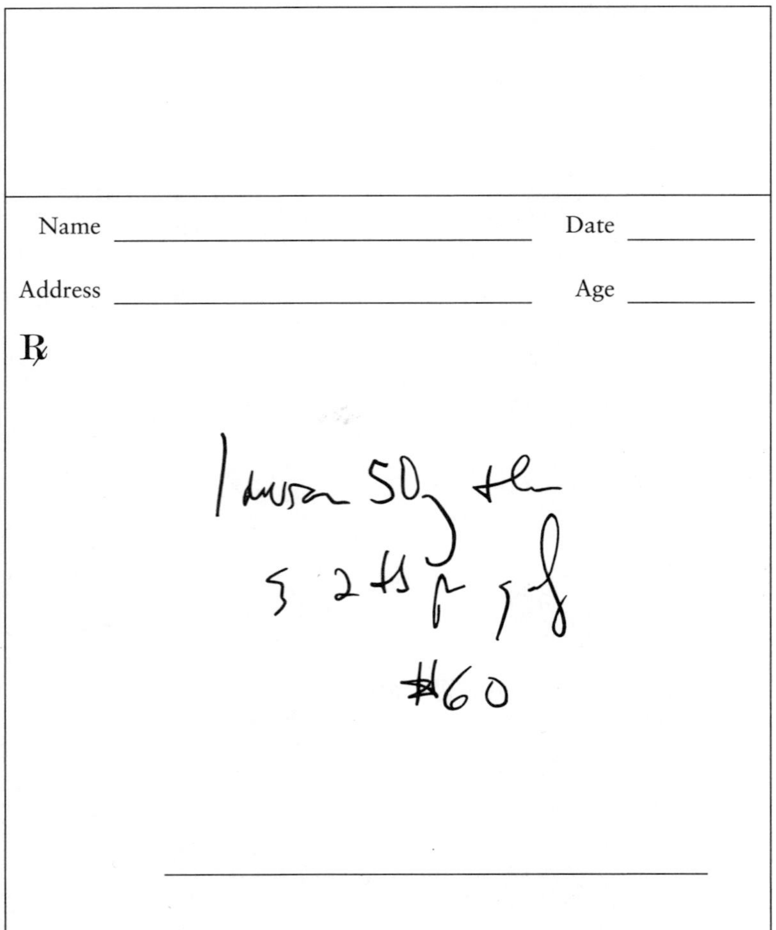
Name ______ Date ______

Address ______ Age ______

℞

______

B.11

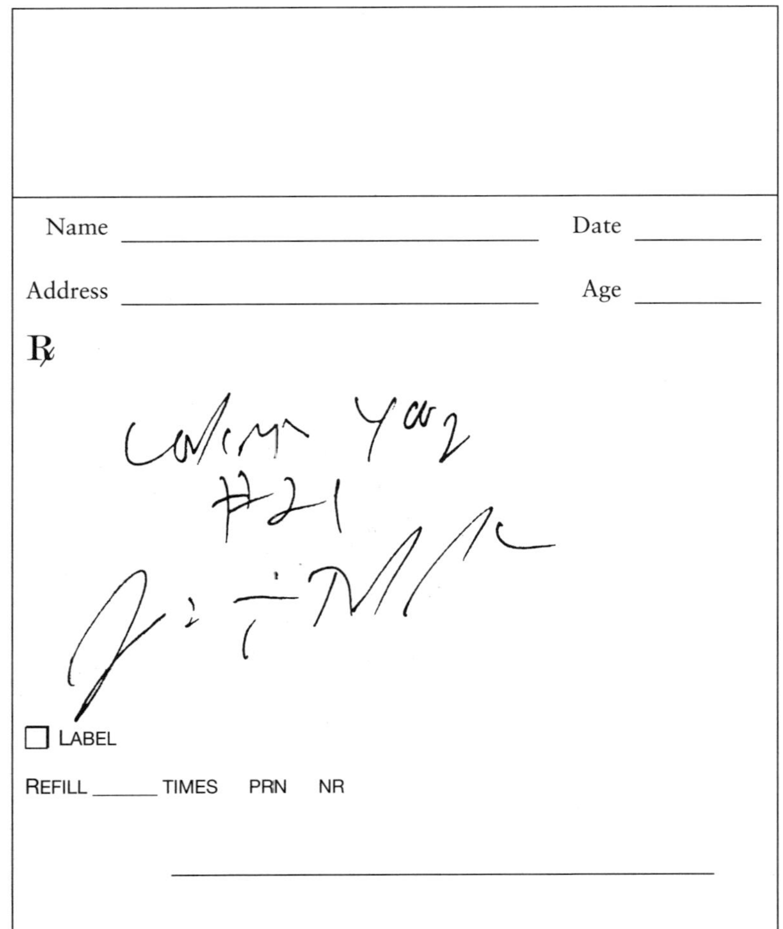
Name ______ Date ______

Address ______ Age ______

℞

☐ LABEL

REFILL ______ TIMES PRN NR

______

B.12

Appendix B

Name ______________________ Date __________

Address ______________________ Age __________

℞

ENTER...NAME AFTER ℞ ON LABEL	MG./CC	QUAN.
Tamoxifen Take # tab po bid	10	60

____

B.13

Name ______________________ Date __________

Address ______________________ Age __________

℞

Poly VoS-1 – ear drops

____

B.14

Appendix B

Name ____________________ Date ________

Address ____________________ Age ________

℞

OPIUM TINCTURE
10 gtts P.O. q
4hrs PRN diarrhea
do not exceed 40 gtts/day
T̄ OZ

____

B.15

Name ____________________ Date ________

Address ____________________ Age ________

℞

Hygroton 50 g.
#30
Sig: 1 QID

____

B.16

Appendix B

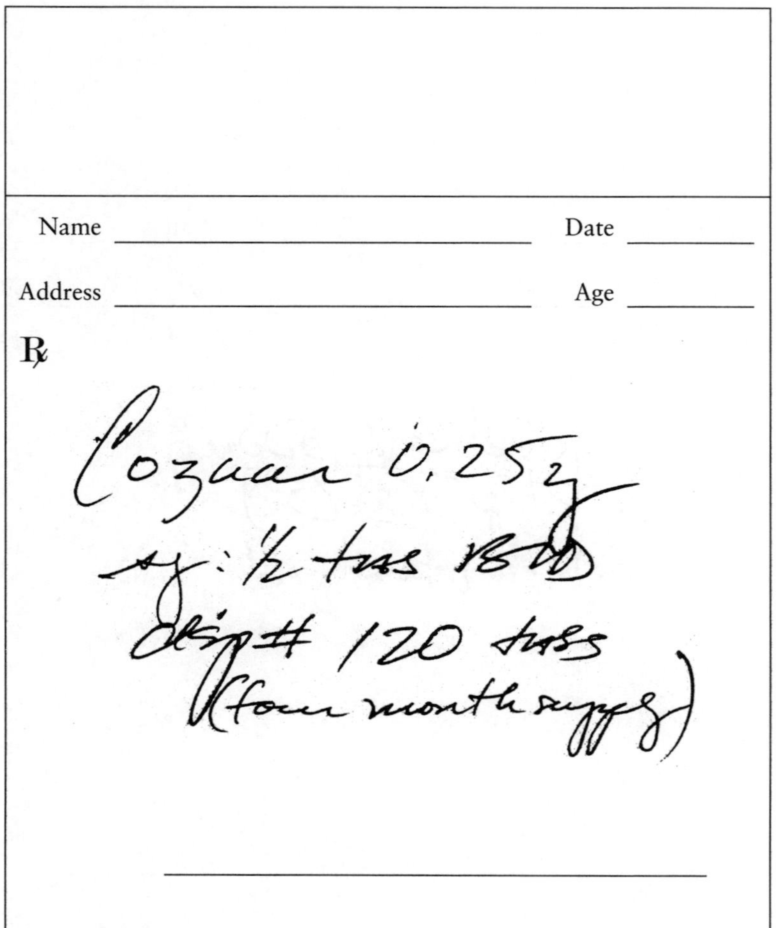

B.17

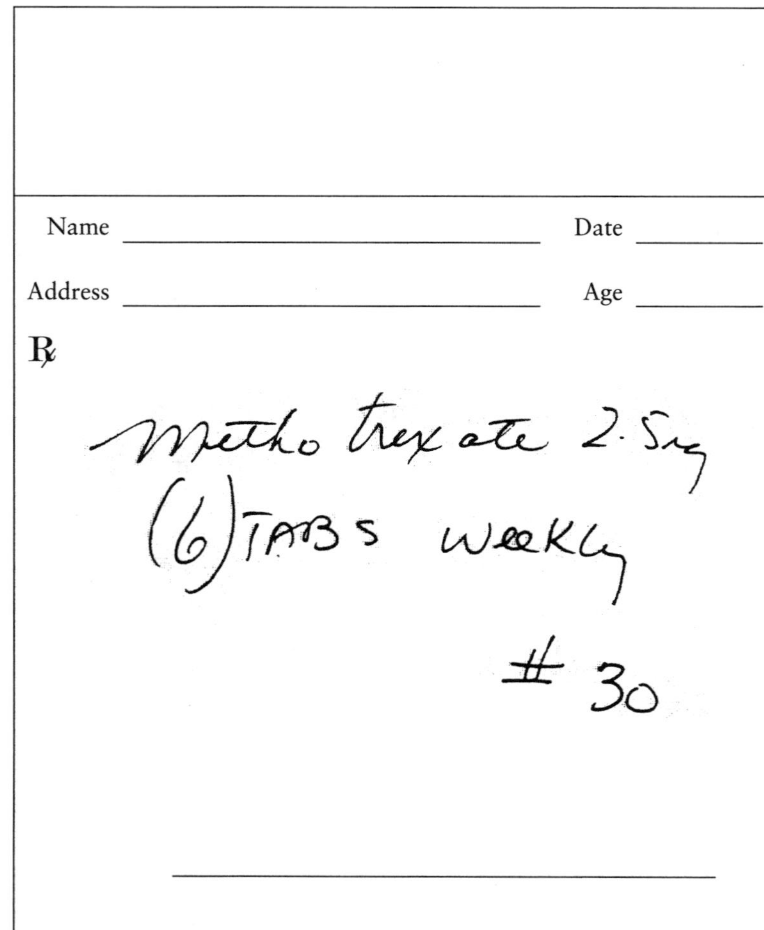

B.18

Appendix B

Name ______________________ Date __________

Address ______________________ Age __________

℞

IMIPRIMINE 150mg TAB #90

Sig iii PO QHS

B.19

Name ______________________ Date __________

Address ______________________ Age __________

℞

Amox. 500mg.

Disp. XX (20)

Sig: i tab qid

B.20

Appendix B

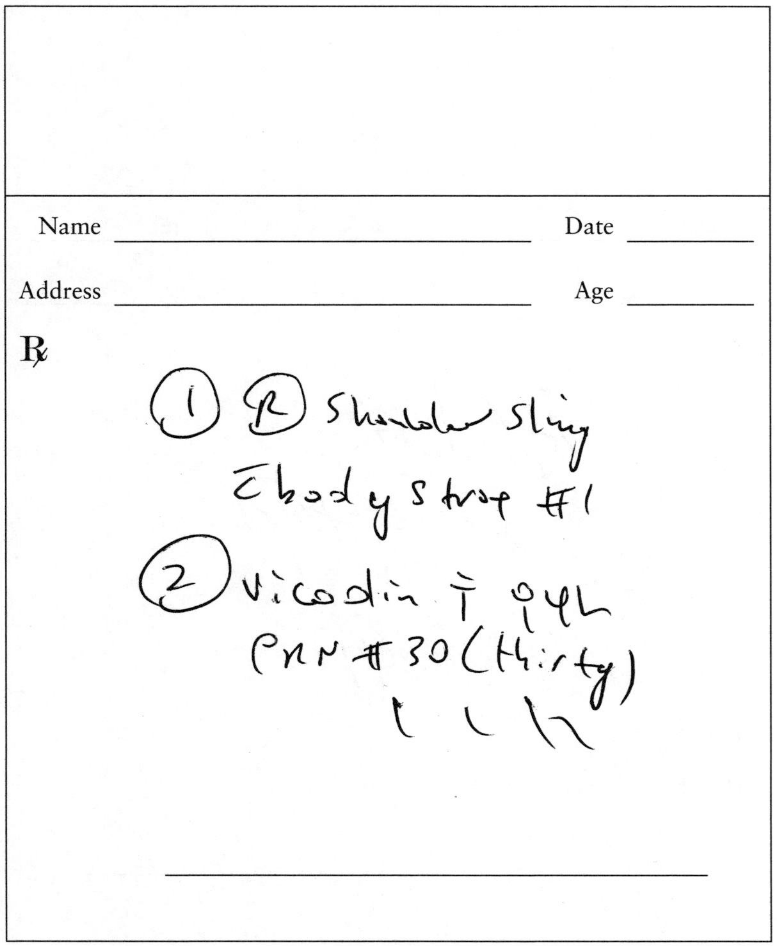

B.21

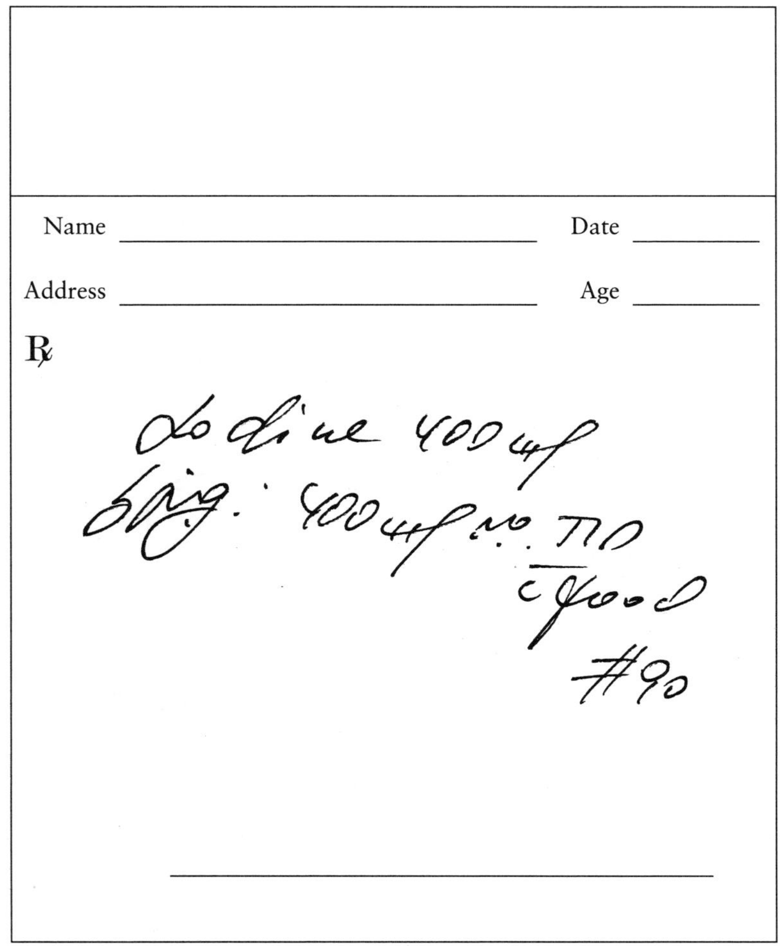

B.22

Appendix B

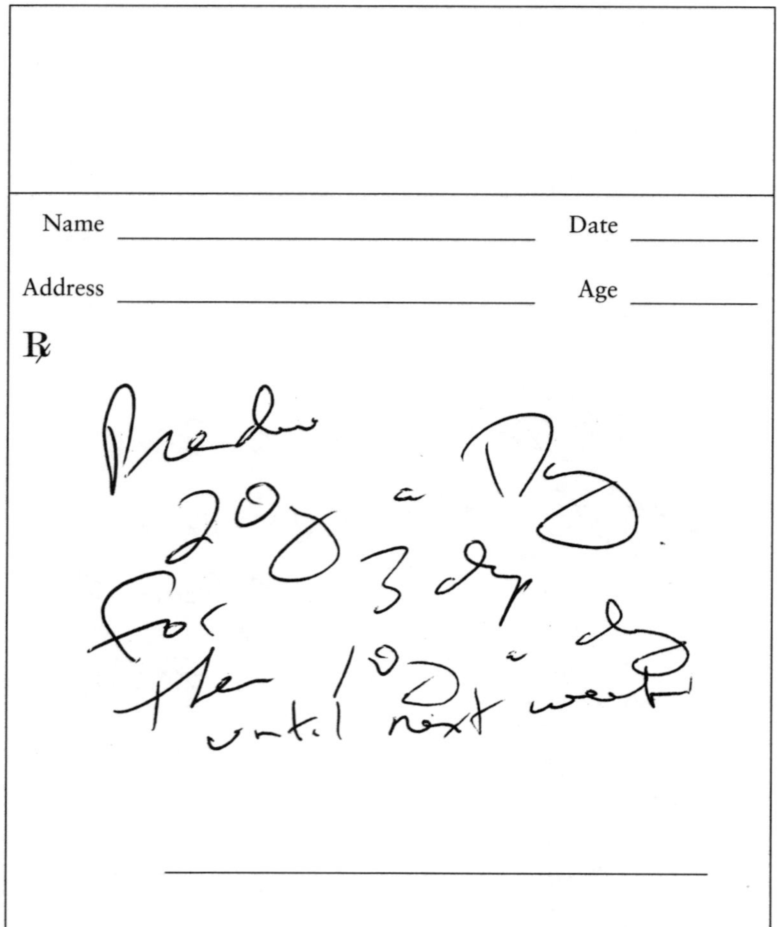

B.23

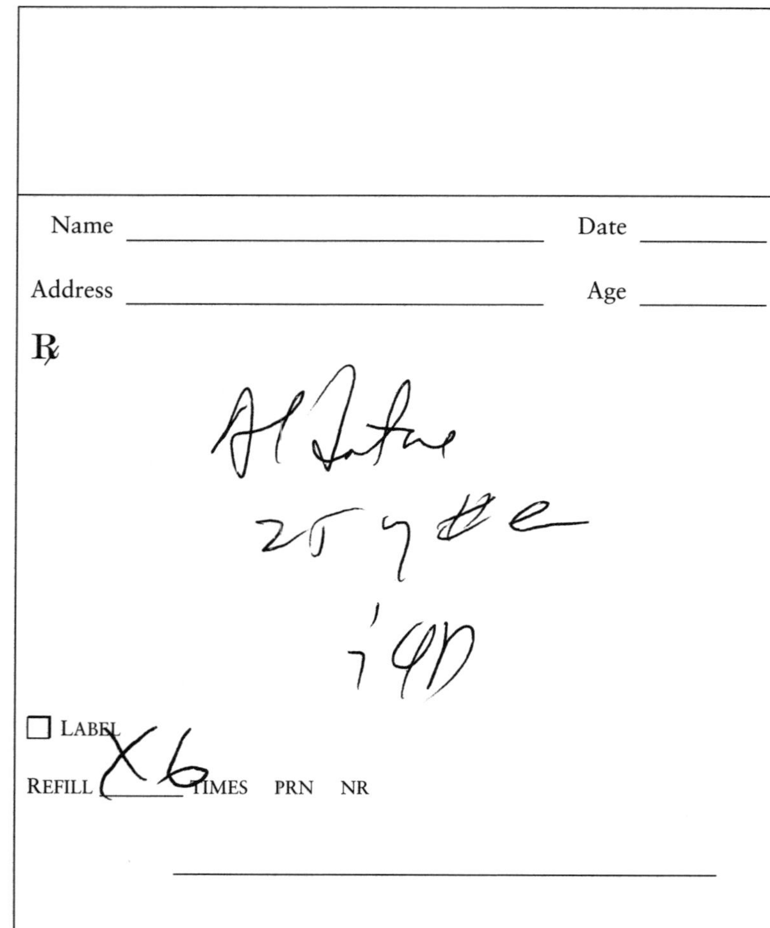

B.24

Appendix B

Name ______________________ Date ________

Address ______________________ Age ________

℞

Viscous lidocaine 30cc
Milk of magnesia 30cc
Benadryl elixir 30cc
Dilute to 500ml c̄ saline
Sig: 30cc oral rinse
Q2 PRN pain

Label

Refill 1 times

____

B.25

Name ______________________ Date ________

Address ______________________ Age ________

℞

Premarin
cream ī gr
Ⓞ hs 2x/week
#1 tube

Label

Refill (1) times

____

B.26

Appendix B

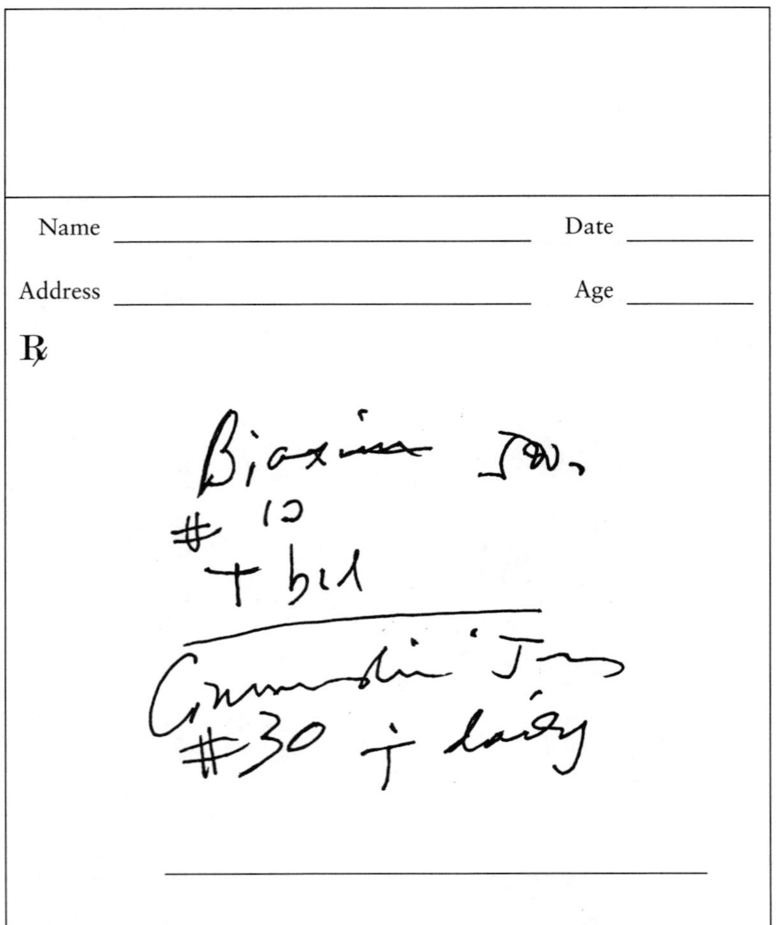

B.27

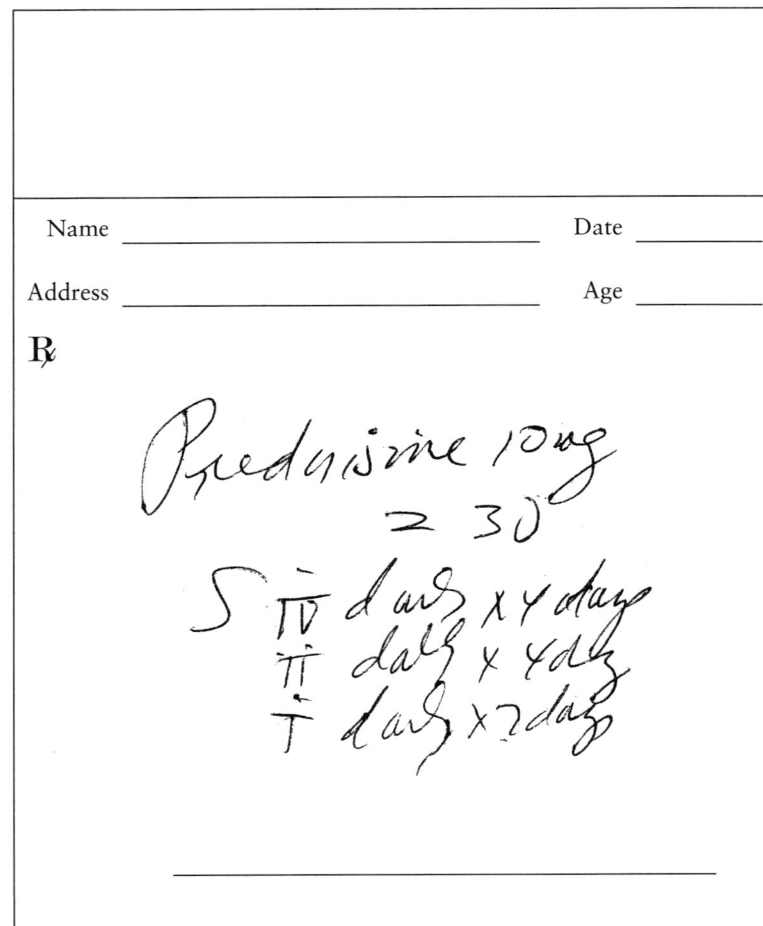

B.28

Appendix B

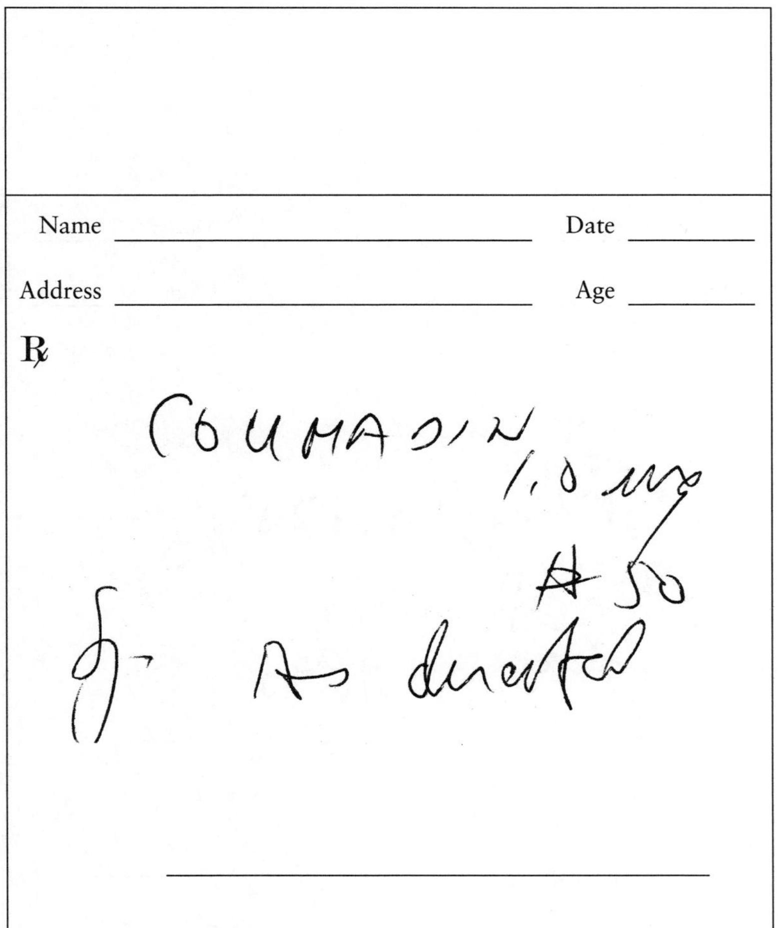
Name ______ Date ______

Address ______ Age ______

℞

COUMADIN 1.0 mg

#50

Sig: As directed

B.29

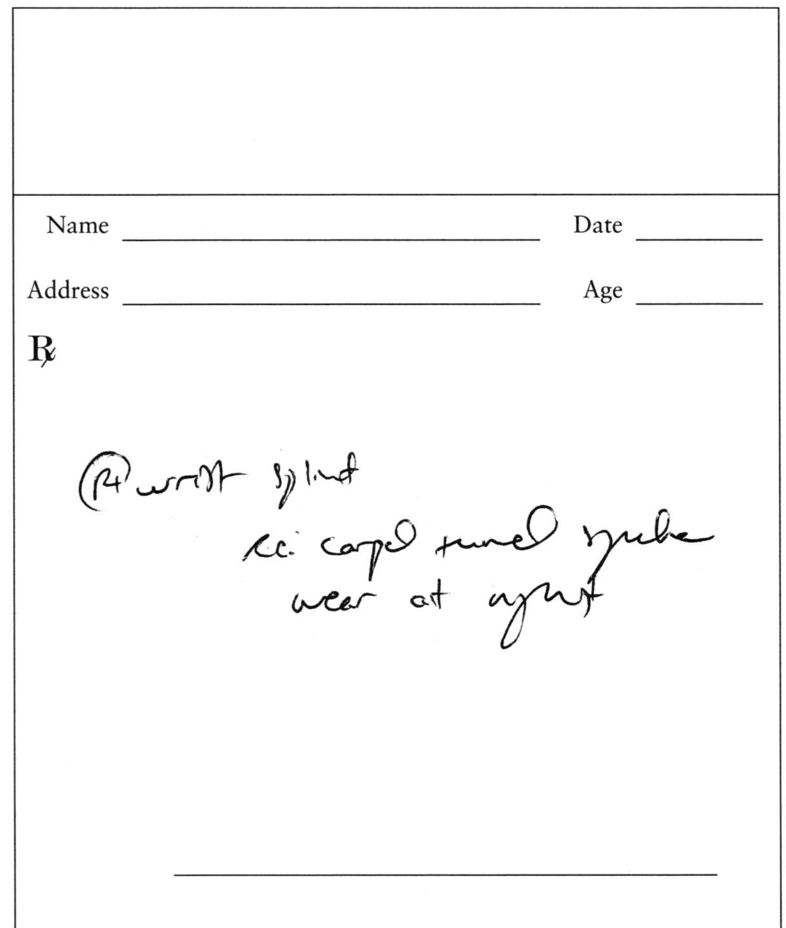
Name ______ Date ______

Address ______ Age ______

℞

(R) wrist splint

Dx: carpal tunnel syndrome

wear at night

B.30

Appendix B

Name ______ Date ______

Address ______ Age ______

℞

[illegible] Augmentin 600
250/[illegible]

5 cc TID

[illegible] Phenobarbital 60
5 cc TID

______

B.31

Name ______ Date ______

Address ______ Age ______

℞

Digoxin .125 mg
#50
Sig T q day

______

B.32

Appendix B

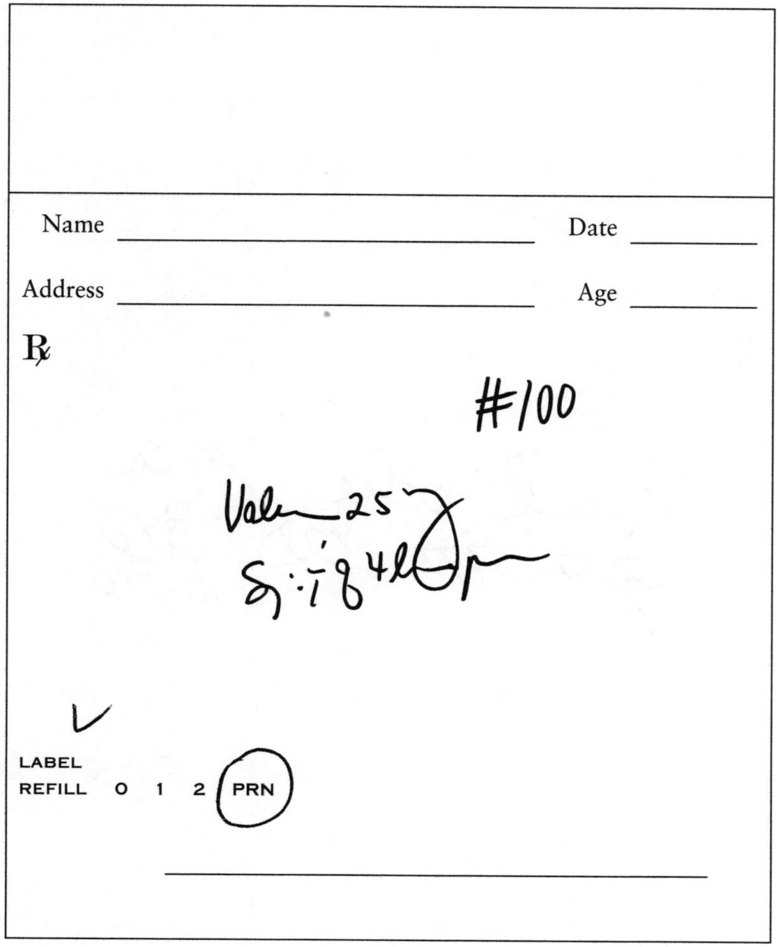
Name ______ Date ______
Address ______ Age ______
℞
#100
LABEL
REFILL 0 1 2 PRN

B.33

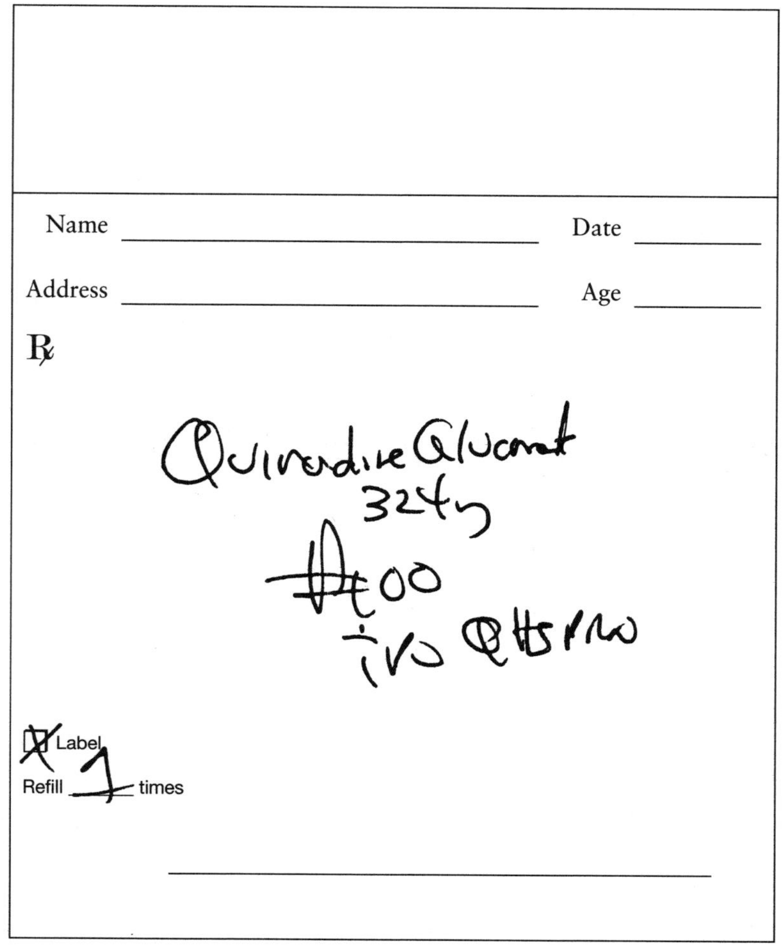
Name ______ Date ______
Address ______ Age ______
℞
Label
Refill ______ times

B.34

Appendix B

Name ____________ Date ______

Address ____________ Age ______

℞

Clonidine HCL
0.3 mg Patch Q.D.
#12

____

B.35

Name ____________ Date ______

Address ____________ Age ______

℞

Vosol otic 10cc
gtt iii OD BID to TID

____

B.36

Appendix B

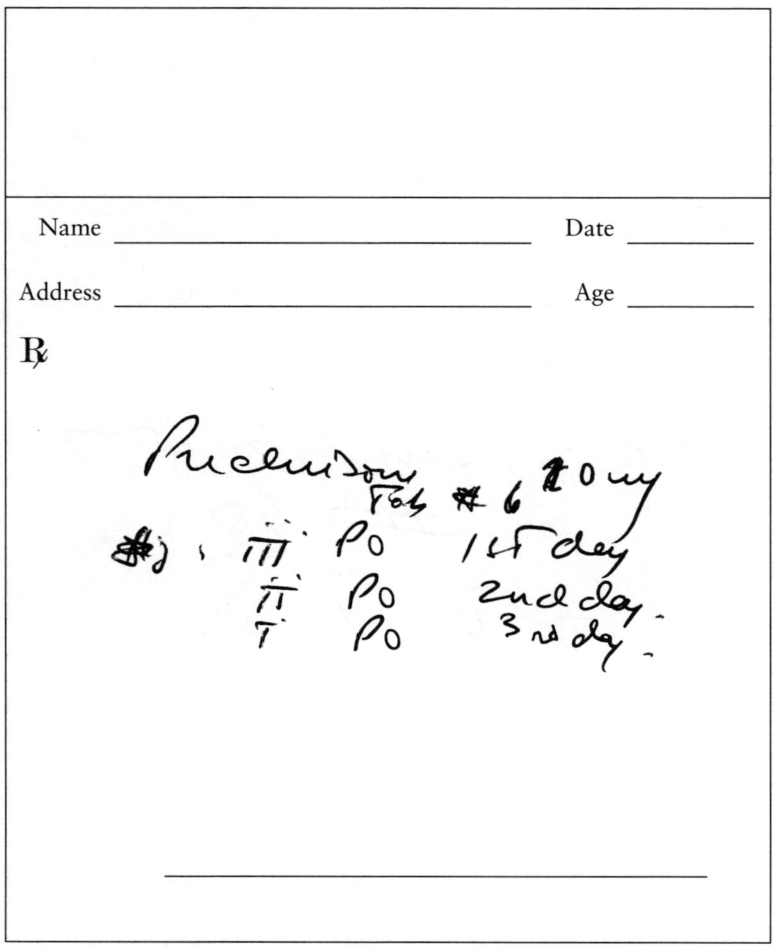

B.37

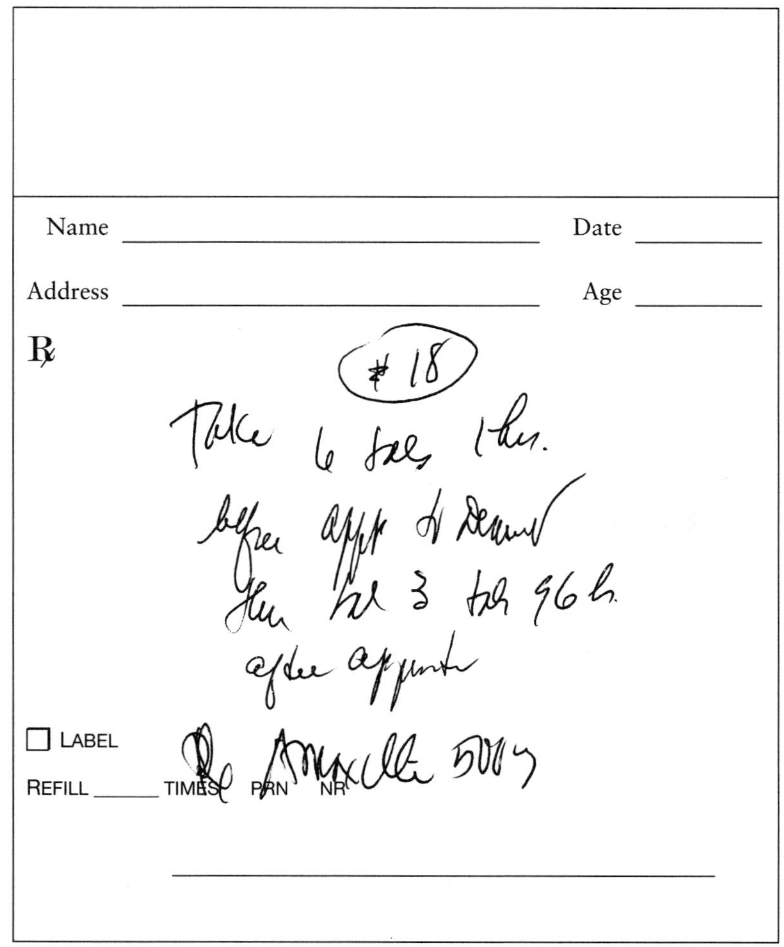

B.38

Appendix B

Name ____________ Date ______

Address ____________ Age ______

℞

Mira Forte gtt

S.i ī gtt OS Q2h

Disp: 1 bottle

____

B.39

Name ____________ Date ______

Address ____________ Age ______

℞

Tamoxifen tab 10 mg

#60

ī B.I.D.

____

B.40

Appendix B

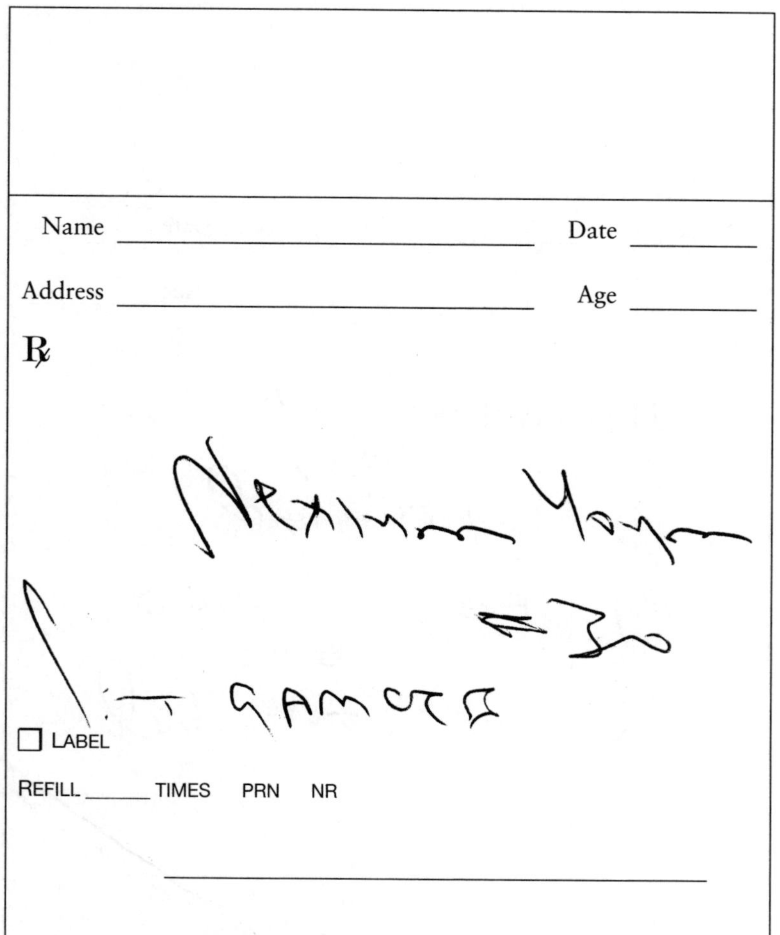
Name Date
Address Age
℞
☐ LABEL
REFILL ______ TIMES PRN NR

B.41

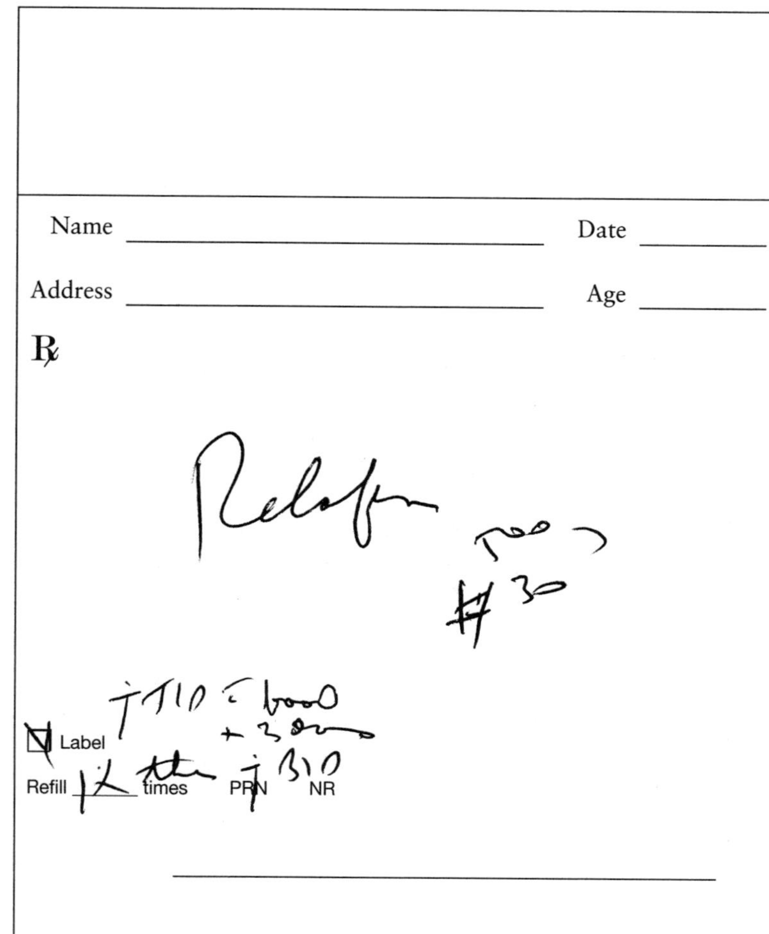
Name Date
Address Age
℞
Label
Refill ______ times PRN NR

B.42

Appendix B

Name ______________________ Date __________

Address ______________________ Age __________

℞ Methotrexate for injection
25 mg/5 cc

Disp: 10 cc

Sig: Squirt 1 cc into juice and drink once a week

☐ LABEL

REFILL ____ TIMES PRN NR

____

B.43

Name ______________________ Date __________

Address ______________________ Age __________

℞ 1) Protonix 40 mg
#30
1 tab q.d.

2) Fergon tab
#100
1 tab b.i.d.

____

B.44